THE SCENT OF EROS

To Janmet

GREAT

meeting

+

speaking with

you —

James V. Kohl

THE SCENT OF EROS

Mysteries of Odor in Human Sexuality

James Vaughn Kohl
and
Robert T. Francoeur

Authors Choice Press
San Jose   New York   Lincoln   Shanghai

The Scent of Eros
Mysteries of Odor in Human Sexuality

Authors Choice Press
an imprint of iUniverse, Inc.

For information address:
iUniverse, Inc.
5220 S. 16th St., Suite 200
Lincoln, NE 68512
www.iuniverse.com

Originally published by Continuum

ISBN: 0-595-23383-X

Printed in the United States of America

CONTENTS

ACKNOWLEDGMENTS

I wish to thank Bruce McEwen and Robert L. Moss, for their reviews, comments, referrals, supporting documentation, and encouragement; Robert T. Francoeur, my co-author, for his friendship and belief in a newcomer; Heino Meyer-Bahlburg, for his painstaking review of the initial conceptualization and challenges; F. Robert Brush, for his review, support, and challenges; Anne Perkins, for her review, support, and animal model; John Kohl, my brother, for his insight and support; Helen Fisher, for her kindness; Ben Oswald, for his friendship and support; Ann Judith Silverman, for her challenges; Elizabeth Allgeier, for her inspirational interest in and support of the concept; Timothy Perper, for his challenges and advice; Marlene Schwanzel-Fukuda, for her referrals; Donald Pfaff, for his review and referrals; Theodore Jacobs, Parvin Modaber Jacobs, Loring Jacobs, Leslie Jacobs, and William Shoemaker, for their patience, understanding, and medical expertise.

I also wish to thank Adam Aguiar, Fred Beeman, Toby Bieber, Eli Coleman, William F. Crowley, Jr., Bob Dennis, Richard Doty, Richard C. Friedman, Lori Gallanger, Thomas Landefeld, Ellen Laura, Stephen Mason, Michael Meredith, John Morgenthaler, Sara Newman, Stephen Newmark, Carole Ober, James Prescott, Gopalan Rajendren, Howard Rupple, Alan Schwartz, Andrew Shenker, Richard Simerly, Leonard Storm, William J. Turner, Tj. B. van Wimersma Greidanus, James Weinrich, Russel Whitaker, Ruth Wood, and Charles Wysocki.

—JAMES V. KOHL

I am particularly grateful to Barbara Garris for making this book more readable with her careful copy-editing and helpful suggestions when we were in midstream and as we approached the finish line. And I thank my long-time friends and colleagues Tim Perper and Martha Cornog for their penetrating insights, true-to-life advice, and ideas for a new opening chapter which they shared so generously with us and our readers.

Finally, both James Kohl and I acknowledge and appreciate the invaluable advice and efforts of Jack Heidenry, our editor at Continuum, who worked with me on books in the 1960s, was my editor at *Penthouse Forum* in the 1980s, and reappeared at just the right moment to become the editor for *The Scent of Eros*. We also thank Evander Lomke and Martin Rowe for coordinating our production and publicity at Continuum.

—ROBERT T. FRANCOEUR

FOREWORD

Many different genes contribute to our physical characteristics, and many different genes play their roles in human behavior. But genes do not act alone. Both our physical and our behavioral characteristics also depend quite heavily on our environment. During the development of our unique characteristics, our environment may be more important than our genes. Our genetic "nature," predisposes certain characteristics. Our environment acts on this genetic predisposition. Simply put, nature initiates; environment determines the outcome.

Sunlight is an environmental influence on genes. Exposure to ultraviolet rays alters genes in skin cells. For those who are genetically predisposed, the result of too much exposure might be a readily visible skin cancer. For others, the result might simply be what we perceive to be the look of weathered skin. In either case, underlying this "look," are genetic changes in cells that we cannot see. But we do not need to see these changes, to know that they occur.

Other people are part of our environment. This *social* environment is often referred to as "nurture." Many years of scientific debate have focused on whether genetic nature is more important than social-environmental nurture. Most scientists agree that both nature and nurture are important to the vast majority of human characteristics.

What is true for characteristic diseases, like skin cancer, also applies to personality characteristics and behavior. News reports about "discoveries" of how behavior is affected by genes are often misrepresentations. For example, in the news from several years ago there was a claim that a gene for male homosexuality had been found. If a clear link existed between a gene and sexual orientation, we could expect a similarly timed news report would tell us that a gene for heterosexuality had been found. There was not, and has not been, any such report. That's because it is most likely that a group of genes determines whether we prefer males or females: our sexual orientation. It is even more likely that the environment influences those genes, and allows for differences in sexual orientation. In a similar manner beauty, intelligence, weight, or even height are the product of countless genes that interact with the environment in ways we do not yet understand.

Our environment influences our genes from long before we are born. While still in our mother's womb, the environmental influences that affect her, also affect us. For example, cigarette smoking has been linked to low birth weight in infants. This is an example of how "second hand smoke" can affect someone else. But, in this case, the "someone else" has not been born.

Low birth weight has been linked to male homosexuality. If reports linking cigarette smoking to low birth weight, and reports linking low birth weight to homosexuality received equal media attention at the same time, we might expect to see the newsworthy, but ridiculously unscientific headline: "Cigarette smoking causes homosexuality."

Media affects us, through representations and through misrepresentations of science. Other media representations link second hand smoke to diseases and conditions later in life. These individual studies are believable. It is easy to understand such links, because we can readily see the smoke that is affecting us. On the other hand, we tend not to think about what we cannot see, and how such invisible forces affect us.

There are many unseen chemicals in our environment that affect us just as much as the chemicals we can see, like smoke. Even though we cannot see or smell the dioxins in our environment, these chemicals have been linked to changes in hormones and to disease processes. Many hormone changes also are linked to behavioral changes. If a chemical from our environment causes hormonal changes, it may also cause changes in behavior. These changes may be very subtle, even unnoticeable, but they do occur.

Unnoticeable changes can, over time, cause changes that are very noticeable. If you want to get to the root of a change, it is as necessary to pay attention to the things that affect us immediately, as it is to pay attention to the things that only affect us over long periods of time.

Unfortunately, a degree of complexity is added to observations of things that not only affect us immediately, but that also affect us over time. People might joke about someone whose bizarre adult behavior they attribute to being dropped at birth. In this case, the joke provides an example of how we can expect an environmental insult: being dropped, to immediately affect us, and also to have later effects on behavior.

If we were able to determine how every environmental insult that ever occurred affected a person's genes, we would have a good idea of how that person developed to become the person he or she is today. We could also attempt to explain differences between people based on differences in genes and differences in their environments. Unfortunately, we can not continuously observe the complex interactions between genes and the environment. Besides, dramatic environmental insults are far less common than the routine environmental effects of normal everyday living.

We are continuously exposed to chemicals, sunlight, noise, and other sensory input. We are affected by exposure whether or not we are aware of this exposure at the time it occurs. So, how can we know whether a particular condition, disease or behavioral trait is genetic or environmental, or both? To make this determination we must try to determine how the environment affects our genes. We may find that traits that we expected to be genetic are actually due largely to the environment in which a person grows, and vice versa. Examining the complex relationships between genes and our environment will challenge myths about the influence of genetics, and also challenge myths about the influence of our environment.

How do we know whether a particular human trait is genetic or environmental or both? Other animals often are used as models. We have the ability to manipulate the genes of other animals, and their environment. We can also observe other animals closely for longer periods of time. This ability is used in attempts to explain the relative contribution of genes and the environment to behavior.

Humans are mammals, and in other mammals pheromones affect genes in cells that secrete a very important hormone. Pheromones are present as chemicals in the natural body odor that we produce. Our pheromones are part of our social environment, and they are used in many species to communicate information. Human pheromones cause changes in hormone levels in other humans, and hormones affect human behavior. Do human pheromones affect human behavior? We think that the answer is very obvious. Yes!

Scientists are prone to overstating the importance of their own discoveries, and I certainly would not exclude myself from such criticism. When I discovered that pheromones were the most likely link between the nature and nurture of human behavior, predictions were made. Other scientists believed that many of these predictions were overstated. Initially, with the 1995 publication of this book, there was scientific criticism that what Dr. Robert Francoeur and I presented extended far beyond the available scientific data. Scientific criticism is no longer common. Data from human studies now fully supports the link between human pheromones and behavior, or simply put, between sex and the sense of smell. This is why we felt it was time to release our book with an epilogue. For non-scientists and for other researchers, the epilogue helps to detail additional information on the links among pheromones, hormones, sex, and the sense of smell.

JAMES VAUGHN KOHL

Introduction

Raspberries and the
Birth of This Book

A good friend of ours is a discussion leader for singles groups. Actually he's an expert on the singles scene and knows enough about why men and women find each other interesting emotionally and sexually to write a book on *Sex Signals: The Biology of Love*. A while back, he shared with us his experience of asking a group, "How do you know if someone you've just met is interested in you?"

One man said it was how she smiled. A woman said she could tell by how close he stood to her. Another woman told the group she knew how interested a man was by how much he looked at her—if he was very interested, he looked at her all the time; if he wasn't that interested, he barely glanced at her. "Good answers," our friend said. But he was quickly interrupted by another man.

"I can tell by how she smells," he said.

Everyone stirred uneasily. No one seemed to like this observation, and they certainly did not know what to make of it. And yet, sometimes odor *does* communicate a great deal about our emotions to other people, especially to people who notice odors—as this man clearly did. But it is also true that many odors, particularly intimate odors, make us uncomfortable in modern superclean America. We spend millions of dollars on soaps and showers and deodorants. In all this cleanliness, are we losing something important about ourselves?

Our mutual friend—the singles group leader—told us another story, one he had to admit ever so slightly embarrassed him. He happened to be driving a date to a restaurant in the country. "Hmm," he said. "There's a raspberry field nearby. Aren't they luscious!"

His friend shook her head. "I can't smell anything in this traffic!"

"But I'm *sure* I smell raspberries!" Our friend glanced at her and realized it was not raspberries he was smelling, but probably her scented feminine hygiene deodorant masking whatever natural genital odor she might be producing.

No, nobody says that true love blooms amid the stench of dirt and filth. No, that is not what we mean at all. We mean something else, something that modern science is discovering about the sense of smell and about the role of odors in that most intimate of all emotional domains, our sexuality.

FRANCOEUR'S STORY OF THIS BOOK

In the summer of 1992 the daily mail brought me a thick brown envelope from Las Vegas. The name of James Kohl in the return address was not familiar, and with a pressing deadline threatening, I only glanced at the cover letter. The writer asked me to read his enclosed twenty-page manuscript on "Luteinizing Hormone: The Link Between Sex and the Sense of Smell" and advise him whether I thought it would be suitable for presentation at the next meeting of the Society for the Scientific Study of Sex (SSSS).

"Interesting. Might be something about pheromones and sex attractants. I'll look at it later."

A week later, I had managed to plow through this very dense, highly technical text. "Quite interesting. Creative and inventive? Yes, but to be honest, this sounds a bit quirky." Still, Kohl's argument that odors and the sense of smell very much influence human sexual behavior stuck in my mind.

Weeks later, while talking with Timothy Perper, the singles expert who smelled raspberries, I mentioned the paper and learned that Perper had received a copy of it as well. As Perper and I discussed the manuscript, we became genuinely interested in Kohl's ideas. Neither of us were quite sure about his evidence and conclusions, but we agreed there was something intriguing and persuasive about his argument. Perper and I were both reminded of a comment of John Money back in 1971. Arno Karlen, a mutual friend of ours, was interviewing this international leader in sexological research when Money did a jump cut from the topic, ". . . few people in the world [are] studying human smell. . . . We don't know what the sense of smell has to do with human sexual development. For all we know, the underarm smell of an infant's father may be crucial in his life! You're laughing, and I'm almost joking. But almost no theory is too wild as we've been learning."[1]

At the same time, we were puzzled that no one in SSSS, so far as we knew, had ever heard of James Vaughn Kohl. His letter indicated he was a clinical laboratory scientist who managed a small clinical laboratory for a group of physicians in Las Vegas, but there was no Ph.D. or M.S. after his name. Undeterred, we decided to see where this curious paper might lead. We encouraged him to submit an abstract for review by the scientific program committee for the next SSSS conference and see if they too found merit in his paper.

At the 1992 SSSS meeting, we met Jim Kohl and looked forward with mixed expectations to his presentation. Both Perper and I were well aware of the kind of blunt, skeptical, no-nonsense biologists we knew would be in Jim's audience. They were there, but strangely quiet and intent during the presentation.[2] Afterward, their questions were probing, obviously indicating they took Jim's evidence and argument quite seriously. Then, during lunch, I listened as he handled some pointed and more detailed questions from several SSSS members who sought him out.

For our 1993 SSSS meeting in Chicago, I asked Jim to join a panel I moderated on "The Brain and Sex: New Advances."[3] Anne Perkins, a reproductive behavioral scientist spoke on hormones and the sexual behavior of male sheep—what insiders call "duds" or "gay" rams—on the range in Idaho.[4] Eli Coleman from the Human Sexuality Program at the University of Minnesota spoke on the therapeutic use of different neuroactive drugs in treating compulsive sexual behavior.[5] Jim Kohl elaborated on a sequence of events linking odors, the sense of smell, and hormones to human sexual behavior.[6] This time, however, he was able to combine the support from Anne's model—the hormones and the behavior of the rams she had been studying—with Eli's human studies. As a result, his argument that odors and the sense of smell are a strong influence on human sexual behavior, was taken even more seriously. And again, none of the neuroscientists in the audience disagreed with the connections he suggested between odors and sex. The next day, Jim tested his ideas one on one with a number of people from varied scientific backgrounds, in a well-attended poster session.[7]

Soon after the 1992 San Diego meeting, Jim and I began discussing the possibility of collaborating on a book called *The Scent of*

Eros. My part would be to translate Jim's intimidating and technical material into popular terms that the ordinary reader would find interesting and understandable.

Doing this has been one of the most difficult writing assignments I have undertaken, even though I have a strong background and teaching experience in human embryology and sexuality. Part of the problem was that Jim has been working intently on this subject for over eight years, mostly by himself, reading everything he could find even remotely related to the subject, synthesizing, and generating new insights and connections. Perhaps because he has been working on his own, he has been able to synthesize seemingly familiar material in innovative ways. Working alone, he has not been influenced by the standard paradigms young scientists absorb as they work their way through graduate school.

I have listened as Jim discussed his ideas with traditionally trained neuroscientists, and it was quickly obvious that there are two ways in which science progresses. Most scientists work within existing and known models or paradigms: endocrinologists study hormones, geneticists study genes, and so on. This path yields good, solid, and detailed knowledge. But this path can also lead to stagnation if not supplemented by the second path. This second path requires the thinker to break out of the standard models and ways of thinking and explore new, innovative, and challenging possible connections and syntheses. Listening to the exchange between Jim and several established giants in neuroscience, I got the hint that he was inadvertently suggesting some new ways to organize our knowledge. "Maybe that would be an interesting way to go."

Now, no one ever works entirely on his own. Science does not work that way, because today's science is not made up of individuals making breakthroughs on their own, but a cooperative effort, like our space missions. Still, we need individuals to contribute to that mission by suggesting new ways of organizing facts, which suggest ways to uncover new facts.

So what is James Vaughn Kohl suggesting? What are his ideas about sex? In a couple of sentences? Subliminal odors, known to scientists as pheromones, are major influences on genes in nerve cells that secrete a hormone which regulates the sexual development and the sexual behavior of animals from insects to mammals, including humans. Despite this common pattern among animals, scientists have generally ignored the possibility that odors and pheromones may also influence human sexual behavior, even though we share similar genes and hormones with other mammals. And even though a nerve cell is a nerve cell in any species.

A good friend and colleague who read this manuscript just before we sent it to the publisher said, "You know, Jim's argument is like a Brillo pad. I cannot follow all the individual strands, but it seems to hold together." Working with Jim was difficult because he likes what filmmakers call "the jump cut" —where suddenly the scene changes and new things are happening. Jim makes sudden, unexpected transitions to new ideas, and these *can* be difficult to follow. Do not be thrown off when you encounter one of these "jump cuts." That is the way I found Jim thinks, and to some extent it is the way I often think. Ideas stimulate other ideas, and the mind jump-cuts to a new theme.

That is the way most of us think. Still, though, when I agreed to collaborate on this book, I realized that I would have to rearrange much of the material so it would flow smoothly. My task was to provide greater continuity—with Kohl's permission, of course—and we had some heated debates about it! I could not remake the movie of his argument, so we have preserved his sometimes quirky style of thought.

Is that the "right" thing to do? When you think about it, it certainly is not the way science is normally written for the general public. Usually, scientists arrange their ideas and evidence in a nice orderly fashion, as if they were building a case in a courtroom trial. But this book is not a courtroom trial. We are dealing with ideas here, not with evidence in a lawsuit! And I wanted very much to preserve his thinking style, with all its complexities, without trampling on the subtleties of ideas.

Still, our readers deserve a guide to the jump cuts in this book. Several key threads run through our chapters. We often refer to a variety of sexual behaviors and responses that are shared by different animals and humans. We also explore similarities in the enzymes, hormones, and receptors that affect animal and human sexual development and behavior, and similarities in the genes that allow cells to make these enzymes, hormones, and receptors.

In our first chapter, we set the stage for our argument and ask why the uniqueness of being human has been a factor in ignoring the possibility that odors may in fact affect human sexual behavior. In chapter 2, we weave together some fascinating examples of animals, including humans, who use odors to communicate, build their societies, and reproduce. Chapter 3 traces the development of the sense of smell from one-celled organisms to humans, while chapter 4 describes how we detect odors and decode their messages. Chapters 5 and 6 link folklore about using odors to influence sexual behavior with scientific evidence of how odors may affect menstrual synchronization and suppression, bonding between mother and infant, recognition of friends, strangers, and lovers, as well as the popularity of oral sex and the origin of some fetishes.

Chapters 7 and 8, the foundation of our argument, trace the development of the sense of smell in the womb and explain how similarities humans share with other mammals in the web of genes, enzymes, hormones, receptors and nerve cells underlie many aspects of sexual development and behavior in humans and other mammals.

Chapters 9 and 10 focus on the roles the three human brains—reptilian, limbic, and thinking minds—play in our emotional and erotic lives, and the role natural amphetamines, opiates, and bonding hormones play in our love lives. How we make subtle odors called pheromones and how we use them to communicate with others are dealt with in chapters 11 and 12. Chapter 13 explores the world of people with an impaired sense of smell and describes the results of an international smell survey conducted recently by the National Geographic Society. Our final chapter looks at the healing power of odors, their many uses in marketing and environmental engineering, and the implications of all this for our lives in the next decade or two.

We have included endnotes in an appendix for readers who want to know who did this or that research, who said what, or where one can get more information on a particular point. We also provide a glossary with brief, simple definitions and a complete bibliography and index.

As I have already suggested, this book is unusual in style and imagination. Some colleagues will react suspiciously because it is not written in "proper scientific style." But if that is the only objection, fine. The content of this book is much more important than its style.

Is there enough support for the idea that odors and the sense of smell influence human sexual behavior? We certainly think so, but we cannot prove that the concept is true. We know the argument is long and complex. When we scientists actually do our work, instead of performing the way we are depicted on television or in the movies, we are not certain that our ideas are true. That is why we call them "hypotheses," tentatively held ideas, ideas that are interesting to think about, ideas that need to be tested and reshaped to lead us to deeper understanding.

Many people misunderstand scientists because they think we sit in laboratories and libraries, thinking about an idea until in a flash of genius we announce "We Have Found the Truth!" Science is a lot harder to effect than that. Science proceeds by presenting tentative ideas, suggestions, hypotheses, guesses, and then seeing if (1) the existing evidence fits and (2) we can gather new evidence to tell us more about these ideas.

In this book, *the reader will see science as it is actually done.* You are reading about how two colleagues interact with each other's ideas, sometimes critically, sometimes enthusiastically, but always with interest and curiosity about how odors and our sense of smell may influence our sexual behavior. We hope the book will be worth reading for that insight alone. If the reader also finds in these chapters that thinking about modern science can be exciting and fun, as well as serious thinking, then so much the better.

A book like this on odors, the sense of smell, and sex *invites the reader to add her or his own thoughts and observations and experience* to the process as it unfolds. *We expect our readers to say:* "Hey, that's right!" and "Oh, I don't agree!" and "I never thought of that before!" And our subject, sexuality, is surely something that most adults know a good deal about. This is not high tech science about atomic structure or quarks or the taxonomy of tropical spiders or designing new, high-power superconductive ceramics. Without doubt those are interesting and important topics, but too often they do not invite the average reader to participate.

Sex, on the other hand, is democratic. Everyone has ideas and opinions about sex, and in reading this book, we hope our readers will play with the ideas we have been piecing together during the past few years and will join us as we try to make sense out of some intriguing aspects of our human sexual experience.

—R. T. F.

1

THE MYSTERY
OF ODOR

For many years, very few scientists expressed an interest in figuring out how we detect odors or in exploring the ways in which the sense of smell might influence human sexual development and behavior.

That situation has changed radically in the past decade as a few pioneering scientists have made some major breakthroughs that have exploded many assumptions about the relative unimportance of the sense of smell. This new evidence has revealed some startling connections between the sense of smell and human sexual development and behavior—so startling at times that as John Money, director of the renowned Psychohormonal Research Unit at the Johns Hopkins University Medical School, sees it, we are facing what promises to be a veritable explosion of knowledge of how we experience our sexual and erotic nature. "This new knowledge will, in all probability, enforce a complete rewrite of the differentiation and development of human sexuality and eroticism early in the twenty-first century."[1]

Earlier in this century, a few scientists did in fact recognize the importance of exploring the possible connections between the sense of smell and sexual behavior. For instance, eighty years ago, Havelock Ellis, a British psychologist, wrote that "for most mammals not only are all sexual associations mainly olfactory, but the impressions received by this sense suffice to dominate all others."[2] Ellis found enough evidence that the sense of smell influences human sexual behavior and relationships to fill sixty-eight pages of fine print in his classic *Studies in the Psychology of Sex: Sexual Selection in Man*. "There can be no doubt," he maintained, that "the extent to which olfaction influences the sexual spheres in civilized [sic] man has been much underestimated."[3]

Half a century later, Irving Bieber confessed that psychologists had almost totally ignored the role odors and the sense of smell play in human sexual development and in our sexual relationships. He pointed out that this prejudice was not based on a lack of evidence or experiments showing that odors, the sense of smell, and sex have little or no connection. Instead, he laid the blame on a cultural bias that makes research on possible links between the sense of smell and human sexual behavior socially unacceptable. This bias, at least in part, can be traced to our modern obsession with cleanliness and the assumption that a lack of cleanliness causes sexual and other body odors. Bieber maintained that his own extensive observations and reading confirmed Ellis's contention that "smell is an important component in the total organization of many particular experiences . . . a powerful sexual stimulus."[4]

More recently, in the prestigious *New England Journal of Medicine*, Lewis Thomas, former president of the Memorial Sloan-Kettering Cancer Center, again focused on the importance of research on the sense of smell. "I should think we might fairly gauge the future of biological science, centuries ahead," he wrote, "by estimating the time it will take to reach a complete, comprehensive understanding of odor. It may not seem a profound enough problem to dominate all the life sciences, but it contains, piece by piece, all the mysteries."[5]

Research in recent years has confirmed these prophetic insights. Almost weekly, experts in different fields of research report new findings documenting how our sense of smell and specific odors influence how we develop as sexual beings, how we find our mates, how and why we bond with certain persons and reject others, and how and why bonds develop between children and family members. Odors influence our choice of persons with whom we have sex, and how often. New research also suggests that odors influence our learning and memory, our emotions and moods. It may well be, as Thomas suggested, that our future progress in understanding odors will be a good indicator of other more sensational and headline-grabbing discoveries in biology and medicine.

Some casual observations and questions may provide us with initial clues to the possible links between the sense of smell and sex. We will explore these observations later, but for the moment consider the following.[6]

- Mary Brown and her neighbor have noticed that their daughters menstrual cycles are synchronized with their own cycles, and that all the women in Mary's office have their period at about the same time.

- Some women have told us they can tell what stage of the menstrual cycle a woman is in by her smell. And many women report experiencing an increase in sex drive in the middle of their monthly cycle when they are fertile—the same time some men report finding a woman most alluring.

- What is it about close dancing that makes it an important element in the courtship rituals of many cultures?

- Many women report their sensitivity to the smell of their partner changes during their menstrual cycle, along with the ease with which they reach orgasm.

- Why do many women find the sweaty sports hero or sun-tanned "macho" man so irresistibly sexy?

- Why are some men so strongly attracted to large-breasted women, and might this have anything to do with the scent producing glands in the breasts?

- Why does a sex drive decline in older men and women sometimes coincide with a decline in their sense of smell?

- Does the recently reported increase in the popularity of oral sex owe anything to our emphasis on reducing natural body odors and the difficulty of eliminating natural vaginal odors?

- If variety enhances the spice of one's sexual life, as folklore suggests, what is it in the novelty of a new partner that is so enticing?

- Does the assumption that blond women have more fun have anything to do with male preferences in hair color? And if so, might this be connected with the observation that blondes, brunettes, and redheads smell differently?

- Why do girls and boys report that their odor preferences change after they enter puberty, and what are the sexual consequences of this?

- Why is a reduced sex drive, delayed puberty, and infertility in women often associated with a reduced sense of smell?

- Why does Joanne end up sleeping on her husband's side of the bed, or wear his shirts or robe while he's away?

- Why do many children object vehemently when their mothers try to put their security blanket or teddy bear in the wash?

An answer to this last question may well be related to the previous one about why Joanne sleeps on "his" side of the bed and wears his shirt when he is away. The familiar body odors picked up by the child's blanket or stuffed toy play an important role in her or his bonding experience and sense of security. Wash a child's favorite security blanket or cherished stuffed animal and you remove the familiar body odors associated with emotional closeness and destroy the feeling of being safe and secure.[7] Similarly, the body scent of a lover on the bed, a pillow, or shirt can provide a reassuring subliminal reminder of an absent lover.

Unfortunately, smell is still the least understood of our five senses. We are just beginning to probe the mysteries of how we smell and what impact odors may have on our development, our health, our moods, our behaviors, and even our abstract thought processes.

Part of the problem in talking about how odors may influence our sexual lives is a language problem because these odors do not fit our usual definition of that term. When we talk about odors, we usually think about the fragrance of flowers, a vine-ripened melon or strawberry, or a perfume. Or we think about some repulsive odor that makes us wince at first breath. These odors we consciously recognize because sensory neurons in the nose and our main olfactory system routinely detect and process these odors in conscious circuits of the brain.

But can something have a scent, fragrance, or aroma, that affects us even if we do not consciously detect and identify the odor? Scientists have discovered that some odors are not processed by the main olfactory system. Instead, these chemical messengers are processed subliminally, below the conscious level, in an accessory or secondary olfactory system.[8] This second kind of chemical signal, known as a pheromone, is defined by *Webster's Unabridged Dictionary of the English Language* as "any of a class of hormonal substances secreted by an individual and stimulating a physiological or behavioral response from an individual of the same species." Pheromones are chemical messengers, odors that convey information subliminally between two or more individuals of the same species. Because some pheromones affect sexual behaviors, they are sometimes referred to as sex attractants, even though most pheromones do not affect sexual behavior.

But if pheromones operate below the level of conscious perception, should we refer to them as odors or scents? The dictionary defines an odor as "that property of a substance which affects the sense of smell." Pheromones are detected by the accessory *olfactory* system in warm-blooded animals, so apparently they do qualify as odors, smells, and scents.

We also have considerable evidence that pheromones affect humans although we do not understand the anatomy behind their detection. Hence the title of our book, *The Scent of Eros: Mysteries of Odors in Human Sexuality*. Because our focus is on pheromones that affect our hormone levels, the development of our brains, and many of our sexual behaviors, we will refer to these subliminal chemical signals as scents or odors.

HOW HUMAN ARE WE?

Immanuel Kant, whose effort to define precisely the superiority of humans is a landmark in Western thought, constantly deplored any suggestion that noble humans could be influenced by anything so base or animalistic as odors. For Kant, smell was "the most dispensable and ungrateful of all the senses." To suggest that odors might influence human emotions and behaviors, he claimed, would be to deny human free will. Being human meant being fully conscious and above the kind of gross, reflex reactions animals experience.[9]

Obviously, we disagree and find Kant's assumption totally illogical. To begin with, Kant assumed that humans have only one mind, a conscious, thinking, analytical—soft-wired in computerese—brain with the freedom of choice lower animals cannot experience. He ignored the possibility that the brains or minds other animals use to process and react to information from their bodies and surrounding environment might persist and comfortably coexist with the conscious brain and free will unique in humans. In all animals with internal skeletons, including humans, odors influence the hard-wired mind of the brain stem or reptilian brain and the emotional circuits of our limbic mind. While they operate below the level of consciousness, the reptilian and limbic minds control our life-sustaining reflexes of feeding, fighting, fleeing, and mating.

The presence of these ancient minds and their behavioral responses is as much a part of human nature as is the very sophisticated conscious brain sitting on top of them. Without such primitive triggers as touch, taste, and smell sparking our automatic, hard-wired behaviors and emotions, we would be disembodied spirits, not humans able to adapt to rapid changes in our environment without wasting time to analyze the situation and weigh our options. In fact, humans have reptilian, limbic, and conscious brains that work together to make us the unique creatures we are.[10]

Kant is also wrong because he spoke as an armchair philosopher who never bothered to test his theory against reality with scientific experimentation. When a scientist thinks about odors and their possible effects on humans, she or he starts by asking a question. The question becomes a hypothesis that can be tested experimentally. Looking at the experimental findings we will discuss later, we arrive at the position that Kant was totally wrong: odors do very much influence human sexual development and behavior. Of course, the ramifications of this broad conclusion are obvious in the kinds of questions scientists have asked themselves as they pursued the idea that odors play a role in our sexual lives.

Are human hormones broken down into pheromones the same way pheromones are produced by dogs, bulls, cows, and other mammals? Are the effects of these subliminal odors on sexual development and behaviors in any way similar in humans and other animals? Do pheromones influence the way our genes work? Do they affect production of the hormones that direct and control our sexual development and behavior? Are neural pathways in the brains of men and women affected differently by the same pheromone? Do gender differences in these reactions result in different messages being sent from the brain back to the body for translation into sexual behavior? Do pheromones affect the primitive, emotional circuits of our brains? Do some pheromones play important roles in our emotion-laden sexual behavior and relationships? Do odors affect learning and memory?

One reason why a "yes" answer to any of these question would not surprise a biologist is that biologists operate on the tested premise that biological processes are usually fairly consistent from one species to the next, even though there are often tremendous differences. One basic element in this consistency is that we share similar genes that determine the structure of enzymes, hormones, receptors, and other proteins that determine the anatomical structures and physiological processes we share with other animals. Thus it is reasonable to assume that, if the sexual behavior of other animals is influenced by the chemical messages in odors and the sense of smell, then our own human sexual development and behavior might be similarly influenced by the subliminal odors we call pheromones.

Not long ago it was widely held that what made humans uniquely human was our ability to make tools, think abstractly, and talk. We now know that we share tool-making abilities with other animals, especially chimpanzees and apes. Other animals besides humans can and do show altruism, courage, intelligence, invention, curiosity, and forethought, as well as friendship, love, fidelity, and many other characteristics once thought to be uniquely human. Dolphins, whales, chimpanzees, and other mammals cannot challenge our verbal skills, but they do have some fairly sophisticated ways of communicating.

If we look for absolute differences between us and other mammals, no clear distinguishing characteristics for our species emerge. Differences do exist, but they appear to be relative or quantitative rather than qualitative and essential.

In defense of human uniqueness, some deny our "animal" nature altogether and try to create a solid wall between animals and humans. The mythic creation story of Genesis, for instance, draws a clear distinction by giving man dominion over all the animals. Some philosophers, psychologists, and scientists attempt to put as much distance as possible between us and our animal origins, downplaying the fact that we share 98 percent of our genes with other higher primates. That 98 percent of our genes we share with our closely related animal relatives makes some similarities and connections between animal and human behavior unavoidable and undeniable.

Even though human sexual interactions are much more complex than the mating of other animals because we can mix love with hormone-driven lust, this does not mean that factors like odors and pheromones that influence the mating of other warm-blooded animals no longer function in humans. In the brains of the earliest land animals, the olfactory system became intimately associated with mating and reproduction, and those early connections between odors and sex have persisted even as brains became more and more complex and conscious.

In the higher primates and among humans, the sexual drive and sexual behavior are no longer limited to reproduction. Humans have added pleasure, recreation, playfulness, exploration, curiosity, and love to the expression of our sexuality, even though we still talk about biological clocks ticking away in women and our genes being driven to perpetuate themselves.

With or without contraceptives, we know that humans around the world increasingly engage in sex for reasons other than making babies. The World Health Organization estimates that in one day, two hundred million men and women around the globe engage in vaginal intercourse. Less than a million of these sexual unions result in pregnancies, so obviously reproduction is not the main motive for human matings. In terms of species survival, humans are far less efficient in their matings than other mammals where the female periodically comes into sexual heat and is receptive to mating only when she is fertile and likely to become pregnant. On average, two humans copulate a hundred times to produce a single pregnancy. (This does not take into account the time and energy humans invest in self-pleasuring, oral sex, and other non-coital erotic pursuits.)

The "World Health Organization Score Board" clearly shows pleasure/play winning over baby-making, by a score of 99,090,000 to 910,000! With easier-to-use, more effective contraceptives coming on the market and growing concern about overpopulation and AIDS, the score is likely to be even more lopsided in the near future.[11] But admitting that humans increasingly engage in sex for pleasure, recreation, bonding, or love far more often than we do to make babies does not mean that odors and pheromones no longer influence our sexual behavior and pairbonding.

Claims of human uniqueness and moral superiority are in fact based on social designs custom-made by humans who assume that our human sexual behavior has transcended the primitive, animalistic drives of the lower animals. The fallacy of the moral superiority assumption is revealed by scientific evidence that odors may, as we will see, activate genes in the neurons that regulate the cycles of human sex-hormone production, which in turn strongly affect our sexual behavior, regardless of conscious motives like tension release, sensual pleasure, mutual desire, love, or reproduction.

THE CONSISTENCY OF LIFE

Biological science is based on the assumption that a basic logic and efficient consistency pervades the way all living organisms, from one-celled animals to humans, have developed to carry on the processes of living. Biological logic tells us that the information encoded in the functional units of DNA (deoxyribonucleic acid) we call genes is responsible for both the similarities and the differences we find among individual humans and between humans and other primates.

Specific genes are responsible for the structures and processes that produce hormones in animals and humans. Some of the hormones produced by primates and our four-legged distant cousins are so similar we can use animal hormones to remedy a hormone deficiency in humans. The final link in the chain is the fact that hormones clearly influence behavior (including sexual behavior) in the lower animals, in mammals, in primates, and in humans.

This evidence cuts across many traditional disciplines. In the past, geneticists, endocrinologists, embryologists, psychologists, anthropologists, and others pursued their questions and tested their hypotheses about possible connections between odors and sex in their own narrow discipline. Today we know the questions and hypotheses are so complex that it will take more than the discipline-bound scientists working on their own to make real breakthroughs.

We need a new science that brings different specialists together in a team approach. The new science, known as psychoneuroendocrinology, is already born and growing like any healthy, robust infant. Ten syllables and twenty-four letters is impressive, but hardly indicative of the creative minds that this new approach brings together. The strength of this new science is its integration: *psycho*—for "behavior"; *neuro*—for "nerve cells," the nervous system and the brain; *endocrin*—for "hormones" and the genes that direct their production; and *ology*—for "the study of." There you have it, psycho-neuro-endocrin-ology, the study of how hormones affect the nerve cells that affect behavior.

Before we go any further, we need to clarify the concept of a hormone. Hormones are chemical messengers secreted by ductless or *endocrine* glands, like the pituitary, ovaries, and testes. Hormones circulate in the blood and are picked up by receptors in the target cells where they control gene activity, cell processes, and development.[12]

In psychoneuroendocrinology, the logic of cause-effect, "this" produces "that," is not always a straight line. One gene can have several different effects, just as a single hormone like testosterone or estrogen can have many different effects in different organs of the body.[13] The relationships between genes, nerve cells, hormones, and behavior, especially the sexual behaviors of humans involved in bonding, love, commitment, altruism, and spirituality, are more complicated than a simple, single linear cause-to-effect. In this new science, we are dealing with many causes—odors, genes, hormones, and neural circuits—interacting together to produce several different effects and behaviors, at different times, in different degrees, and in different parts of the brain. This is a major, but not insurmountable, problem for psychoneuroendocrinologists.[14]

While psychoneuroendocrinologists cannot experiment directly on humans by manipulating their genes and hormones, they can often find evidence in animal research that suggests tentative, cautious insights and theories about humans. Animal studies can never account for all of human variability, but evidence from animal studies can provide new insights into possible parallel or similar links between odors, genes, nerve cells, hormones, and behavior in humans.

In many species of animals, odors are produced and detected by males and females in ways that clearly influence their courtship, mating, and parenting behaviors, as well as the social structure and interaction of individuals in the family, hive, colony, or herd. We know a good deal about these effects on animal behavior, but we are just beginning to understand how odors influence human sexual behavior. We have many bits and pieces of research with animals, and some with humans, that fit together and suggest a big picture that is biologically consistent but also allows for important differences between different animal species, and between other animals and humans.

Here, biological consistency suggests we jump-cut to a connection between odors and the immune system that makes us the unique individuals we are. Early in the research on organ transplants, scientists learned that all cells carry a unique protein signature on their surface that enables a donor's immune system to identify and reject a transplanted organ. These identifying protein tags are produced by a group of genes located in a region known as MHC or Major Histocompatible Complex. But the MHC genes are also responsible for the distinctive body odor litter-mates share in common. This identifying body odor enables a mouse to quickly tell whether an approaching mouse is a family member or potential enemy that needs to be driven off.[15] "One of the most exciting recent developments in the study of individual odors is the finding that several primate species, including humans, may have the ability to distinguish between individuals by [their] odors."[16] Yes. some humans can apparently tell whether two mice come from the same litter or from different strains based on the identifying odor of their urine and feces.[17] In a similar way, dogs can discriminate between the smell of garments worn by non-identical twins, but cannot detect a difference when the garments were worn by identical twins.[18] In all animals, the many different systems work together so that the sense of smell and the unique identifying odors a body produces are part of the whole system, and connected more or less with their survival and sexual behavior.

In addition to the obvious survival advantage this ability gives a mouse when it is approached by a potential enemy, this ability to detect body odor gives mice another advantage. Biologists have long known that inbreeding—mating between closely related males and females—increases the risk of severe, often lethal conditions in the offspring. If an individual happens to have a single defective gene, she or he will not show its effects provided the gene is "recessive" and requires two copies to be expressed. A person with one defective recessive gene will be normal but can pass the defective gene on to an offspring, who will also be normal provided it does not receive a matching recessive gene from the other parent. Unfortunately, when both parents are closely related, their offspring is more likely to receive the same defective gene from each parent and to suffer serious consequences.

Some ten thousand years ago our distant ancestors discovered this aspect of sexual reproduction when they started capturing and keeping wild animals as livestock. Breeding these animals to produce more docile beasts of burden, more wool or milk, and better hunting and guard dogs quickly became a major preoccupation. Smart breeders observed the advantages and risks of inbreeding close relatives and outbreeding with a stud or prize female in a neighboring herd. Shared observations produced a hypothesis, a theory, and finally, a conclusion. They could test this conclusion by carefully comparing the offspring produced by breeding closely related and unrelated males and females.

Anthropologists, following the lead of Claude Levi-Strauss, do not believe this understanding of the genetics of breeding cattle, sheep, and dogs played a significant role in the origins of human taboos against incest. For many anthropologists like Levi-Strauss, social rules about marriage are what makes us different from other animals. These regulations determine who officially mates with whom and they appear to be more designed to reduce kinship conflicts and to promote the exchange of women between male lineages.

Wild animals, mice, dogs, and cats do not have the ability to create a hypothesis about the risks of their breeding with close kin. And yet, given a choice, most animals in the wild will not mate with litter-mates. Why? Mice appear to have some kind of neural program for recognizing odors that allows them to welcome litter-mates and respond to a strange odor by attacking an outsider. While the ability to distinguish litter-mates from non-litter-mates by their odors triggers clan bonding and nest defense, it also seems to trigger a negative reaction, based on the same odors, that prompts them to avoid mating with a familiar-smelling litter-mate while being attracted to the unfamiliar odor of unrelated mice. Both behaviors obviously promote survival for mice and other animals that share similar odor-based mechanisms for recognizing kin and stranger.

And what about humans? Closely related humans grow up more or less sharing the same home space for many years. Family members also share very similar MHC genes, and a daily familiarity with the unique odor associated with those shared genes. Given the harmful effects of inbreeding and the benefits of diverse genes that come with marrying outsiders, the logic of biological systems might favor development of emotional and mating circuits in our brains that promote bonding with familiar-smelling kin, and falling in love and mating with the different-smelling stranger. Basing such tendencies on the interactions of our genes, sense of smell, and neural circuits would be efficient and could improve our genetic health.

TESTING THE FLAME

Jump-cut for a minute from this discussion about odors and incest to testing this hypothesis.

Whether we are talking about how odors influence human behavior, or about the role black holes played in the origins of our universe, we do know that all of our knowledge is conditional. We are constantly expanding, revising, redrawing, and updating our pictures of human behavior. An incurable curiosity drives us to an endless search for better answers to questions that are never quite answered to our satisfaction.

A major problem in this endless quest for understanding is the difficulty we have in proving that a particular event or behavior—"this"—is caused by some other particular factor—"that." We build our picture of how things in our world function on a scaffold of ideas, theories, hypotheses, and laws designed to connect the "this's" and "that's" of our world into a meaningful structure. If these connections make sense, and if our evidence supports the different conclusions, we can fit the different hypotheses together into a bigger picture that makes sense of our world. And that is what all science and human wisdom is about, trying to make sense of the incredibly complex and confusing world we live in.

A hypothesis may start out as nothing more than a guess, a mere idea. Or we may tease it out of exquisitely detailed scientific experiments. Whatever its origins, a scientific hypothesis stands or falls on logic and on the strength of the evidence we gather to justify calling this idea an observation, a hypothesis, a theory, or eventually a law of nature.[19] In this knowledge system, the logic of evidence and the way we prove something are independent of where we get our original idea. Whether or not one has been educated as a scientist, the important thing is to ask logical, analytical questions about the connection between "this" and "that."

The first time a child puts a hand into an open flame and finds out what "hot" or "burn" means, he or she is well on the way to forming a hypothesis about the connection between cause and effect, in this case, between the flame and pain. The child may need more than one similarly painful experiences before she or he realizes that the cause and effect connection is more than just a hypothesis, and that some kind of law of nature comes into play when flame contacts skin.

This is how the painful observation that a flame burns was expanded into a law of nature that includes burns from all hot surfaces, electromagnetic radiation, X-rays, and sunlight. But the scientific venture also requires that scientists constantly test and challenge what is considered a biological law or law of nature.

A WORKING HYPOTHESIS

In other animals, odors are a major factor in the interactions between genes, nerve cells, hormones, and neural pathways during development. Odors also affect the circuits and pathways within the brain that influence learning, memory, and behavior. Since humans share many of their biological systems with other animal species because we are animals, it seems logical that odors and the sense of smell probably play a much greater role than we commonly think in human social interactions, sexual attraction, sexual arousal, mating, bonding, and parenting. Briefly stated, this is the hypothesis we propose to examine in this book.

2

ON THE
DARKEST NIGHT

E arly in this century, the French naturalist Jean Henri Fabré
brought home an unusual cocoon he found while walking in the
woods. When a large beautiful female emperor moth emerged, he
put it in a cage in his office. The next morning, forty males were fluttering around the cage, drawn from the outside world through an open
window by some unknown lure.

Over the next few nights, more than 150 males came to court the
caged female. Curious about what was attracting the males and sus-
pecting it might be some kind of chemical signal or odor, Fabré con-
fined his female under a glass bell jar and found that males ignored her
presence.

Experts on insects have since learned much about this and similar
chemical signals. We know, for instance, that insects have the most
acute sense of smell in all nature. Male moths can detect and follow the
sex attractant (pheromone) produced by a female two miles away on
the darkest night.[1]

This ability makes the female gypsy moth's pheromone or mating
scent the perfect bait for traps designed to lure male gypsy moths before
they can mate. Reflecting on why we fear the power of such odors,
Lewis Thomas reported that, theoretically, if a single gypsy moth were to
release all her sex scent in one burst, she could attract a trillion mates.[2]
Similar scents make population studies of moths, butterflies, roaches,
and other insects quite easy for naturalists and environmentalists.

The power of such sex attractants is undisputed. Male moths
could care less about the sensual fluttering, feathery antennae, and
beautiful colored wings of a lovely female. Their overwhelming

compulsion is to mate with whatever emits that irresistible mating scent, even if it is the abdomen of a decapitated female of their species.

In a similar fragrant fashion, a newly hatched queen bee announces her readiness for a nuptial flight to drone males with a sexy scent from a gland in her mouth. When scientists harvested this scent and sent it aloft on a balloon, drones piled on trying desperately to mate. Another type of pheromone from the same gland identifies the queen to her hive workers and drones. Select worker bees collect this pheromone from the queen and pass it on to all the female workers to prevent their ovaries from developing. No new queen can be produced in the hive until the queen dies and no longer produces this scent which in effect sterilizes other bees as they develop.

Other types of pheromones from the queen bee also control the social structure as well as the feeding and grooming behaviors within the hive. At the entrance to the hive, guard bees check every bee trying to enter. If it does not have the proper scent that identifies it as a member of the hive, it is driven off or killed. Stingers left in a foreign bee, or in an intruding human hand, contain a pheromone that invites other bees to attack.

The natural aggression of ants is also suppressed by a pheromone they share with their nest mates. Foreign ants are easily recognized by their odor and attacked. If ants are deprived of their odor-detecting antennae, they attack any member of their species, nest mate or not.

Ants also use a pheromone to mark the trail back home when they leave the nest in search of food. Invariably it is a wandering search and not always successful. But whether or not food is found, the ant knows it can follow its trail back home. If food is found, other ants will set out along the fresh trail. But then a curious thing occurs. Despite the original meandering trail, the ants quickly lay out a straight-line, shortest-distance path to the food. The second ant does not do this right off, but starts the process by taking a couple of short cuts when the original meandering odor trail doubles back on itself. Each subsequent ant shortens the distance, laying down a fresh pheromone trail that overpowers the scent of old meandering loops. In recent years, Dr. Bert Holldobler in Würzburg, Germany and colleagues have discovered at least twenty-five glands that ants use to produce two dozen different pheromones. Coupled with tactile and visual clues including different dances and threatening, tender, and directional signals, these scents help coordinate the activities of every individual ant with the tasks of all the other ants in the colony. Pheromones keep every ant continually tied into its colony's version of Internet.[3]

The insect's extraordinary, highly specialized sense of smell makes them the most successful animals in hostile surroundings. Pheromones enable insects to locate one another, stimulate courtship and mating, warn of impending danger, and direct others to suitable food, egg-laying, and resting sites. Their robot-like response to these odors makes them much more attractive to animal communications specialists than researching similar chemical signals and responses in other species, including humans. It is much easier to find links between odor and behavior in insects than to pursue similar links in algae, nematodes, spiders, crustacea, fish, salamanders, snakes, and mammals.[4]

MESSAGES OF EXCITEMENT

Until 1959, these behavior-controlling scents were called "ecto-hormones," short for "external hormones."[5] Hormones, like testosterone and estrogen, are chemical messengers produced by organs in the body and transported by the blood to various organs and systems in the body, including the brain. Hormones act on genes in cells to stimulate and direct the development of tissues, organs, and organ systems and their many functions. Early researchers settled on the label "ecto-hormone" because these aromatic chemical messengers are produced in the metabolism or breakdown of hormones and, like hormones, act on the genes to control various behaviors. Adding the prefix "ecto" indicated they were different because their messages were carried by the air from one animal to another instead of by the blood to different organs within the body of one animal as hormones are.

By 1959 it was clear that there were more differences than similarities between hormones and these behavior-controlling scents. The term "ecto-hormone" gradually lost favor and was replaced by a new term, *pheromone*. The new term, pronounced *fair'-uh-mohn*, was derived from the Greek *pherein* "to transfer" and *hormon* "to excite."[6] Expanding on our earlier description, we can now add that, as hormone-derived aromatic messengers, pheromones influence the sexual development and behavior of all individuals within a particular species of animal.[7]

Pheromones have two distinct but related effects. In the hypothalamus, they influence the production of gonadotropin-releasing hormone

(GnRH) that is responsible for starting the cascade, pulses, and cycles of sex hormones that originate in the pituitary gland and involve the adrenal glands, ovaries, and testes. The hormone cascade from the pituitary, adrenal glands, ovaries, and testes affects all sexual development, physiology, and behavior. But pheromones also trigger production of some GnRH that acts as a neurotransmitter. This GnRH affects activity in neurons that also influence sexual development and behavior.[8]

Pheromones are derived from hormones produced by specialized cells and passed into the animal's surroundings as either liquids or gases. Some pheromones are too heavy to evaporate into the air and must be passed by physical contact and picked up by the tongue which passes them to the neurons in the olfactory system. Even though pheromones produce their effects without passing through the conscious circuits of the brain, we still commonly refer to them as scents or odors because the neurons in the olfactory system convert their chemical messages into nerve impulses which are sent along to the brain for decoding and processing. In high concentrations, some pheromones do have a detectable odor—musk, civet, and castoreum, for instance.[9]

Another distinguishing characteristic of pheromones is that their message is usually only effective with other members of the same species. Male silkworm and gypsy moths completely ignore the mating pheromone of the female emperor moth. Only drone and worker honey bees, not bumble bees, pay attention to the queen honey bee's aromatic messages. In contrast, many hormones are not species-specific. Testosterone, estrogen, progesterone, growth hormone, and insulin obtained from other mammals may be used to treat human hormone disorders or deficiencies.

Some exceptions to this species-specific character of pheromones do exist however. Pheromones from some mammals are quite effectively used in perfumes—castoreum from beavers, civetone from the civet cat, and musk from the musk deer.[10]

While early pheromone research concentrated on insects, the potential for profitable applications to improve the breeding of cattle, sheep, pigs, and other domesticated animals has been a strong lure for many scientists to extend their research to higher animals. Since most beef and pork comes from artificially inseminated cattle and pigs, knowing when the female is fertile and when insemination is likely to be most productive becomes an important business consideration. In some animals, the female shows obvious physical signs of being sexually receptive and fertile. This is not the case in cows and sows. Randy bulls and boars must investigate the female's scent before they attempt to mount and mate.

Pig breeders use a whiff of canned boar pheromone to check a sow's readiness for artificial insemination. The aerosol spray contains synthetic versions of androstenone, the sex pheromone that gives a characteristic odor of urine to boars. A whiff of androstenone, accompanied by pressure on the back, and a sow in heat will arch her back downwards to present her hind quarters for mounting. Sows not in their fertile period are indifferent to the spray. Given the proper response of arching the back and presenting, the hog breeder knows which sows to artificially inseminate with semen from a champion boar.[11]

French gourmets have long known that sows have a special ability to detect truffles, a rare edible fungus, three feet underground. The odor truffles emit is almost identical to the odor of androstenol, another of the pig's own sexual attractants. From the time of the Romans, through Napoleon to the present day, truffles have been praised and treasured as a formidable aphrodisiac, even though scientists have not documented any substance as a true aphrodisiac for humans.[12] The more urinous-like smell of androstenone has also been detected in parsnips and in the roots of celery which were once reputed to be "the poor man's truffles and aphrodisiacs."

In the early 1970s, new efforts to improve the mating of endangered animal species in zoological parks and game preserves added to the biologists' growing interest in mammalian pheromones.[13]

Dogs and cats have a notorious compulsion to mark outdoor objects, particularly trees, as part of their territory with the pheromones in their urine. Owners of unspayed bitches are well aware that male dogs are quick to pick up on the sex pheromones of a bitch "in heat" from as far away as three miles.[14] Dogs, cats, and other mammals also use similar chemical messages to indicate rank and dominance, much as bees, ants, and termites use pheromones to maintain social order.

The pheromones of billy goats, rams, and boars have other functions besides signalling females. Kid goats, lambs, and piglets mature sexually much more quickly when exposed to an appropriate male priming pheromone. Once these males are sexually mature, a natural selection game comes into play when the adult male with the strongest pheromone effects a kind of psychological castration on his rivals. This reduces the competition and lets the dominant male share his genes with as many available females as possible without wasting his energy on combat.

Specialists in animal communications and behavior now talk about two types of pheromones in mammals: signaling and priming pheromones. Signaling pheromones cause a more or less immediate change in behavior, probably by acting on genes in the cells that produce neurotransmitters. Priming pheromones, on the other hand, trigger GnRH production which in turn regulates the level of different hormones, which then affect development, metabolism, and various behaviors including mating and reproductive behavior.[15]

Signaling pheromones can carry different messages. Some send an alarm, like the pheromone in a bee sting that tells other bees to attack the enemy.[16] Some mark a trail to food. Some help individuals recognize members of their own family or group and identify strangers. Others contribute to that unique, identifying scent that tells the bee, ant, or human it is home. The unique scent that identifies a particular house or apartment as home is created by signaling pheromones in the sweat, dead skin cells, and other secretions left on the furniture, beds, and carpeting as family members go about their daily routines. The sex attractant Fabré's female emperor moth produced is a classic example of a signalling or "seducer" pheromone. Like the androstenone that triggers the sow's receptivity to mate when she is in heat, seducer pheromones enhance libido and sexual interest.

The end result of chemical messages in primer pheromones is to regulate hormone and neurotransmitter production in various regions of the brain.[17] This control starts with a priming action that produces "releasing hormones," so named because their sole function is to turn on and control production of a variety of other hormones that regulate the growth and functioning of organs and systems throughout the body. Some of these other hormones, for example, regulate the onset of puberty or sexual maturation, the development of secondary sex characteristics like breasts and facial and body hair. Ultimately, priming pheromones trigger production of hormones that control sex drive, regulate the menstrual cycle, and control egg and sperm production.[18]

HUMAN ODORS

Every body, including human bodies, has a personal "odor signature," as distinctive as our fingerprints, voice, and personality. One of the strongest human odors is androstenone, a major component in the acrid, gamy smell of perspiration. This is not the watery sweat that covers our bodies after a good workout, but the particularly strong scented pheromonally active secretions of the apocrine glands associated with the hair follicles all over the body but concentrated in the armpits and groin.[19] In ancient Greece, Hippocrates, the father of medicine, reported that the apocrine glands become active at puberty. Today we know that the secretions of the apocrine glands have little or no odor until particular strains of bacteria on the skin converts this delicate secretion into the gamy smelling androstenone and other pheromones.[20]

Havelock Ellis maintained that our individual odor signature is actually a combination of several different odors. Most important, for Ellis, were (1) the general skin odor, "a faint, but agreeable, fragrance often to be detected on the skin even immediately after washing;" (2) the smell of the hair and scalp; (3) the odor of the breath; (4) armpit odor; (5) foot odor; (6) perineal odor; (7) in men the odor of smegma under the penile foreskin; and (8) in women the odor of the mons veneris, the smegma of the clitoris and vulva, vaginal mucus, and menstrual odor.[21]

Commenting on the specific body odors of various peoples and the ability to distinguish individuals by smell, Ellis noted that:

> In approaching the specifically sexual aspects of odor in the human
> species we may start from the fundamental fact—a fact we seek so
> far as possible to disguise in our ordinary social relations—that all
> men and women are odorous.

Ellis then summarized reports on the odors of various groups including Australian blacks, African blacks, Chinese, Nigrito natives in the Bay of Bengal west of Malaysia, Monbuttus, Europeans, Japanese, negroes from the Congo, South American Indians, and the Indians of central Chile. The body odors reported for individuals and groups ranged from "ammoniacal and rancid," or "like the odor of the he-goat" to a phosphoric character, a musky odor, the odor of garlic, a slight and agreeable hazelnut, and a strong Gorgonzola perfume, with some odors quite distinct and strong while others were faint.[22]

A Japanese anthropologist reported that the odor of Europeans was:

> a strong and pungent smell—sometimes sweet, sometimes bitter—
> of varying strength in different individuals, absent in children and
> the aged, and having its chief focus in the armpits, which, however
> carefully they are washed, immediately become odorous again.

This same Japanese anthropologist found that the sweat glands are larger in Europeans than in the Japanese, and that the Japanese take such offense to "armpit stink" that it can disqualify a young man from service in the army.[23] One possible explanation to this strong negative reaction to body odor might be the long tradition of arranged marriages that forced Japanese men and women into close contact with partners they found unappealing.[24]

Ellis tried to maintain the reportorial objectivity of a social scientist, but he could not escape some of the ethnic insensitivity characteristic of Victorian Europeans when he wrote that:

> ... savages are often accused more or less justly of indifference to bad odors [as perceived by Europeans]. They are very often, however, keenly alive to the significance of smells and their varieties, though it does not appear that the sense of smell is notably more developed in savage than in civilized peoples.[25]

One might well speculate about how the natural order of human relations is altered by advertisers promoting an American obsession with deodorants and antiperspirants out of a profit interest. Or the effects of the American Puritan tradition of "cleanliness is next to godliness" on male-female relations.[26] Whatever the origins and variations of body odors and reactions to them that have existed and currently affect human interactions, the statement that "all men and women are odorous" cannot be denied.[27]

The French poet Charles Baudelaire once remarked that the essence of our soul resides in our erotic sweat. The imaginative and emotional significance of odors is a recurring theme in *Fleurs de Mal* and many of his *Petits Poémes en Prose*. Odor was to Baudelaire what music was to others.

In her provocative exploration of *The Anatomy of Love*, anthropologist Helen Fisher notes that Napoleon frequently confessed his abiding interest in erotic sweat. Once he reportedly wrote his beloved Josephine: "I will be arriving in Paris tomorrow evening. Don't wash." The novelist Joris-Karl Huysmans, another nineteenth-century Frenchman, used to follow women through the fields, smelling them. The scent of a woman's underarms, Huysmans reported, "easily uncaged the animal in man." Small wonder French prostitutes would dab vaginal fluid behind their ears to help waft their "wares" to potential customers.[28]

3

A BALL OF STRING

According to an ancient Greek myth, when King Minos faced a revolt, the sea god Poseidon sent a giant bull to him as a sign of divine approval. Unfortunately, once Minos had put down the revolt, he neglected to make the appropriate sacrifices to the bull. In revenge, Poseidon gave Minos' wife an irresistible passion for the bull. Queen Pasiphae then persuaded the architect Daedalus to build her a wooden cow so she could satisfy her lust for the bull. When Pasiphae gave birth to the Minotaur, a monster with a human body and a bull's head, Daedalus built a great stone maze to imprison the Minotaur.

Every nine years, the Minotaur had to be fed fourteen youthful maidens from Athens. When King Theseus of Athens visited Crete, King Minos' fair daughter, Ariadne, fell in love with him. Determined to end the slaughter of his fellow Athenians, Theseus resolved to find a way through the labyrinth and slay the Minotaur. If he was successful, he would have to find his way out, or die in the maze. Ariadne provided him with a ball of string to guide him out so she could marry him.[1]

To understand and appreciate the role of pheromones in our sexual lives, we need our own Ariadne's thread to trace the development of the sense of smell from its most primitive forms in bacteria to its latest degree of sophistication in the human nose.[2] Our ball of string is the logic and consistency we can find in living organisms. All life forms, from the simplest, earliest one-celled organisms to humans with billions of cells in their bodies, start life as a single cell. Inside every cell is biology's thread of consistency, the spiral double helix of DNA with thousands of genes that turn raw materials into proteins and produce organs that then create the symphony of a living, eating, moving, sensing, communicating, and reproducing organism. That genetic information lets individuals find a niche where they can survive in an ever-changing world and produce offspring who pass the genetic code from generation to generation. Individuals inevitably die, but the information in DNA—the thread of life's processes—passes from one generation to the next. Within each of the fascinating varieties of life produced by random mutations and tested by natural selection is the thread of our genetic heritage.

The very simplest forms of life survived because they developed two links to the outside world: an ability to respond to physical contact with the outside environment based on the experience of pressure, injury, and temperature, and the ability to react to chemical messages from a distance, or smell. "Among organisms that swim, fly, or stride, the oldest and most common language is composed not of sounds or gestures but of chemicals."[3] The ability to see and hear came much later in the history of life.[4]

Throughout the history of life, touch and smell have been essential, not just for living, but also for reproducing. From bacteria to humans, the sense of smell alerts living organisms to danger, warns them of poisons, helps them locate food, and identifies mates. The difference between the sense of smell in bacteria and humans is that humans possess specialized sensory cells to sort out these chemical messages and pass them on to very sophisticated neural circuits that can analyze, compare, and interpret the information consciously against the memories of past experiences.[5]

The olfactory neurons that enable higher animals to detect odors are unique. They are delicate giant cells, stretching out several inches long. Like other neurons in our body, they have a central cell body with a nucleus and ultrafine branches called dendrites. Sensory dendrites with specialized receptors pick up sensations from outside and convert them into electrical impulses which pass through the neuron body and into a long axon branch.[6]

At the far end of the long or short axon branch, the electrical impulse produced by hearing, tasting, seeing, or touching jumps across a synapse to one or more nearby dendrites of other neurons. In sensory neurons, the message passes from neuron to neuron, across one synapse after another, until it reaches the reflex arcs of the spinal cord or enters a decoding circuit in the brain.

Our sense of smell has a simpler elegance. When we inhale, the dendrites of the olfactory neurons pick up aromatic molecules from the outside on the delicate, mucus-covered surface of our nasal passages.

On the other end of each olfactory cell, an axon connects directly to smell centers at the base of our brain. This gives the sense of smell a direct connection between the incoming message from our environment and the brain so that we can react without taking time to think when survival may depend on an immediate response. Once an odor is decoded by the brain, it may trigger a visible reaction such as a sneeze to expel toxic air or a hand reaching to pick a flower.[7]

The ability to smell developed very slowly, in countless minute experiments, most of them dead ends but with enough successes to produce a beautifully varied tree of life.

The sense of smell started as an elementary but efficient form of chemical communication at a distance, in the first one-celled organisms, the ancestors of today's bacteria, yeasts, and fungi. Olfactory nerves very likely developed from the chemical receptors of ancient one-celled organisms. As the nervous systems of animals became more complex and they developed a central nervous system and ever more complex brains, these chemical receptors became connected with olfactory bulbs, a dominant part of the earliest brains.

Along the way through the olfactory maze, Ariadne's thread reveals four crucial turning points that help us understand what smell means for humans.[8]

Despite their infinitesimal size—ten million bacteria lined up end to end would stretch only three feet—bacteria are elegant life forms. Their simplicity has a marvelous efficiency that allows them to produce billions of offspring in a few hours given a favorable environment, and to survive the harshest demands. The genetic material of bacteria has mutated to survive, packaged in round balls, tiny rods, and spiral corkscrews with a whip-like flagellum for swimming. Packed inside a protective cell wall and membrane are various storage granules and ribosomes that convert food to energy and new protein.[9]

Bacteria have a primitive nucleus, an area containing the genetic material essential to support basic life functions and reproduction. To reproduce, most bacteria copy all their genes at regular intervals and then split into two identical but smaller bacteria each with a complete set of genes. There is no opposite sex, no need to rely on any sensation, including a chemical sensation like smell, to find a mate.[10]

Finding food is another matter. Bacteria absorb elements, gases, and tiny molecules of organic debris dissolved in their liquid world.

Inside the bacteria, these simple substances are broken down and recombined into the proteins needed to support life. Some elements, like oxygen, carbon, nitrogen, and sulphur, pass through the bacterium's cell wall rather easily, but nutritious organic debris has to be identified and sorted out from useless or harmful material before being "swallowed."

How does the bacterium "know" what organic matter it needs to live? The membrane enclosing the bacterial cell contains about twenty-five different chemical receptors—proteins with structures designed to catch chemicals—that help it sort between useful and toxic organic debris. Each receptor has a specific shape, like a lock waiting passively for a molecule, a key, with a matching shape to drift by and flip its cylinder open. In the case of a sensory neuron, the union of a receptor and its matching molecule creates a chemical reaction and electrical message. If the bacterium has one or more whip-like structures or flagella, the electrical message may start this structure whipping back and forth, or spinning like a propeller mounted on the outside of the cell. The bacterium then moves toward molecules that sustain its life, or away from toxic substances, depending upon the chemical message it receives.

All this depends on a favorable environment, with enough food to support more of the particular species of bacteria. Some bacteria react to chemical messengers that tell them when there are too many bacteria for the available food supply. Why reproduce when your offspring are doomed to starve? Bacteria stop reproducing when the level of pheromones indicates the environment cannot support any more bacteria.

Some bacteria have developed a very primitive form of mating that allows them to exchange their genetic material and produce offspring ever so slightly different from themselves. Most of the time, bacteria rely on the trial and error of chance encounters. But some bacteria seem to have found a way to communicate their "need to mate" with simple chemical messengers. Microbiologists call this response a form of "chemotaxis," movement of an organism toward or away from a chemical stimulus.[11] For bacteria blessed with a flagellum and capable of swimming, this chemical communication—smelling without a nose—is an effective way to find food or a mate.

Although chemical messengers that appear to function as pheromones have been identified and analyzed in some bacteria, the question remains whether the term pheromone applies, if we define a pheromone as a chemical signal that influences the way an animal functions and behaves.[12] Since bacteria do not engage in true sexual reproduction, there is little need for highly specific sexual communication or any particular behavior.[13]

Are other one-celled organisms attracted to each other by pheromones? We know that they require chemical cues to find food, and that mating requires the cooperation of two individuals, so this question is not unreasonable. However, if attraction is defined as one individual's positive response to a chemical messenger produced by another organism, a response that results in moving toward that organism, then again the answer is "no"—at least for the common brewer's yeast, which has no means of moving toward a pheromone source.[14]

Most of the time yeast cells reproduce asexually. Individual cells copy their single set of chromosomes and "bud" or split into two identical cells. Despite this, yeast cells are not all alike. They come in two different "mating types." Mating types A and B yeast cells are not like males and females in more complex organisms, because each yeast organism has only one cell and no sexual anatomy. Occasionally, however, when a type A and type B yeast cell are ready to exchange their genetic material, they may release a chemical messenger that allows them to stick together if they bump into each other. They can then combine their genetic material, much as sperm and egg cells in higher organisms combine their DNA at fertilization.[15] This new yeast cell then undergoes cell division to produce four offspring, each with a single set of genetic material. These then resume reproducing asexually until the next chance encounter.[16]

This occasional "mating" of yeast cells does depend on a chemical messenger, a "pheromone," secreted by the mating A and B cells. While this chemical communication in yeast does not meet our strict definition of a pheromone as a chemical messenger that enhances sexual attraction, we have to admit that, unlike bacteria, yeast cells do reproduce "sexually," and a chemical messenger—a pheromone—is essential to their mating!

More authentic pheromone interactions are found in a species of aquatic fungus that has a whip-like flagellum that enables it to swim around and move toward another when it encounters a sex attractant molecule. A spreading bread mold also relies on chemical communications at a distance to guide its wandering branches to branches of a nearby fungus of a slightly different mating type. Fungi, like the bread molds, are not developed enough to have males and females, so mycologists call their mating types the + strain and the − strain. When the branches of a + and a − fungi approach each other and make contact, the tips swell into reproductive cells, fuse, and the DNA from both cells joins in a single cell that goes dormant for a while. When the embryonic cell wakes up, it reverts to the old standby of asexual reproduction.[17]

So Ariadne's thread of consistency, our ball of string, leads us back millions of years to the first one-celled organisms that developed a sensitivity to chemical messengers we sophisticates now label aromas, odors, smells, and pheromones.

ON TO JELLYFISH

Eventually some ancient blue-green bacteria took the next step to one-celled marine algae and animals like the paramecium and amoeba, with some minor improvement in the sense of smell.[18] When the eggs of marine brown algae are ready to be fertilized, they release a pheromone, a seductive molecular song that prompts sperm attached to nearby algae to break away from their slimy home and swim toward the eggs.

Brainless, spineless jellyfish, and their relatives, the corals and sea anemones, represent the next major advance in the organization of colonies of specialized one-celled animals. Whether they are carried along by ocean currents or sit on ship bottoms, pilings, or reefs, these animals wait with outstretched tentacles for food to drift by. In their "skin" simple sensory cells wait, alert for the scent of a potential meal or enemy. A toxic or enemy scent sends the pulsating jellyfish or anemone into withdrawal or pulsating retreat. A food scent sets the tentacles into predatory action.[19]

When a meal blunders into the swaying tentacles, the reaction is swift and deadly. Stinging structures, each a loaded harpoon with a very sensitive trigger, cover the tentacles' surface. An enemy or potential meal instantly causes the release of a barrage of barbed harpoons that pump poison into the enemy to scare it off or into prey to kill it. Once the scent of food is clear, the dead prey can be slowly maneuvered into a waiting mouth.

The odor receptors and nerve net of a jellyfish, anemone, or coral are not nearly so efficient as our nose and brain, but they do have an advantage over one-celled organisms.

With the passage of time came the "cross-eyed" planarians or flat-worms, popular in high-school experiments with regeneration. These animals tie their odor-sensing cells into the first true nervous system with a pair of nerve cords channeling sensory input to a central switch-board or primitive brain. This development allowed them to coordi-nate their muscle movements for moving, feeding, and mating, based on information from chemical messengers.[20]

The olfactory system of mollusks like snails, clams, and oysters marks another turn in our maze. Drop a piece of crushed mussel into the water of a salt marsh and a mob of hungry mud snails and minnows soon gather. Crush a mud snail and other mud snails turn tail in a slow motion retreat into the protective mud.[21]

Chemical communication in clams and scallops involves both contact reception through special cells that are similar to taste buds, and distance reception through neurons connected directly to the brain that are similar to olfactory neurons.[22] This new ability to separate the chemical senses of "taste" and "smell" is very important. Especially con-sidering that what any animal smells is a large part of what it experi-ences when it tastes something.

Scavenger catfish can detect amino acids leaking from a distant dead minnow with their chemical-sensitive whiskers. Having found the dead minnow, the catfish tests the chemical "taste" of the minnow with its whiskers before swallowing or rejecting it. If you injure a minnow, its damaged cells emit a fear pheromone that sends fellow minnows dart-ing in evasive retreat. And it takes but a couple of molecules of a chemical message to get a reaction. Young sockeye salmon, for instance, can detect concentrations of chemicals from food mixed with water at ratios of one part in eighty million.[23]

Today's salmon roam thousands of ocean miles before returning to the river of their birth to spawn. A similar homing instinct seems to help frogs and salamanders locate their native ponds and sea turtles return to their nesting beaches. How do they find their way back home? As best we know now, it is all a question of smell and a strong memory for the chemical stew in the water back home.

The brains of the hatchling salmon are imprinted with the unique, complex scent of the soil, plants, and algae that surrounded them in their young life. Scientists believe this complex scent imprints a powerful memory in a neural template in the limbic system. Because the limbic system, a specialized collection of nerve circuits in the floor of the cerebral hemispheres, also regulates the basic drive to mate and reproduce, this memory template is activated when the mature salmon is driven to reproduce. Why take chances on just any stream or river when this memory template can lead the salmon back to their original birth place?[24]

Fertilized Coho salmon eggs can be raised in the controlled environment of a hatchery and the fingerlings exposed to carefully monitored scents. If a specific scent is added to the water, the olfactory memory circuits of the fingerlings imprint to that scent the same way other young salmon imprint to the odor of the stream where they hatch and spend their first weeks of life. After these scent-imprinted fingerlings are turned loose in the ocean and grow to adults, they can be enticed by the scent to migrate up foreign rivers to the waiting hooks of expectant fishermen.[25]

If we can isolate pheromones from female salmon, would we be able to use them to trap male salmon the way we use female gypsy moth pheromone to trap male gypsy moths?[26] While scientists have yet to isolate a species-specific pheromone in salmon, female goldfish produce a potent chemical sex pheromone that stimulates males to spawn.[27] So do female rainbow trout.[28]

The brains of the first arthropods in the oceans, the ancestors of today's lobster, nautilus, and crab, and the early land insects were little more than computerized decoders of smells and mechanized pursuers of odors. Lobsters taste with their feet and smell with their antennules, which they wave constantly to sniff the waters.

Land snails have developed two sets of antennae, one for smell, the other for taste. Curious scientists have tested the snail's sense of smell and its connection with long-term memory by training snails to follow and remember different smells for up to three months.[29]

The behavior of insects, by far the most successful and numerous form of life, relies heavily on their brains which are little more than central processing units linking olfactory responses with appropriate survival behaviors. Insects have separate senses of taste and smell. They smell with antennae and rely on taste receptors around their mouth, and on their feet and wings.[30] The mosquito's antennae can detect carbon dioxide exhaled by its next victim, allowing it to home in like a heat-seeking missile.

A parasitic wasp looking for a caterpillar in which to lay its egg can detect the pheromone of a wasp larva in an already occupied caterpillar and continue its search for a suitable host. Harvard University's Edmund Wilson, the founder of sociobiology, notes that one milligram, a thousandth part of a gram, of the trail scent left by the leaf-cutter ant is strong enough to lead a small column of ants three times around the world.[31]

In California, the bolas spider relies heavily on pheromones to trap its meals.[32] This small spider produces a silken lasso with a sticky loop at the end. It then adds a siren molecule that mimics the pheromone of a female moth to lure a male moth into its trap. The bolas spider has a repertoire of at least sixteen different counterfeit but effective pheromones, so it can choose for its meal from at least sixteen different species of moths simply by changing its pheromone order.[33]

Even more impressive is a parasitic wasp that deposits its eggs on the caterpillar of the army beetworm to assure its offspring a steady meal when they hatch. The caterpillars produce no distinctive odors or pheromone of their own that the parasitic wasp can use to locate the prey. However, when the caterpillar begins to munch on the leaves of a corn stalk, their saliva somehow triggers the plant to produce volatile chemicals similar to terpene, which gives turpentine its distinctive odor. This terpene odor, consumed by the caterpillar with its green meal, acts like a pheromone, guiding the wasp to its prey. Cutting the corn leaf with a knife does not result in terpene production; only the caterpillar's saliva does that.

When the beetworm egg hatches as the sun sets, the tiny new caterpillar immediately starts munching away. But the corn plant does not add terpene to the caterpillar's meal until the following morning when the parasitic wasps are ready to take off in search of suitable hosts for their eggs. Mysteriously, the corn plant matches its peak production of terpene to the times during the day when the wasps are out hunting. How the corn plant developed this ability to synchronize its terpene production with the wasp's peak hunting times invites wide speculations because scientists have no answer to this incredible combination of behaviors.[34]

MORE SOPHISTICATED BRAINS

Although few animals can equal the odor sensitivity of the insects and their computer-like hard-wired links between smell and behavior, the warm-blooded vertebrates have added an important new element. Over all, the ability to receive and process chemical messages in land-dwelling vertebrates—animals with internal skeletons—and warm-blooded mammals serves the same purpose as it does in animals without backbones. In more complex animals, the influences and effects of odors on all behavior, including sexual behavior, is likewise much more complex.[35]

In land-dwelling, air-breathing vertebrates, the nasal cavities have been separated from the mouth to serve as breathing passages that extend up to half the depth of the skull. This contrasts sharply with marine vertebrates like fish in which water flows through a combined nasal cavity and mouth. In land mammals, the nasal cavity is lined with mucous membranes, which moisten and warm the incoming air. On the moist mucous membranes, many hairlike structures or cilia capture dirt that might block the flow of air and disrupt the olfactory nerves waiting to pick up chemical messages carried by the incoming air.

Unlike cold-blooded reptiles which mate unemotionally when turned on by the "right" sex pheromone, only warm-blooded mammals can decode, interpret, and link odors with memories and emotions. Only mammals link their olfactory systems directly with structures in the conscious and unconscious processing centers of the brain that are essential to both memory and emotions.

Mammals range from alleged super-smellers like pigs and dogs to the primates and humans who seem on the surface to pay more attention to visual and sound signals than to smell. What does it take to be a super-smeller? In the past, the ability to detect odors was believed to depend only on the number of chemical or olfactory receptors present in a particular animal species. From this perspective, bacteria with their twenty-five or so chemical receptors are at the low end of the scale. At the other end are dogs, which have about two hundred million olfactory receptors in their noses, twenty times as many as humans.[36] If our sole criterion to qualify as a super-smeller is the number of odor receptors, then dogs win out.

This initial impression does not hold up however because some odor receptors can respond to different odors and generate distinctly different patterns of activity in neurons. These patterns of activity are decoded in the brain. Larger, more complex brains mean a greater ability to decode, process, and transform odor cues to behavior. Since the size and complexity of the brain determines the number of different behaviors an animal is capable of, the focus now shifts from the raw number of olfactory receptors to the complexity of the brain circuits.[37]

Since primates, including humans, have much more complex brains than dogs, they also have a much greater ability to make use of their sense of smell. Because of our cerebral skills, we may make better use of our sense of smell than any other species and qualify as the ultimate super-smellers![38]

Still, the olfactory skills of dogs are impressive. Dogs, especially males dogs, are dedicated sniffers. One writer on the subject described his best friend as "a nose propelled by a Labrador retriever."[39] Since we seldom consciously call on our sense of smell for much more than savoring a dinner or sniffing an occasional flower, we assume our pet dog makes a similarly simple use of his sense of smell. We assume our dog sniffs around only because he is checking out the territory, finding out if a male has invaded his turf, or sniffing for a possible playmate, a bitch in heat. In reality, a good sniff may well tell your dog what brand of kibbles or canned food the earlier visitor had for breakfast, how his/her kidneys are functioning, whether he or she is feeling good or depressed, and what its sex life has been of late.[40]

We often rely on the olfactory skills of dogs, training them with rewards to do what we cannot do. The natural gas that enters our homes has a pungent distinct odor added so we can detect a dangerous leak. German shepherds can be trained to detect that same odor in a leaking pipeline buried under eighteen feet of frozen ground.

Trained dogs are widely used to sniff out explosives and illegal drugs. Drug runners have unsuccessfully tried every way they can think of to outsmart the trained canine. They seal cocaine or heroin in vacuum cans and hide it in a tank full of gasoline. A good dog finds it. They remove a piston from the engine of a car or truck and replace it with cocaine. A good dog sniffs it out. Even disguising drugs with chocolate, pepper, perfume, or garlic does not fool a well-trained dog.

Would such a disguise fool a well-trained person? There are many anecdotes in the literature attesting to the fact that, "What human beings lack in acuity . . . they make up in powers of discrimination, which rival those of any other mammal."[41] One of the authors has personal experience with a woman whose ability to smell leaking gas outperforms the detection equipment of the gas company and any gas-sniffing dog. The gas company's initial response to her concern over the pervasive odor was typical. They attempted to detect the leak in and around her home with sophisticated sensors. No leak was found on two different occasions. Still, on the woman's insistence, the gas company inspectors returned a third time, and detected a leak outdoors, several hundred feet from her residence, and far from where anyone might have imagined a human could smell it. Could the same women have smelled gas leaking from a pipeline buried under eighteen feet of frozen ground? Fortunately, we have trained dogs.

The individualized body odor of every man, woman, and child, composed of sweat, flakes of dead, decomposing skin cells, cologne, smegma, and pheromones, marks the clothes we wear, the chair we sit in, and the car we drive. A trained dog can easily pick up on these scents if they are not more than a few hours old. Scent trails are delicate and quickly fade, especially in hot dry weather and when the sun hits the trail. Cool, moist weather forms ideal conditions for preserving a scent trail.

Some people make their living creating perfumes, or designing odors to enhance the sale of products of all kinds. Cigar and pipe devotees dwell in their own world of fragrances. Four-star chefs can sniff a bouillabaisse and tell you all its subtle ingredients. And many wine connoisseurs can challenge the legendary James Bond in detecting the vintage and vineyard of a particular wine. "Estimates vary considerably," one expert tells us, "but the consensus among investigators seems to be that, after some training, a healthy person can distinguish between ten thousand and forty thousand odors. Among professional perfumers and whiskey blenders, the number may approach a hundred thousand."[42] Beyond these sensual delights of life, smell can be crucial to our survival. It can alert us to fire, gases, and the pungent odors of spoiled foods.

Human responses to odors are not driven with the hard-wired certainty of the insect's response. The conscious circuits of our mind also take us beyond the rapid-fire response of dogs to specific odors, as any drowsy morning pet-walker knows when he is unexpectedly yanked off his feet. We react to smells, but we do not seem to be as driven by them as other animals. Or are we?

4

THE ANATOMY
OF SMELLING

"When we smell another's body, it is that body itself that we are breathing in through our mouth and nose, that we possess instantly, as it were in its most secret substance, its very nature. Once inhaled, the smell is the fusion of the other's body and my own. But it is a disincarnate body, a vaporized body that remains whole and entire in itself while at the same time becoming a volatile spirit." At least that is the way Jean-Paul Sartre saw it in his 1963 biography of Baudelaire.

Scientists are much less poetic when they ask how we can inhale the essence of another's body. How do we detect, sort out, identify, decode, and interpret the uncounted aromatic messages we suck into our nasal passages and then quickly expel?

Only seven of the 105 natural chemical elements—fluorine, chlorine, bromine, iodine, oxygen (ozone), phosphorus, and arsenic—have an odor. Odors are characteristic of organic molecules that contain carbon atoms as a core with atoms of other elements attached to that basic structure. In the case of a pheromone, the molecule might be a few carbon atoms linked together in a chain with other atoms attached as side branches.

The process of smelling starts with any molecule that is volatile, so tiny it is hardly affected by gravity's pull. Such molecules can drift aimlessly in the ebb and flow of the winds. Every breath we draw pulls such particles through our nasal passages into our lungs where oxygen and carbon dioxide are exchanged. This express route runs from the nasal openings straight back a few inches to the opening of the throat at the back of the mouth and down to the lungs. While some eddies may reach the upper chamber of our nasal passages, this express route allows us to inhale and exhale quite efficiently twelve to fourteen times a minute.

Two branches of a trigeminal nerve reach from the brain to nerve endings widely distributed throughout the nasal cavities where they screen for dangerous or irritating odors passing through the express route. Chemical receptors associated with this nerve react to irritating odors with a prickly sensation that causes us to sneeze. A whiff of ammonia will trigger this reflex, expelling harmful air before it damages the delicate tissues of our nose, throat, and lungs. After a reflex sneeze, fresh air rushes into the lungs, helping to revive a person in a faint.[1]

Above the nasal passage's express route, in two narrow chambers just below the brain and behind the nasal bridge, are three ridges of spongy tissue that warm and humidify incoming air. Faced with a potentially dangerous situation, with a fragrant rose or the buttery, garlicky bouquet of shrimp scampi, we can sniff the air up into these recesses. There the aromatic particles land on a pair of mucus-bathed patches of skin, smaller than a dime where *ten million* olfactory neurons wait with delicate branches floating in the mucus, waiting to be activated when their receptors find matching aromatic molecules brought in on the air we inhale.

The olfactory neurons have two main differences from the sensory neurons we use to see, hear, and feel. Neurons in the eye's retina react to light only after it passes through the cornea, lens, and two masses of gelatinous material. The neurons in the ear's spiral cochlea react to sound vibrations after they have hit the ear drum and been converted into mechanical vibrations by the bones of the middle ear. Touch neurons in the skin pass their messages through several connecting neurons to the spinal cord and up the cord to the brain. Chemical messengers, on the other hand, are "hot-wired"—picked up directly by receptors in the olfactory neurons and sent straight to the olfactory bulbs and processing centers in the brain.

The second unique trait of olfactory neurons is their ability to regenerate. Unlike neurons in our spinal cord, eyes, and ears, olfactory neurons constantly replace themselves, as a team of neuroscientists at Florida State University led by Pasquale Graziadei, Lloyd Beidler, and Michael Meredith, have documented over the past ten years.[2]

While Meredith has investigated neural pathways in the olfactory systems of hamsters and sharks,[3] Graziadei prefers studying the relationship between the development of the brain and nose in frog and chicken embryos. Constant exposure to damaging, sometimes toxic molecules in the air, Gradziadei has discovered, kills most olfactory neurons in only four to eight weeks. Over the years, this devastation could wreak havoc with our interest in food and sex. Fortunately, our olfactory neurons can reproduce and replace themselves as they wear out.

This ability is an important factor in survival. A blind or deaf rat can still survive and mate to stay alive and keep the species going. A rat that cannot smell is much worse off. It cannot smell a poison in what looks and tastes like a great meal. It cannot discern the sexual readiness of a mate, or detect the scent of a cat waiting in ambush.

Beyond everyday survival and mating, the olfactory neurons play an early and major role in guiding the development of the fetal brain and setting up the production of hormones in the hypothalamus, pituitary gland, and ovaries and testes that are responsible for our sexual development and behavior in later life.

By the end of the fourth week of pregnancy, two thick plates of cells develop on the face of the fetus. Cells in these olfactory plates quickly migrate inward to become the olfactory bulbs and connect with the brain, particularly with the future hypothalamus and the limbic region. Some of these cells actually migrate into the future hypothalamus while others form a loose network scattered through the developing olfactory and limbic systems. These cells, known as GnRH neurons, quickly begin to produce GnRH, Gonadotropin-Releasing Hormone, the "starter hormone" that controls the cascade of hormones from the pituitary, adrenal glands, ovaries, and testes that influence all our sexual development and behavior.

Male fetuses end up with more GnRH-secreting neurons in their hypothalamus than do females. Down the line, this means males produce more luteinizing hormone (LH) and more testosterone than female fetuses. More testosterone causes male fetuses to develop male sexual anatomy externally—and internally, in the connections between nerve cells (synapses) in the brain.

Without the timely and proper migration of these GnRH neurons, many things can go wrong in fetal development. The sense of smell, for instance, can be impaired and, more crucially, the hypothalamus will not produce the GnRH needed for normal sexual development and sexual behavior. Some brain development may even be affected.

In humans, Kallmann's syndrome offers a good illustration of this effect. In boys and girls with Kallmann's syndrome, the hypothalamus does not produce normal levels of GnRH. Without this hormone trigger, the pituitary cannot produce the hormones needed to turn on production of androgens, estrogens, and progesterone in the testes or ovaries. As a result, teenagers with this condition have a delayed puberty, often have trouble falling in love, and delay marriage. They may marry, but in an arranged sort of way without falling in love. Behind their impaired sexuality and lack of a sense of smell lies a failure of the GnRH neurons to migrate properly and trigger normal brain and sexual development.[4]

This connection between GnRH neurons and brain development makes sense when we look at some experiments with tadpoles which are at the same stage of embryonic development as mammalian fetuses before they are born. When Gradziadei surgically removed the nose of a tadpole, it developed into a frog with no forebrain. Gradziadei suspects that the GnRH neurons in the olfactory system play a similar major role in guiding development of the human embryo's brain.[5] Some neuroscientists even maintain that our forebrain and the two hemispheres of our brain where we consciously process information from the outside world actually developed from the paired olfactory bulbs.

When Graziadei removed the olfactory bulbs in the brain of a mouse, new neurons were produced to recreate the bulbs. Even when he removed 90 percent of the bulbs, the animal could still smell quite well, evidence that the olfactory bulbs are very good at compensating for injury and continued their essential function of passing on aromatic information to the brain from the outside world.

When Graziadei transplanted the very early embryonic structures of the olfactory system from one tadpole to another, his test animal not only developed two olfactory systems, but the stimulus produced a much larger than normal brain in the tadpole. When he removed the early nose and transplanted it to another part of the tadpole's body, the brain developed but with striking abnormalities. Comparable tests transplanting the tadpole's early eye structure showed few similar dramatic effects.[6]

Graziadei's more recent work with chicken embryos takes us another step closer to understanding the importance of the olfactory system before and after birth. One important link, according to Graziadei, is the fact that "We see human babies born with anencephaly [with the brain's twin hemispheres missing], and in every case, the babies also have no noses. Why is that? Obviously, there is a very fundamental, chemical connection here, and we want to find out not only what it is, but how it works."[7]

A Bridge to Inner Space

In the main olfactory system with which we are most familiar, aromatic molecules are caught in the moist mucus on the ridges of the upper nasal passages. Each of the millions of odor-sensitive cells in these ridges has a tassel of six to twelve hair-like cilia floating in the mucus.[8] Scattered in the surface of these microscopic cilia are pockets formed by chemical receptors, similar to those that bacteria and one-celled animals use to detect food and toxins. When an aromatic molecule encounters a receptor pocket that fits its molecular shape, the two join up, like a key slipping into a lock.[9]

The union of an aromatic molecule with its proper receptor triggers a minute change in the electrical balance of the cell membrane that "fires off" an electrical message through the long branch or axon leading to the olfactory bulbs in the base of the brain a few millimeters above the passages.[10]

That electrical message originates in the base of the receptor pocket where some fifty G-protein molecules are attached. When the right odor comes along and fits into its receptor pocket, the receptor twists just enough to release these proteins into the cell material inside the thread-like cilium. When the freed G-proteins interact with other proteins inside the cilium, they open up channels in the membrane of the receptor neuron. This allows sodium ions—sodium atoms with a positive electrical charge—to pour into the body of the neuron. When the positive charge builds up to a critical level, the neuron "fires" an electrical pulse along its long thread-like axon to the olfactory lobes in a process that takes only a few thousandths of a second.[11]

In addition to being able to discriminate between the molecules that can activate its receptors, the olfactory neurons must have a mechanism that modulates the intensity of each response. The size and duration of an impulse is fixed, but its frequency varies. Decoding the neuron's response means decoding the frequency of the nerve impulse.

Linda Buck, a Harvard University neurobiologist, has added another piece to our understanding of how we smell when she identified the genes responsible for as many as a thousand different receptors in the mammalian nose. Even though some of these genes may act in concert to produce the thousand receptors, it may be that close to one percent of our hundred thousand or so genes are devoted to creating our odor-sensitive receptors. Only three of these hundred thousand genes are responsible for producing the receptors for the three primary colors entering our eyes as light. And that says something about the relative importance of the two senses of smelling and seeing.[12]

Although we may have only a thousand different odor-detecting neurons in our main olfactory system, some humans can recognize ten thousand distinct odors. How can the brain distinguish so many odors with only a thousand receptors? Buck suggests that while each neuron may carry only one kind of receptor and send only one message to the olfactory lobes and brain, the brain can distinguish between different odors if they trigger more than one receptor and different combinations of receptors. In other words, if we are dealing with four different receptors—label them A, B, C, and D for convenience—a lemon molecule may bind with the A, B, and D receptors to send a triple message to the brain decoding circuit. An orange molecule may activate the A, C, and D receptors, a tangerine odor the A, B, and C receptors, and a grapefruit the B and C from this set plus another receptor, say a G receptor. Combination messages from the thousand different receptors could account for our brain's ability to identify ten thousand odors.[13]

This model makes sense for complex odors especially when, in our example, some of the receptors activated by orange, lemon, tangerine, and grapefruit odors are the same for all citrus scents. Buck admits that a neuron may carry more than one kind of receptor, and that the coding scheme may be more complex than the model she has suggested.

Once triggered by the appropriate aromatic molecule, an olfactory neuron sends an impulse along its axon branch through a thin bony layer directly into the paired olfactory bulbs just above the nose in the floor of the brain. These extensions of the brain contain bundles of neurons, each capable of processing impulses from about twenty-six thousand receptors. These bundles filter out the trivial static and send essential signals along to other regions of the brain.

Like other biological processes, the olfactory system includes a thermostatic feedback loop that keeps the system from running amuck if we get carried away with a particular aromatic stimulus. When messages from your stomach tell your brain it is full, this message is passed along to the olfactory bulb, toning down the impact of that second fragrant piece of homemade, fresh-from-the-oven apple pie nestled against all-natural vanilla ice cream.

There are also times when a particularly strong, noxious odor is unbearable. In short order after being assaulted with the overwhelming stench of a slaughter house or cesspool, the brain reacts by refusing to process any more messages of that particular odor. Nasal fatigue provides an important defense mechanism against sensory overload.

Hidden behind these obvious reactions to various odors is a much more subtle and powerful double reaction. Our olfactory system uses G-protein activity in the olfactory receptors to convert odors and pheromones into electrical signals. These signals are converted into a chemical signal, GnRH, which acts as both a neurotransmitter and a hormone. As a neurotransmitter, GnRH may directly influence our behavior.[14] As a hormone produced in the hypothalamus, GnRH regulates hormone production in the pituitary gland.[15] Because hormones from the pituitary flow through the blood to every organ and system in the body, smell plays a major role in regulating all kinds of functions essential for life, from growth, body metabolism, maintaining proper fluid balances, insulin production, stress management, sexual development, mating, milk production and breast feeding, to fighting, fleeing, feeding, and more.[16] All this means that odors and pheromones processed by our main olfactory system clearly affect and influence our sexual development and behavior.

Messages from the olfactory bulbs are also sent along to the olfactory cortex in the brain which helps distinguish odors based on past experiences. This enables us to tell the smell of burning leaves from the quite different smell of a burning cloth pot-holder. Messages also travel from the olfactory bulbs to the memory and emotional centers of the brain, and to the thalamus which appears to connect limbic odor messages with higher thought functions in the thinking part of the brain. The conscious brain caps this process by relating odor messages to messages and memories from the other senses.

SNAKES AND THE VNO

So far, in talking about how we smell, we have concentrated on the *main* olfactory system, located in the nasal passages and main olfactory bulbs. But some animals also have an *accessory* olfactory system (AOS), which is specialized for detecting the subliminal signals of pheromones. Scientists have known about this AOS in reptiles and mammals since the early 1800s, but only recently have they begun to look for it in humans.

Research on how we see and hear has always taken precedence over research on how we smell, but the fact that in other animals the AOS processes pheromones which operate below the conscious level and affect the emotions and sexual behavior may in part explain the reluctance of researchers to probe into this aspect of how humans smell. If we were to get philosophical about the lack of research on pheromones and the AOS, we might suggest that researchers and the public have been turned off by the possibility humans might rely on an olfactory system that is dominant in the life of snakes and reptiles. In addition, the ancient Hebrews viewed the serpent as the disrupter of the peace in the mythic Garden of Eden when it allegedly seduced the first couple. In many cultures, but especially in the West, snakes trigger fear and revulsion. That forked tongue continuously flicking in the air seems somehow threatening and satanic.

In reality snakes, like other reptiles and mammals, test the air for aromatic clues to danger and food.[17] As the tongue darts back and forth between the air and the snake's mouth, it captures heavy aromatic chemicals and dumps these into a pair of odor-sensing sacs, the vomeronasal organs (VNO), which sit in the roof of the mouth beneath the main olfactory system. The snake's forked tongue and paired VNO allow it to take two slightly different scent samples and send a stereoscopic message to the brain. By comparing the strength of the two scents, the snake knows the potential mate or meal is straight ahead, or more or less to the right or left, much the way we tell the direction of a sound by messages from our two ears.[18]

Early in the history of the vertebrates, reptiles developed the VNO/AOS to handle odor messages that are too heavy to be sniffed, even though their messages may be vital to an animal's survival. In the VNO sacs, a sensory epithelium similar to that of the main olfactory system begins decoding the pheromone messages and converting this information into electrical impulses.

In other animals, pheromone messages from the sensory neurons of the VNO feed through a maze of neurons directly to a tiny organ called the accessory olfactory bulb (AOB) buried just below the frontal lobes of the brain. Electrochemical signals to other neurons increase production of GnRH that enhances the olfactory responses and speeds up neural transmission with or without altering other hormone levels. After some additional decoding in the AOB, nerve impulses go directly to the amygdala, an area in the limbic system concerned with a variety of behavioral mechanisms and emotional responses.[19] From the amygdala, the signals are fed to the GnRH-producing circuits of the hypothalamus that regulate sex hormone production, sexual differentiation, and sexual behavior. This includes control of the body's basic Four F's—feeding, fighting, fleeing, and mating.[20]

The VNO is essential to reproduction in other animals. Without its response to pheromones, production of key sex hormones would be disrupted.[21] Without trigger signals from the VNO the hypothalamus would not start, stop, or cycle the levels of its production of GnRH that regulates production of several hormones in the pituitary master gland.[22] It also facilitates mating behavior, especially in males with low testosterone or impaired sensations from their genitals and in females whose hypothalamus is not up to par in triggering the cycle of sex hormones.

Blocking input to the VNO of a male garter snake will completely eliminate any sexual behavior. Blocking its main olfactory system has no effect on mating.[23] Male snakes respond to sex pheromones secreted onto the skin as a prelude to courtship. During courtship, the male snake increases its tongue-flicking as it rubs its chin up and down the female's back in a sort of full body massage. However, some male snakes, known as "she-males," produce sex pheromones that make them smell like females to other males. This trick misleads competing males into trying to mate with them. While the confused male tries to court the "she-male," the "she-male" wastes no time and immediately mates with the available true females.[24]

Both the snake darting its tongue and the bull licking the vulva of an estrous cow are picking up pheromones that are pumped into the VNO. In both cases, with variations allowing for the differences between snakes and cattle, this sets up a chain reaction from the VNO to the olfactory bulbs and hypothalamus, which then controls sexual development and behavior.[25]

The way the AOS is put together varies quite a bit from one species to the next. Researchers have found the VNO sacs in humans, tucked inside the bony area, near where the hard palate and nasal septum meet behind the nostrils. But they have not been able to find other components of the mammalian or reptilian accessory olfactory systems in humans. Nor have they been able to trace the neural tracts that logically must exist to connect the human VNO with some region of the limbic brain.[26]

Embryologists have long admitted that the VNO does develop early in human fetal life, but they claimed it degenerates and disappears long before birth.[27] If traces of the VNO remained after birth, it would be obvious that they could not function in the noble, rational human. How could we admit that something so primitive, instinctive, or reflexive as the VNO and pheromones could play a part in human mating?[28]

This picture changed unexpectedly and dramatically in 1991, at an international symposium on advances in mammalian pheromone research held in Paris under the sponsorship of EROX Corporation, an American company pioneering research on human pheromones. David Moran and colleagues reported they found vomeronasal pits in nearly every one of two hundred persons they examined.[29] Their examination of these VNO structures with light and electron microscopes provided new details on the cells in the human VNO that are "unlike any other in the human body." Another report by Garcia-Velasco and Mondragon found vomeronasal structures in nearly every one of the one thousand subjects they examined.[30] Stensaas and colleagues confirmed the presence of two kinds of "potential receptor elements" in the human VNO.[31]

Suddenly, what scientists had believed did not exist in humans did in fact exist. Suddenly, the VNO emerged as an important part of the human sensory system. Equally important, the newly discovered human VNO appears to function much the same way as it does in other animals.[32] Researchers began to suspect and explore links between the human VNO, pheromones, and human behavior, learning, memory, and emotions. Once again, scientists have found another of Ariadne's threads linking humans with our animal ancestors.

Meanwhile, neuroscientists have proposed more than sixty hypotheses, models, and theories to explain how nerve cells detect and sort out odors in animals and humans. The model described earlier in this chapter is the latest description of the anatomy of smell, but it certainly will be challenged and refined as the research continues.

While the mystery of how the brain works to control behavior is the supreme question confronting all neuroscience, Meredith, a co-director of the Florida State University Program in Neuroscience, believes the answer may first come from those who are tracking how the brain receives, interprets, and identifies the constant barrage of messages that come to our brains through our noses from the outside world. Recent research into how we smell is bringing us tantalizingly closer to some real answers. Before long, this mystery may be solved.

5

LOVE APPLES
AND THE NOBLE
PERFUME OF VENERY

Back in Shakespeare's time, it was the custom for a woman in love to tuck a peeled apple in her armpit. When it was saturated with her scent, she offered this "love apple" to her paramour to inhale so that hopefully he would be turned on.[1]

In some areas of Greece, the Balkans, and other Mediterranean countries, men still carry a handkerchief under their armpit during festivals so they can flutter this odor-bearing token under the noses of the women they invite to dance. They swear by the results. Women in ancient Egypt and eighteenth-century France varied this custom by carrying a delightfully scented little bag nestled in the vulva between their legs.[2] Some American immigrants from the Caribbean have their own recipe for a more meaty "love apple." The recipe calls for a hamburger patty steeped in one's own sweat. After cooking, it is served to the loved one in expectation he will find the cook irresistible.[3]

Behind these tidbits of anthropological folklore are bacteria working on the odorless secretions of apocrine and sebaceous glands associated with hair follicles. Bacteria work on hormones which are the by-products of the metabolism of cholesterol secreted in underarm sweat and around the genitals, turning some of them into pheromones.[4] Men and women differ in their pheromone production and distribution because they produce different ratios of androgens, estrogens, and progesterone. Women produce fewer androgens and more estrogens and progesterone than men, and men have a reverse ratio with more androgens. The androgens (from the adrenal glands and testes) are converted into androgen-dependent pheromones, while estrogens and progesterone from the ovaries and testes are converted into a number of chemical compounds that act as pheromones.

In 1974, John Cowley asked some psychology students at Hatfield Polytechnic in England to rate the leadership abilities of three men and three women who were running for student office. Each student was given a surgical mask to wear, ostensibly to hide their facial expressions from the six candidates. Half of the masks were secretly dabbed with a tiny sample of either androstenone or vaginal aliphatic acid secretions. Male students using the scented masks did not rate the six candidates any differently from the control male students. Women wearing the vaginal-scented masks gave higher leadership ratings to candidates with self-effacing, shy personalities and lower ratings to assertive, confident candidates. Women wearing the androstenone-scented masks gave their highest rating to an aggressive, positive candidate.[5]

In 1978, research psychologists at the University of Manchester in the United Kingdom also tested the human reactions to androstenone. Test and control males were asked to rate the attractiveness of women in a series of photographs. Before rating the women, the test males sniffed a sample of androstenone; the control males were exposed to a non-pheromone scent. The men who sniffed the pheromone consistently rated all the women much higher on the attractiveness scale than did the control males. The obvious explanation is that androstenone may evoke erotic memories, stir the libido, and/or trigger something else in the erotic centers of the test males' brains so that they saw the women in the photographs as sexier, warmer, and more attractive than did the non-sniffers.[6]

At the University of Warwick, Michael Kirk-Smith used alpha-androstenol, a musky sweat aromatic, in two similar experiments. In his first test, men and women reacted to a series of photographs of women. When he added a minute trace of alpha-androstenol to the air, both men and women rated the photographs of the women as sexier, warmer, and more attractive than they did when the air did not contain alpha-androstenol. In Kirk-Smith's second experiment, men and women were asked to evaluate several men. Some of the men were secretly given a dab of alpha-androstenol on the face. The women consistently upgraded the males with the sweat pheromone while the men invariably downrated the same males.

These kinds of experimental tests suggest some intriguing questions about the effects that subliminal chemical messages from hidden armpits and vulvas might have on men and women in the office, classroom, bedroom, and home. Do these subliminal scents influence, in any significant way, the casual everyday interactions of men and women? Does the effect vary for women depending on where they are in their monthly cycle? Women are at least one hundred times more sensitive to odors at the midpoint in their monthly cycle. How might variations in the balance of androgens and estrogens at different times in a woman's monthly cycle alter her pheromones and affect the reactions of men to her? Does the sensitivity of women vary with age?

It will take scientists years to find answers to such questions, but we already have some provocative observations and experiments suggesting that pheromones can normalize irregular menstrual cycles, synchronize or suppress menses and ovulation, and perhaps even synchronize the hormone cycles of men and women and gay men living together. Pheromones also enable us to recognize family members and strangers by their scent alone. They trigger aggressive behavior and appear to play a role in oral sex and some fetishes.

A word of caution, though. Human behavior is far from simple to analyze, and identifying the nature and effects of odors and pheromones is equally difficult to decipher. So, as we add experiment to experiment and our case for a strong connection between odors and pheromones influencing genes, hormones, and human sexual development and behavior becomes stronger, there is a temptation to get carried away by the provocative, sometimes startling, picture emerging from the scattered pieces of research. We have to remember that it is not a simple matter of linking "this scent" with "that behavioral outcome" and labeling "this" *the* cause and "that" *the* effect.

Some of the better-known pheromones have been used for centuries, but scientific tests of their actual effects on humans are a new adventure.

Civet or civetone, for example, has long been valued as an aphrodisiac scent. Since early times, this oily yellow secretion has been harvested from the anal glands of the ferocious civet cat found in Burma, Thailand, and two small coastal areas in Africa. If inhaled undiluted, civet is so strong it can cause nosebleeds and sometimes death. When properly diluted, it has a much more refined scent, more floral than musky. Another reputed ancient sex attractant is castoreum from the anal glands of European beavers. Finally, we should mention a common chemical compound that is an active ingredient in a number of powerful aphrodisiacs or sex attractants. Indole is found in aromatic extracts of lilac, madonna lily, narcissus, privet, orange blossom, tuberose, and civet. It is also produced by human scent glands. Inhaled in small quantities, the scent is sweet and pleasing. Too strong a dose produces nausea, headaches, and depression.[7]

Since musk has long been praised as "THE perfume of venery," we will explore this pheromone in detail later in this chapter.

TESTING THE SEXUAL ESSENCE

One of the more impressive effects of pheromones like musk, "male sweat," and vaginal scents is their ability to influence our behavior by priming the production of hormones in the midbrain's hypothalamus and pituitary. By affecting hormone production, odors can influence the onset of puberty and the timing and length of the menstrual cycle. Pheromones can trigger aggression in other species[8] and either prevent or end a pregnancy in rodents and in humans.[9]

Martha McClintock, a Boston undergraduate major in psychology in the early 1970s, became curious about a common folk tale involving menstruation and women living together. McClintock designed an experiment that confirmed anecdotal reports that the random menstrual cycles of daughters and mothers living together, nuns in convents, and college women in dormitories began to occur at the same time after they had lived together for a few months. In addition to confirming this "dormitory effect," McClintock found several subjects who reported that their menstrual cycles became more regular and shorter when they dated more often.[10]

By chance, McClintock's paper appeared in the prestigious British journal *Nature* shortly after a paper by an anonymous male scientist. Living alone on an island, this scientist had noticed that his beard grew more rapidly when he left for the mainland and enjoyed contact with women and his sexual partner. Blessed with a quantitative mind, he confirmed his casual observation by measuring the dry weight of facial hair left in his electric razor after each shave.[11] For males, apparently, contact with the other sex can stimulate production of androgens, which affect beard growth and pheromone production.

A few years later, Michael Russell at Sonoma State Hospital in California decided to test these observations and that of a female colleague who noticed that her own cycle seemed to pull that of other women she worked with into synchrony. Russell asked "Genevieve" to wear sterile cotton pads under her armpits to collect her perspiration. Then, three times a week for four months, he dabbed the "essence of Genevieve" on the upper lip of eight female volunteers and plain alcohol on the eight control females. The menstrual cycles of the eight control women were not affected, but after four months the gap between the cycle-starts of the eight test women had narrowed significantly. Russell did not publish the results of his mid-1970s research for ten years, so it had no effect on the debate stirred by McClintock's brief paper.[12]

Twenty-five years ago, the idea that a woman's scent could alter the menstrual cycle of other women was heresy. Scientists quickly challenged any suggestion that humans might produce pheromones and be affected by them, especially when their own findings did not confirm McClintock's results.[13] The debate was finally resolved in the mid-1980s by several independent studies.

At Philadelphia's Monell Chemical Senses Center, Preti, Cutler, and colleagues exposed ten women with normal random cycles to the underarm sweat of other women. Every few days they dabbed perspiration from donor women on the upper lip of test women. Within three months, the menstrual cycles of the test women began to coincide with the cycles of the sweat donors.[14]

When female mice are housed together in small groups of four or five with no males around, they tend to develop false pregnancies induced by the enhanced female scent.[15] When larger numbers of female mice are kept in relatively crowded conditions, their estrous cycles gradually lengthen and then stop.[16] In both cases, the female mice will return to their normal estrous and fertility cycles if exposed to the urine of a normal male. The urine of a castrated male, whose lack of testes reduces his testeosterone and hence whose pheromone production is very low, cannot reverse these effects produced by female scent.

Again, we are left with more questions than answers. If women produce an aromatic substance strong enough to synchronize the menstrual cycles of other women with whom they associate closely, can these or similar odors reach out to affect a man across a crowded room? And do woman likewise react to the "chemistry" of a man?

Ten years ago, at Washington State University, Jane Veith and colleagues found that women who spent two or more nights with men during a forty-day period ovulated more often than women who slept with a male only one night or not at all in the forty days. It did not matter how often the women had sexual intercourse or what their sleeping arrangement was. The researchers could not determine what caused this reaction, but they did have a strong suspicion that it was some kind of pheromone.[17]

At the University of Pennsylvania, Winifred Cutler confirmed McClintock's observation that women with a regular sexual life tend to have shorter and more regular cycles than non-dating women. She also reported more regular and shorter cycles in women who work with natural and synthetic musks, which are related to testosterone, the hormone responsible for sex drive and for beard growth in the anonymous scientist.

The next step was to try to find out what effect androstenone might have on women. Cutler's group asked some men to wear absorbent pads in their armpits for several days. After extracting "male essence" from these pads, they mixed it with alcohol, froze and stored it. Later the thawed essence was dabbed on the upper lip of women who came to the clinic three times a week. After being exposed to this "male essence" for three or four months, some of the women who began the project with irregular menstrual cycles found their cycles had shifted to a normal 29.5 day cycle.[18]

The fact that exposure to pheromones can normalize or block the menstrual cycle can have important consequences for a woman's fertility or lack thereof. One intriguing application might involve the use of pheromones to help infertile women with irregular cycles and improve the "natural rhythm method" of birth control approved by the Vatican. Pheromones might also be useful in alleviating some symptoms of menopause.[19]

After comparing these findings with McClintock's and Hopson's research, John Money, director of the psychohormonal research program at Johns Hopkins University, suggested that "the most likely hypothesis to explain synchronization in couples or groups is that it is mediated, perhaps subliminally, through the sense of smell by way of pheromones or odors."[20]

More evidence supporting the hypothesis that pheromones can affect the menstrual and egg production cycles has come from Gisela Epple's research on the behavior of marmosets at the Monell Center.[21] These small South American monkeys dutifully smear aromatic secretions from their genital region everywhere to let other marmosets know their gender, identity, and rank in the local dominance pecking order. This behavior is important in the reproductive life of marmosets because only one female in each marmoset troop is fertile. The dominant female somehow suppresses sexual receptivity and egg production in all the other females, who can only wait and hope she leaves the troop, loses her position, or dies.

The key to this troop fertility pattern is a pheromone in the dominant female's dabbings that biochemically inhibits fertility in the other females. When the scent of the dominant female is decoded and passed on to the hypothalamus of the other females, it suppresses ovulation. In fact, the vaporous contraceptive in the female marmoset's genital smear is a close relative of the estrogenic steroids used in the oral contraceptive.

Ten years ago scientists in India were using a nasal spray to deliver small doses of the same estrogen and progesterone contained in the contraceptive pill via the olfactory system. The nose has also been used by Sven Nillius, at Sweden's Uppsala University, to start up the reproductive system of an infertile woman by spraying GnRH into her nasal passages. In the near future, some new hormonal or pheromonal spritz up the nose may well replace the popular oral and implantable contraceptives and oral hormones for infertile women.[22]

MUSK AND VENERY

Four thousand years ago, in Arabia, Persia, and Tibet, musk was treasured as the most divine aphrodisiac. Musk was a special favorite of the Prophet Mohammed, as well as a powerful medicine and cardiac stimulant. Its name, from the ancient Sanskrit for testicle, clearly indicates the nature and purpose of this pungent aromatic secretion of a gland under the skin of the abdomen of the male musk deer, a small Asian deer. El Ktab, a classic Islamic text, describes musk as "the noblest of perfumes and that which most provokes [men and women] to venery."

When Carolus Linnaeus, an eighteenth-century Swedish botanist, used differences in the sexual organs of flowers to create the first modern scientific classification of plants, he listed musk as the most important member of *Odores ambrosiacae*. Musk deserves its status because, as Linnaeus discovered when he examined specimens of plants and animals from all over the world, musk is "the fragrance of sex."[23]

Everywhere in nature we find musky odors being used to bring males and females together to mate. The recipe for musk and its aromatic strength may vary from species to species, but the essential formula and its effects on males and females remains the same. Its fragrance brings male and female musk ox together in the Arctic wilderness and guides musky moles through dark tunnels to trysts. Several species of muskrats rely on it, as do musk ducks, musk turtles, and musk beetles. In the plant world we have musk hyacinths, musk mallows, musk orchids, musk melons, musk rose, musk thistle, musk cherries, musk pears, musk plums, muskats and muscatels, musk seeds, musk trees, and musk wood, all using this fragrance to attract pollinators.[24]

Among the natural perfumes, musk most nearly approaches the status of "universal aphrodisiac." Often emitted only during the mating season when females are in sexual heat and fertile and males are in rut, the sexual odor of most animals is most frequently some modification of musk.

With the difficulty and cost of harvesting musk-producing glands from the musk deer high in the Himalayas and Atlas Mountains, chemists had a strong commercial interest in identifying the main active ingredient. Having isolated and identified the structure of this aromatic molecule, chemists can now mimic nature's musk with compounds like galaxolide and Exaltolide.[25]

As powerful as musk is as a sex attractant, getting males and females together to mate is too vital for nature to rely on a single aromatic messenger. Rather, it relies on an arsenal of similar sexy aromas that work together. Musk, in fact, is not a very scientific or specific term; it covers many similar aromatic secretions and the many different end-products of breaking down various sex hormones. Androstenol, as mentioned earlier, has a musky scent. Smegma, the waxy secretion of sebaceous glands around the rim of the glans of the penis and clitoris, starts off colorless and odorless. Only when it comes in contact with bacteria under the foreskin does it develop a cheesy consistency and begin to smell musky.[26]

Sweat from the armpit, saliva, and urine contain several phero-mones derived from the breakdown of androgenic hormones that are often described as "musky," although some women describe their aro-mas as "flowery." The "musky" scent of male semen probably comes from the prostatic fluid that makes up a third of semen and contains testosterone and its metabolic products. Human urine also contains "musky" delta-2-androsterone-one-17. In the late 1970s, George Dodd isolated, purified, and synthesized one of the compounds in human sweat, alpha-androstenol. A relative of musks and androstenone, alpha-androstenol smells almost exactly like sandalwood, an ancient and still popular sexy perfume.

Women produce musky secretions, including androstenol, in their underarm sweat, and in similar secretions from the Bartholin's glands near the moist inner labia, from the Skene's glands along the urethra, and in vaginal secretions. Women also produce "musky" smegma around the glans of the clitoris. In addition, progesterone, a hormone that increases in the two weeks between release of the egg and the menstrual flow, contributes another characteristic sex odor.

At least one hundred other identifiable aromatic components contribute to the sexy smell of men and women.[27]

As a pheromone in sweat and saliva, "urinous" androstenone has a mixed reputation. When Birmingham University researchers sprayed it on a chair in an office waiting room, men avoided the chair, especially when it was applied in higher doses. Most women seemed attracted to the chair.[28] When Tom Clark, at Guy's Hospital in London, sprayed "musky" alpha-androstenol in several telephone booths at the London train station, both men and women spent more time on the phone when the same booth was scented than when left unscented.[29]

Most people consider high concentrations of musk, other pheromones, and human body odors repulsive, and avoid them. In low concentrations, however, these same scents enhance fine perfumes and serve as attractive aphrodisiacs.[30] Such dose-related effects and the var-ied responses to pheromones are a clear indication that our main and accessory olfactory systems are highly evolved and have excellent pow-ers to discriminate between thousands of odors, including many we are not even conscious of. Pheromones are a central factor in priming our matings and sexual behaviors.

A hundred years ago, Auguste Galopin summed up *The Perfume of Woman and the Sense of Smell in Love*, when he wrote that "The purest union that can exist between a man and a woman is that created by the sense of smell and sanctioned by the brain's normal assimilation of the animate molecules emitted by the secretions produced by two bodies in contact and sympathy, and in the subsequent evaporation."[31]

6

FRIENDS, STRANGERS, AND LOVERS

Do we like what we smell? Although the question is simple enough, the answer may depend on long-forgotten childhood memories and emotions. For researchers, both the question and the answer stir debate. Are there some inborn tendencies, favored by eons of natural selection, that give us a natural propensity to like certain odors and pheromones? Or do we decide some odor is pleasant when we hear others say it is pleasant? Or is an odor pleasant because we acquire our preferences from experience? Are odor and pheromone preferences based on nature? On nurture? Or a combination of both?

Newborn infants respond to a wide variety of odors. A newborn, even one born two months premature, will grimace and turn its head away from a noxious odor, or turn toward a pleasant odor.[1] Is this an inborn preference, somehow encoded in the neural pathways, perhaps even genetic in origin?

Place a pad with the odor of ginger or cherry inside the crib of a female infant before it is twenty-two hours old, and the next day she will show a preference for the familiar odor.[2] Males, at this early age, do not show a similar preference. Is this inborn, or learned? Or a combination of the two?

After mothers apply a perfume to their breasts before nursing for a day or two, infants between one and two weeks old appear to prefer the familiar scent to a new one. This preference, shared by male and female infants, is unlearned after two weeks during which the mother does not apply any scent.[3] Here we have a learned preference, reinforced by an association with the reward of food.

The mother-infant bond has been celebrated by politicians and sermonizers, sculptors and painters, sociologists, anthropologists, and animal behaviorists, conservatives and liberals, atheists and celibate monks, since the beginning of time. It is also a favorite research topic for psychoneuroendocrinologists and behavioral psychologists. Back when newborns often spent their first six hours in isolation, before the popular trend to natural childbirth that keeps newborn infants with their mothers from birth on, researchers found that mothers could recognize their own babies by smell alone six hours after birth.[4]

We should acknowledge here that for some, any discussion of a "maternal instinct" or the role of pheromones in mother-infant bonding raises the specter of Sigmund Freud's "biology is destiny" dictum. The evidence cited here does not support biology as destiny, but it does clearly suggests a response behavior classically conditioned by pheromones and the interaction of nature and nurture at particularly critical periods in our development. Still, discussions of the existence of some kind of "maternal instinct" tendency linked with hormones and the connections between pheromones and mother-infant bonding are fraught with risks, and somehow "politically incorrect" in this age of gender equality.[5]

The evidence, however, is clear that human infants can and do in fact identify and respond to their mothers solely on the basis of body odor and breast pheromones.[6] At six weeks, sleeping infants turn their heads and suck with their mouths when exposed to a breast pad from their mother. At six days—some researchers say three days—awake babies can discriminate between their mother's breasts and strange women based solely on their pheromones. They ignore or cry when presented with pads from a strange mother or pads moistened with cow's milk.[7] Breast-fed infants also recognize their mother's underarm pheromones, while bottle-fed infants do not.[8]

The independent observations of Michael Russell and colleagues in California and Aidan Macfarlane at Oxford University on the role pheromone signals play in the communication and bonding between a mother and a newborn infant match nicely with studies of mother-infant bonding in rats, mice, rabbits, and other animals. What does this tell us about the role human pheromones might play in establishing the relationship between mother and child?

Might this early pheromone-influenced experience of mother-infant bonding also affect our later sexual behavior? According to John

Money, an important aspect in our sexual maturation is our development of a "lovemap," a personalized "neural template or representa-
tion" encoded in the mind/brain that depicts an idealized lover and the
idealized program of sexual behavior.[9] In our next chapter, when we
explore sexual development in the womb, we will delve into some controversial and provocative research on how the balance and ratio of
maternal hormones appears to affect the newborn's sensitivity/insensi-
tivity to the mother's breast odor which in turn appears to be linked
with tendencies in adult sexual orientation.

While genes, hormones, pheromones, nurturance and sensuality
in infancy and childhood, and preadolescent/adolescent erotic experiences all play their roles in creating our personalized lovemap, John
Money believes a major factor in developing a normal and healthy
lovemap is strong infant bonding. "Mother-baby pairbonding," Money
writes, "is developmentally a precursor of what subsequently is the
male-female pairbonding of mating."[10]

Nursing at the breast exposes the infant to maternal pheromones
from apocrine and sebaceous glands in the underarms and in the dark
tissue around the nipples. These pheromones may well create lasting
memories of sensual pleasure, security, and love in the erotic circuits of
the infant's brain that are awakened years later with sexual maturity
when it encounters similar pheromones in a lover. Psychologist
Anthony Walsh believes we go through a series of stages in developing
our intimacy skills, moving from pairbonding skills we learn in Skin
Love to the family bonding we learn in Kin Love during childhood, to
adolescence and falling In Love.[11]

Many studies, going back to Frank Beach's work in the 1950's, tes-
tify to the importance of pheromones in maternal behavior. Beach
found that mother rats identify their young by smell and can pick their
own offspring out of another litter. Kittens nurse at one nipple only,
having identified it by its unique scent. The survival advantage of this
early neural imprinting is obvious. It also raises the possibility, some
suggest, that the fetal limbic system may be affected by smell and taste
messages contained in the 400 milliliters of amniotic fluid the fetus
drinks each day before birth.[12]

Children can also determine the sex of strangers by scent alone.[13]
Richard Doty, at the Philadelphia Veterans Administration Hospital,
has shown that we can tell people apart by the smell of their hands,

T-shirts, or undershirts. We can even be trained to identify specific people using olfactory cues.[14] We can also distinguish the sex of an unseen person after smelling their breath. Gary Beauchamp and colleagues have shown that humans can learn to discriminate accurately between the urine of men and women, based on its musky scent, even though urine contains at least sixty different volatile ingredients.[15] Gender differences in our musky and urinous tones also enable most of us to tell the difference between a men's locker room and a women's locker room based on odor alone.[16]

Some of our ability to distinguish males and females based on smell may be due to differences in the types of personal hygiene products men and women use. But this ability goes deeper to an inherent difference in the personal odor of men and women present even before an exercise-induced increase in sweat and pheromone production. Scented hairspray, perfumes, deodorants, and antiperspirants cannot wipe out the natural odor difference between men and women.[17]

Children under five years of age are generally more tolerant of odors that most adults find disagreeable. They do not draw back in disgust, for example, when presented with the strong smell of androstenone, the urinous odor in sweat.[18] Older children prefer fruity smells more and floral scents less than adults do. Their ranking of pleasant and unpleasant odors also changes substantially as they go through childhood and start to mature sexually.[19]

Some odors like androstenone are perceived as more pleasant at low concentrations and less pleasant at higher concentration.[20] Children and adults report strikingly different responses to androstenone. As we move through our teen years, many of us become more sensitive to lower concentrations of androstenone and consider it more pleasant. At the same time, the percentage of people who can detect this odor declines throughout adolescence.[21]

The ability to detect the odor of androstenone is, in part, genetically determined.[22] The proportion of males who cannot smell androstenone triples during puberty, the very time boys start producing this pheromone.[23] About half of the men who initially reported they could not detect this odor regained a sensitivity to it after being exposed to it for a time.[24] Interestingly, tests of skin reactions have shown that some people who reported they could not smell androstenone did actually respond to it subconsciously.[25]

As for women and androstenone, they are more sensitive to this scent than men. They are also more likely to describe the odor as unpleasant, at least when it is found in high concentrations.[26]

AGGRESSIVE ODORS AND INFANTICIDE

Pheromones, especially androstenone, may trigger aggressive behavior. While a boar's androstenone-laden urine produces sexual receptivity in a sow, it makes other boars aggressive. Some odor, probably a pheromone, in the urine of male mice also triggers aggression in other male mice.[27]

Normally, female rats that have not given birth will kill and eat the offspring of another female if given the chance. In addition to getting a meal out of this, the aggressive female takes over the nest abandoned by the mother. However, if a non-pregnant female spends some days with the pregnant rat before she gives birth, something happens and she does not attack and kill the newborn. Julie Mennella and Howard Moltz, who studied this behavior at the University of Chicago, concluded that "the mother emits a pheromone during pregnancy which in itself reduces the incidence of infanticide and, in fact, often makes potentially infanticidal females maternal." The maternal pheromones apparently cause a shift in hormone production in the non-pregnant female that increases the level of hormone(s) involved in maternal behavior and decreases the level of aggression-related hormone.[28]

Similarly, the scent of female urine often lessens the risk of attack by strange males. Female rabbits and dogs can wander with little risk through a male's territory because of their pheromones. This allows them greater choice in mating partners. Male rabbits and dogs, on the other hand, press their tails down tightly when frightened to suppress their genital odor and reduce the risk of irritating nearby dominant males.[29]

In some animals, the odor of urine is also important in reducing aggression. Before copulating, a male rabbit will urinate on the female, leaving her with his personal marker odor that signals other males to stay away. Ruth Winter suggests that this behavior may be echoed in a more sophisticated way when a man gives a woman perfume, marking her as his mate.[30]

Might male urinary pheromones have a similar, or a reverse effect on the hormone production and balance in males? And on their behavior?

Because of the difficulty of collecting mouse urine, Ching-tse Lee and colleagues at Brooklyn College substituted human male urine for mouse urine in their test of the response of male mice to the pheromones in urine. Urine from girls, women, and prepubertal boys had no effect on the male mice. But the urine of men produced the same aggressive behavior as the urine of male mice.[31]

Efforts to isolate and identify the compound(s) responsible for this effect continue, but Ariadne's thread of biological consistency suggests that it is likely to be a steroid derivative of an androgen. This consistency led the authors of Sex and the Brain to speculate about the possible role of male scent expressed in the hostile graffiti in men's restrooms and the aggression of men in large groups, as well as on the hockey rink, basketball court, or football field.[32]

When a pregnant mouse is exposed to a strange male's urine, that odor blocks production of a releasing hormone in the hypothalamus which in turn lowers the level of her pituitary hormones. Result? The pregnancy ends in miscarriage.[33] Is this nature's way of reducing the energy cost to a pregnant female whose offspring would likely be turned into a meal by the strange male lurking around her nest if her pregnancy continued and she gave birth without a male mate to protect her young?

If a female mouse is not pregnant, exposure to a strange male's urine odor again shifts her hormone balance in such a way that she cannot become pregnant.[34] On the other side, a female mouse depends on exposure to the urine odor of a familiar male to maintain a normal hormonal cycle and come into sexual heat. In 1956, W. K. Whitten, at the Jackson Laboratory in Bar Harbor, Maine, found that if he dabbed the nose of a female rat with a local anesthetic so she could not smell, her estrous cycle became irregular.[35]

THE AROMAS OF ORAL SEX

While the strong scent of androstenone may trigger aggression in males, a mild androstenone scent may also serve as a sex attractant and turn-on for females. This fact, coupled with the recently discovered sex attractants in primate and human vaginal secretions suggests that we might pursue a very different avenue and ask whether the rising popularity of oral-genital sex might in some way be related to genital pheromones.

Today's high standards of personal hygiene reduce the amount of pheromones secreted by apocrine glands and trapped by the pubic hair. Shaving underarms also removes axillary hair that would normally trap human pheromones. Might this depletion of natural pheromones create a subliminal yearning for the stimulation and excitement of human pheromones, which liberated modern adults satisfy by engaging in oral sex?[36]

When Richard Michael and colleagues at Georgia's Emory University isolated several estrogen-derived aliphatic acids from the vaginal secretions of female rhesus monkeys, they named them "copulins" in the belief that these compounds enticed male monkeys to copulate. Subsequent research showed that female monkeys produce the most copulins when they are fertile and thus clearly more attractive to males. They found that some human females produce similar vaginal secretions, and that women on the pill produce fewer of these secretions. They even showed that human vaginal secretions turned on male monkeys when smeared on the vulva of castrated female rhesus monkeys.[37]

John Amoore, at the Western Regional Research Laboratory, has explored the effects of trimethylamine, an aromatic component in menstrual blood well known to organic chemists who describe its smell as "fishy." Amoore believes there is good evidence that trimethylamine may be an important sex attractant in other mammals, and possibly in humans. While males of other species react strongly to the presence of high levels of trimethylamine in human menstrual products, one wonders what role it might play as a human sex attractant when menstruation occurs fourteen days after the fertile time of ovulation. Among non-human mammalian females where uterine/vaginal bleeding signals sexual receptivity, trimethylamine may promote mating at peak fertility.[38]

Recently, while discussing the possibilities of vaginal pheromones with some graduate students in the Human Sexuality Program at New York University, Francoeur noticed an unexpected reaction from a forty-year-old Nigerian student, Charles, who shared with the class his childhood experience of discovering an older woman making a special soup for her husband. A major ingredient in this soup was vaginal secretions and menstrual fluids. Apparently, if one accepts the hypothesis of vaginal/menstrual aphrodisiacs, the woman wanted to regain her husband's wandering attention by surreptitiously exposing him to a strong dose of her pheromones.

A few days later, when Francoeur shared this experience with Rosie Noble, Director of the Health Careers Program at Montclair State University in New Jersey, she also smiled unexpectedly. The story reminded her of childhood memories of African-American matriarchs rocking on their front porches in Atlanta and elsewhere in the South, talking secretively with a young wife concerned about her straying husband. "What you need, woman, is strong fixin's. Some woman has fixed your husband. Put the strongest fixin's you can get into your man's dinner and you'll win him back." The "fixin's" commonly used around the South, according to Dr. Noble, were, as in Nigeria, vaginal and menstrual products with their aliphatic acids.[39]

A few weeks after Francoeur's discussions with Charles Sekuruumah and Dr. Noble, he uncovered another example of the folk use of vaginal secretions while talking with a Brazilian lawyer. She shared her own recollections of a white magic spiritualist potion popular in the rural areas of Brazil where some women serve a special coffee to a male friend. After brewing, she reported, the coffee is filtered through a woman's well-worn underwear.

More than enough questions about human vaginal pheromones remain unanswered. These are complicated by conflicting results and by the failure to find any direct, clear, and uncomplicated correlation between human sexual responses and the aliphatic acids that Richard Michael and his colleagues isolated and studied.[40]

This lack of solid data, however, does not keep scientists from playing creatively with possibilities, for such creative playing often leads to new hypotheses that can be tested to advance our knowledge. Eighty years ago, Havelock Ellis suggested that "*cunnilingus* and *fellatio* derive part of their attraction, more especially in some individuals, from a predilection for the odors of the sexual parts."[41] What Ellis called "sexual parts" opens the door to some very complicated and as yet undefined interactions between smell and human sexual behavior. "The odors of the sexual parts" includes all kinds of pheromones from armpits, breasts, and nipples, the vulva, apocrine glands scattered among pubic hair, Bartholin's glands, the Skene's glands of females, the male prostate, and smegma from the glans of the clitoris and penis.

John Money suggests that "It is quite possible that some people, male and female, are more responsive than others to erotic odors. Thus, it is possible that some men and women surpass others in their enthusiasm for oral sex. . . . If one partner is intensely dependent on the odors, flavors, and sensations of oral sex for erotosexual arousal, and if the other has an intense aversion to it, compromise may prove unattainable and the partnership may prove unviable."[42]

We might also suggest that, in the natural history of the primate and humans, some scent-producing apocrine glands in the underarm region migrated to a frontal position and subsequently enlarged. Breast development may compensate for women's lack of body hair which normally traps and retains pheromones by providing an additional area for pheromone distribution. At the same time, the pheromone-secreting apocrine glands associated with hairs on the breasts and sebaceous glands in the areolas around the nipples provide a new and attractive erogenous area for males to explore and enjoy orally with their partner.[43]

Equally intriguing and untested is the idea that some fetishes may be linked with pheromones. Years ago Ellis remarked that with some fetishes:

> the odor of the woman alone, whoever she may be and however unattractive she may be, suffices to furnish complete sexual satisfaction. In many, although not all, of those cases in which articles of women's clothing become the object of a fetishistic attraction, there is certainly an olfactory element due to the personal odor attaching to the garments.[44]

There is clinical and anecdotal evidence that some fetishes develop because some nonsexual odor becomes associated with the pleasures of early masturbatory experiences in the emotional, erotic, and memory circuits of the limbic brain. Money and other sexologists have cited numerous cases in which various nonsexual objects, shoes, underclothing, sweat shirts, and other clothing "that come in contact with exocrine or sweaty secretions of the crotch or the underarms" have become fetishistic substitutes for the sexual stimulation of another person. But, as Money has commented,

> One man's meat is another's proverbial poison, and so it is that sweaty, excretory, and menstrual residues valued by an olfactory paraphile are labeled filth in the official terminology, namely mysophilia.[45]

We can also cite anecdotal reports heard over the years at various meetings of the Society for the Scientific Study of Sex. For some men and women the mere smell of wet rubber or leather can trigger sexual arousal and orgasmic satisfaction. In such fetishes, a particular smell appears to have been imprinted on the limbic memory circuits and associated with sexual arousal and satisfaction around the time of puberty.

Ellis described a typical example of this in the leather fetish of a young woman client of his. She repeatedly experienced "a considerable degree of pleasurable sexual excitement in the presence of the smell of leather objects, more especially of leather-bound ledgers and in shops where leather objects were sold." Ellis traced the origin of this fetish back to her strong memory of an early experience masturbating and smelling the strong fragrance of leather.[46]

One of Ellis' more intriguing suggestions connects a heightened sense of smell with asphixophilia, a dependence on partial self-strangulation to achieve sexual arousal and orgasm. He reported that some patients who engaged in partial self-strangulation while masturbating reported a "heightened olfactory sexual excitation" and intensified olfactory sensibility.[47]

THE NATURAL SUPERIORITY OF WOMEN

We know that men have a higher level of testosterone than women, and that this higher level of testosterone reduces and inhibits their sense of smell. Men also produce only a little estrogen, the hormone that enhances the sense of smell. Women, by contrast, have a higher level of estrogen than men, and this higher level enhances their sense of smell. Women also do not produce much testosterone, the hormone that inhibits the sense of smell.

Not surprisingly, then, women after puberty are a hundred times more sensitive than men to Exaltolide, an aromatic compound much like men's sexual musk.[48] Most women can smell mild sweat from three feet away. When they are ovulating and fertile, in mid-cycle, they have an even greater sensitivity to odors, including sweat.[49] Several women friends have told us that they can smell when another woman has her period. Behind this kind of response is a sensitivity to the pheromones derived from the fluctuating hormones in the woman's monthly cycle. Le Magnen maintains that the increasing level of estrogen that evokes a surge of LH followed by release of an egg is the cause of women's midcycle sensitivity, which for some odors increases by as much as a hundred thousandfold.[50] Part of the natural olfactory superiority of women may be found in evidence that higher estrogen levels increase the number of odor-sensitive neurons.[51]

The natural olfactory superiority of women and the links between smell, mother-child bonding, sexual bonding, and mating clearly fits in with the contention of behavioral psychologists that humans live in a world of female choice.[52] This reality brings us back once again to Ariadne's thread of biological consistency. It seems logical and biologically consistent that women should enjoy a greater sensitivity to and a greater ability to decode the subliminal messages in pheromones.

And yet, regardless of gender differences, we all certainly can and do use our sense of smell to our advantage and the advantage of our species.[53] What human beings lack in acuity they make up for in powers of discrimination, which rival those of any other mammal.

DEEP IN THE WOMB

There is a classic, sexist story of how the sperm and egg meet and a new human starts its adventure in the womb. In this drama, the female role is played by a passive, roly-poly, dowdy egg just released from its nest in an ovarian follicle. After the waving finger-like projections of the fallopian tube nudge this shy egg into its funnel-like opening, cilia create a current that pushes it along through the narrow tube to find its destiny, a knight-in-shining-armor, victorious sperm.

Swimming with determination toward this waiting egg are a troop of lead male actors, a hundred or less, hardy, determined sperm. A few hours earlier, these survivors were among five hundred million sperm that spurted from the ejaculation gate. After the shock of ejaculation, millions of sperm lost their bearings and exhausted themselves in the folds of the cavernous vagina or struggling to find their way through the cervical canal leading to the womb. Millions more died in the folds and crypts of the womb, or fell by the wayside exhausted from fighting the current created by the cilia in the vagina and tubes. The hundred or so survivors had cleverly found a thread to guide them through the mucus barrier at the cervical gate to the womb. They had survived the swim through the uterine cavity and were now engaged in the last lap of the fallopian tube, on their way to the egg. At the start of the last lap, they parted company with half the finalists, who took the wrong turn into the other fallopian tube. Like the sperm lost in the vagina and uterus, these sperm also died without ever coming close to the goal.

When the egg finally comes within reach, the few surviving sperm sprint, fighting to find a way through the "radiating crown" of nurse cells protecting the egg, until one determined and triumphant sperm wins the five-inch race. This victor penetrates the waiting egg, and releases its twenty-three chromosomes which embrace the egg's matching chromosomes. This starts the process of cell division that in nine months will produce a baby.[1]

The egg waiting patiently to be fertilized by a determined and victorious sperm! How easy it is to slip into that classic male-skewed tale of a sperm finding its egg!

What really happens is quite different, according to Emily Martin, a cultural anthropologist who has studied how we create images of our bodies and body parts to reflect our cultural prejudices and patriarchal biases.[2] Martin's analysis, based on the latest clinical research in fertility and reproduction, rejects male-skewed adjectives and perspectives when they contradict what we actually know about the behavior of eggs and sperm. The results are intriguing and enlightening. Compare the sperm/egg story above with the following story of egg and sperm inspired by Martin's efforts.

Deep in the seminiferous tubules of the testes, nurse cells are busy towing rafts of up to one hundred immature sperm through the production lines to the central tunnel and on to the coiled storage tube on top of the testes. With hundreds of thousands of nurse cells guiding the production of two hundred million sperm every hour, a thousand every second, quality control is frankly quite poor. One in five sperm is defective, with missing or surplus chromosomes, bent tails, two or three tails, double heads, or no head at all.

Ejaculation dumps a huge swarm of reluctant, feeble swimming sperm into the vagina near the cervix. Shocked by the acidic vaginal/cervical secretions, about half of the half a billion sperm start swimming vigorously, but with no real direction. Their heads thrash side to side ten times more energetically than they push forward. (The last thing you want in a sperm, Martin explains, is a determined, no-nonsense, straight-ahead swimmer who takes off in the wrong direction as it tumbles out of the penis and heads off straight into some vaginal crevasse or burrows into the first solid object it encounters.) Half of the sperm in any ejaculate are either incapable of swimming or are too lazy. They lay around until they die.

Some of the survivors, if they are lucky, bump into a protein thread in the cervical mucus that will lead them through the cervical canal into the uterine cavity. Responding to the new alkaline environment of the cervix, the surviving sperm change their erratic tail-lashing to a smooth spiral movement that propels them along the protein threads and into reservoirs or crypts in the walls of the cervix. Some reproductive physiologists believe the chemistry of the cervix changes with ejaculation to make sure the sperm stop in the crypts and rest their tails.[3]

When the sperm leave the cervical crypts and make their way into the vast cavern of the uterus, they take off in all directions, flopping along, bumping into walls, until the sheer odds of pinball-like action brings a few dozen sperm up close to the egg. There, calcium ions in the oviduct trigger these few survivors to thrash about, a behavior that probably increases their odds of bumping into the egg.

Twenty years ago, researchers found that the eggs of many species of animals produce and release chemical messengers that are critical to guiding the sperm to the egg. Researchers named these egg chemicals *gynogamones*, "gyno" for female and "**gamone**" because these chemical messengers in the female egg or gamete function in some ways like a pheromone. Activated by the calcium in the tube and lured by a gynogamone, the sperm mill about the egg until it selects one good-looking sperm, one with a well-formed head (indicating it has all the essential twenty-three chromosomes) and a sturdy, straight tail (indicating it is healthy). Enzymes in the protective layer surrounding the egg hook into receptors in the head of the chosen sperm and it is reeled in like a trout desperately trying to escape. Once the sperm is pulled inside the egg, its tail is lopped off, the power organelles (mitochondria) in its midpiece recycled, and the chromosomes in its head liberated so they can join with the egg's chromosomes and make a zygote, embryo, fetus, and nine months later a baby.

This is a much different tale of the sperm's adventure, but it is more accurate in view of recent research. For a long time we have known that the eggs of some lizards, insects, crustaceans, and even turkeys can divide on their own to produce offspring without waiting or needing to be fertilized by a sperm.[4] The role of female gynogamones and the changing environment in the female reproductive track are also important in the second story.[5] More to the point of our case, recent research in Belgium suggests that immature sperm cells in the testes have the genetic instructions needed to produce twenty different odor receptors.

> Whether the odor receptors in fact develop and function remains to be seen, but these are the same kind of receptors that allow the nose to smell. That the nose and sperm could have receptors in common

is not unusual. Molecules that work well in one place are often pressed into service for similar tasks elsewhere in the body.[6]

FROM SEX CHROMOSOMES TO MALE OR FEMALE

The union of egg and sperm triggers an unbelievably complex symphony of processes and events that results in billions of highly specialized cells working together to create a living being that can feel, experience emotions, and construct a world based on abstractions. We only have time to touch on a few of the main turning points in our sexual development, and even with these we will concentrate, as we did above with the role of gynogamones in fertilization, on the development of a major hormone system in the fetus that is very much influenced after birth by our responses to pheromones and their interactions with genes and hormones that in turn affect our sexual development and behaviors.

By the end of the first week, the single cell has divided into hundreds of cells. In a few days some cells have specialized into a thin wall that will become the placenta and an inner mass of cells that will become the embryo itself. As this hollow ball and its inner cell mass burrows into the wall of the uterus, some cells specialize to become the skin and central nervous system, others to become muscles, blood, and connective tissues, and still others to line the digestive and respiratory tracts.

Thirty years ago geneticists knew there had to be a set of "form-shaping" genes, morphogens, that tell different cells in the very early embryo to head off in a specific direction to become bone, liver, heart, muscle, olfactory, or some other kind of cell. They also suspected that certain key masses of cells serve as local headquarters that signal and organize neighboring cells.

> The central part of the signalling system, which is essentially the same in all the organisms studied, is a receptor protein embedded in the membrane of the cell with one end protruding outside the cell and the other poking into the cell's interior. Once the outer segment of the receptor protein is triggered by the appropriate chemical signal, it initiates a cascade of events that culminate in switching the cell into a different developmental path.[7]

In 1993, scientists identified structure-forming genes they call hedgehog genes in mice, zebra fish, and chickens, three staples of embryonic laboratory research. Once the hedgehog genes are switched on in a particular set of cells, they make proteins that spread out to neighboring cells. As they spread, they are diluted, becoming less concentrated and their signals less strong. These graduated signals tell each cell its position in the limb or other organ and what its particular role should be. Hedgehog genes that control development of different regions of the brain turn on around fifteen days after fertilization and finish their task about day twenty-eight.[8] A year earlier, scientists reported finding what they called HOX morphogens that operate a little later in embryonic development than the hedgehog genes.[9]

Structure-forming genes like the hedgehog and HOX genes play a major role in developing our male and female sexual and reproductive anatomy. For females, this process starts with two X chromosomes. For males, the usual chromosome pattern is an X and a Y chromosome, with the Y chromosome carrying a special gene known as the testes determining factor, or TDF gene.[10]

If a fetus has a Y chromosome and a TDF gene, it will develop testes in the second month of pregnancy. If a fetus has two X chromosomes and no TDF gene, it will develop ovaries in the third month.

In the second month of pregnancy, a fetus with testes will react to hormone signals from its newly formed pituitary gland and start producing high levels of androgenic hormones, particularly testosterone, along with a low level of estrogens. Hormone production in a fetus with ovaries starts a few weeks later, and the predominant hormones are estrogens, mainly estradiol, with a low level of testosterone.[11]

A high level of testosterone and other androgens causes an embryo to develop internal male sexual structures, including a prostate gland and sperm ducts. A second androgenic hormone known as MIH eliminates internal ducts that could develop into a vagina, uterus and fallopian tubes. A derivative of testosterone known as DHT also directs the formation of a penis and scrotum.[12]

Female sexual anatomy, both internal and external, is triggered by a "default program" in the genes. This genetic program causes an embryo with a low level of testosterone and little or no MIH to develop a vagina, uterus, and paired fallopian tubes. The same genetic program allows a clitoris and labia to develop without any hormone influence.[13]

In the second and third month of pregnancy, various regions and specialized structures and circuits are rapidly developing in the embryo's brain. These include connections with the developing olfactory system, eyes and ears, the limbic system and hypothalamus, and blood vessels to carry hormones from the hypothalamus to the nearby pituitary gland.

Normally, a "barrier" prevents hormones from crossing from the blood into the brain cells because they can seriously disrupt its normal functioning. But testosterone is an exception. It easily crosses the brain barrier and, after being converted into some estrogen, it "masculinizes" various "neural programs" and pathways in different brain circuits, setting up gender-dimorphic neurotemplates for a later puberty and steady production of GnRH in males.[14]

Brain pathways develop differently in male and female embryos because males have high levels of testosterone and MIH and low levels of estrogens while females have lots of estrogens and low levels of testosterone and MIH. These differences in neural encoding eventually result in behavioral tendencies we are now finding more common or stronger in females or males.[15]

With this sketch of our sexual development in the womb, we are ready to delve deeper into the biological basis for the many connections we have already seen between pheromones, the olfactory systems, and our sexual development and behaviors. The basis of these connections we will find in the Hypothalamic-Pituitary-Gonadal (HPG) axis, and in GnRH, the releasing hormone from the hypothalamus that starts and regulates the activity of genes behind the cascade of sex hormones. In contrast with its slow action as a hormone, GnRH can have an immediate effect on sexual behavior when it functions as a neurotransmitter.

GNRH PULSES AND THE HPG AXIS

The foundation of the HPG axis is laid down in the fourth week of pregnancy, before the ovaries or testes start developing. That is when a pair of nasal thickenings form on the face and deepen into pits. In the pits, neurons develop that are capable of producing GnRH. Although we have already mentioned GnRH neurons and GnRH several times and alluded to the crucial roles of GnRH as a neurotransmitter and hormone, we have only hinted at their full importance and pivotal role in the HPG axis regulation of our sexual development and behaviors.

In the fourth and fifth weeks, GnRH neurons in the olfactory plates/pits migrate inward and under the developing forebrain to contribute to the structure and the function of what will become the hypothalamus. They also form a loose network of GnRH producing neurons scattered throughout the olfactory system.[16] Later in life these GnRH neurons will be activated by serotonin, dopamine, and other neurotransmitters, and their complex role in our sexual development will unfold.

During pregnancy, more GnRH neurons migrate into the hypothalamus of male fetuses than migrate into the female hypothalamus. Some gene, possibly a hedgehog or HOX gene, tells olfactory neurons in the nasal plate to migrate to the hypothalamus in the third and fourth week. Genes on the male's Y chromosome may also play a role in sending more GnRH neurons to the male hypothalamus than the female hypothalamus.[17] Whatever triggers this difference, it has many long-term consequences for females and males because the number of GnRH neurons in the hypothalamus determines the speed and strength of the pulses of GnRH production.[18]

Because males have more GnRH neurons, they have a faster GnRH pulse. This causes the pituitary gland to turn out more luteinizing hormone or LH than follicle stimulating hormone (FSH). This, in turn, causes the testes to produce a high level of testosterone and a lower level of estrogens.

More testosterone and fewer estrogens in males has many consequences, the obvious consequence being a penis, scrotum, and male secondary sex characteristics. But hidden in the male brain are more subtle consequences like more synapses between neurons and a male pattern of neural encoding that includes programs for tonic (continuous or noncyclic) production of sex hormones in the HPG axis, later puberty, and a heightened sensitivity to female pheromones. Males may also have a tendency to be more visual than touch oriented, and more compulsive in their masturbation than females.[19]

Because females have fewer GnRH neurons in the hypothalamus, they have slower GnRH pulses that result in a high level of FSH and of estrogens, specifically estradiol, and less LH and testosterone. Anatomically, this results in a clitoris, vagina, uterus, and fallopian tubes, with secondary sex characteristics we label feminine or female. In the female brain, it means development of different synapses and a female organization of neural circuits. The crucial neural program sets up a program for a pattern of GnRH pulses that vary in speed and strength during the woman's monthly cycle. This pattern of varying GnRH pulses regulates hormone production in the HPG axis that is responsible for the female's earlier puberty, higher sensitivity to touch, and lower receptivity to female pheromones.[20]

To create the HPG axis which is at the heart of our sexual development and all our sexual behaviors, the development of our olfactory system, hypothalamus, limbic system, pituitary gland, and ovaries or testes have to be closely coordinated because they are in many ways interdependent and feed back one to the other.[21]

In women, a monthly cycle of pulses of GnRH pulses of varying speed and strength from the hypothalamus and the loose GnRH neuron network outside the hypothalamus cause variations in the production of FSH and LH in the pituitary. In the ovaries, FSH and LH regulate growth and ovulation of the egg, and secretion of estrogens and progesterone to direct the uterine and menstrual cycle. Within the hypothalamus, certain circuits are genetically programmed to monitor the changing levels of estrogens and progesterone in the blood. When these levels do not match the recipe for a healthy monthly cycle in the ovaries and uterus, the proper message is sent along to the pituitary to slow or speed up production of either FSH or LH.[22]

In men, a similar process occurs in the HPG axis, except that GnRH pulses are relatively steady rather than varying in a monthly cycle.[23] In the testes, FSH from the pituitary stimulates production of androgen-binding protein while LH regulates testosterone production. Both androgen-binding protein and testosterone are needed for sperm production. Rising levels of sperm cause other cells in the testes to release a hormone known as inhibin which blocks the continued release of FSH. This keeps sperm production moving along at about two hundred million sperm an hour in the healthy adult male. When the level of testosterone rises too high in the blood, this information is picked up by monitors in the hypothalamus, and GnRH and LH production slows down.

Sometimes this monitoring system is not sufficient. A female fetus, for instance, may be exposed to high levels of testosterone because of the mother has taken a synthetic hormone known as DES to reduce the risk of miscarriage. Or the mother or fetus may have overactive adrenal glands that pump out extra testosterone. This can masculinize a female fetus by influencing the way the HPG axis works. The sexual anatomy may then shift toward the male pattern.[24]

At birth, male babies get a surge of GnRH that results in a LH surge. This is apparently triggered by exposure to the mother's pheromones.[25] This LH surge keeps the testes pumping out a high level of testosterone which further masculinizes the brain by destroying or altering connections between nerve cells and creating male circuits.[26] By the age of eighteen months, all the infant's brain nerve cells are present and organized, although synapses will continue to develop.[27]

In newborn females, on the other hand, the GnRH pulse keeps production of FSH, LH, and estradiol high. One of the many effects of estradiol is to promote and maintain the growth of neurons and their connections in the brain.

In the womb, hormones—especially estradiol and testosterone—appear to alter how well neurons transmit signals to the hypothalamus. Whether the estradiol comes from the fetus, from the mother, or from an outside source, it can change the speed and strength of the GnRH pulse because it is the interaction between the transmission of nerve impulses and levels of GnRH that regulates the development of the male and female hormone control systems that form the biological core of mammalian reproduction.[28]

This link between hormones, the transmission of signals to the hypothalamus, and the response of GnRH neurons that regulate the cascade of hormones from the pituitary to the ovaries or testes is the key to our sexual development and behavior. But it is very difficult to get direct evidence of these complex and varied connections. Fortunately, the effects of pheromones in triggering menstrual synchronization or suppression, courtship and mating, and aggressive behavior in animals provide indirect evidence that olfactory input causes variations in the speed or strength of the GnRH pulse. In some of the animal experiments mentioned earlier, the level of LH production increased when adults of the same species came in contact with the pheromones of the opposite sex. Exposing a female to male pheromones can in fact cause a surge in the level of LH that is characteristic of normal ovulation in females. Conversely, exposure to the pheromones of other females seems to suppress the LH surge that accompanies ovulation. In all these cases, the LH surge has to be triggered by a GnRH pulse. This means that whatever can influence the speed and strength of the GnRH pulse in the long run may well affect our sexual development and/or behavior.

The hormones in the HPG Axis—GnRH, LH, FSH, androgens like testosterone and estrogens like estradiol—are much the same in both males and females. It is only their proportions, their shifting ratios, that differ. In males, the negative feedback from levels of testosterone and estradiol in the blood keeps the production of GnRH in the hypothalamus and LH and FSH in the pituitary nicely balanced. One hormone stimulates production of the other that in turn suppresses the first when it gets too high. Everything runs smoothly, and the pattern of GnRH production in the hypothalamus is steady and continuous, not cyclic.

In females, the situation is different because three hormones are involved, progesterone being the added factor. Balancing three hormones requires a positive rather than simple negative feedback system. Positive feedback occurs when one hormone stimulates production of a second hormone that does not suppress the first until a higher level of a third hormone allows a balance to be achieved. Because three hormones are involved, and the balance is not maintained, only achieved on a regular basis, and this pattern is cyclic by nature.[29]

During childhood, in the years before puberty, and during puberty, the pituitary glands of girls consistently release more FSH and less LH than males do as a result of GnRH signals from the hypothalamus.[30] Males, on the other hand, release more testosterone and fewer estrogens than females, while females release more estrogens and less testosterone. Conclusion? It takes less GnRH to trigger production of FSH and estrogens than it does to produce LH and testosterone. That means that it takes more than blue booties to make a male; it takes a hypothalamus with faster GnRH pulses during fetal development, in childhood, and during puberty. On the other hand, pink booties are also not enough to make one female. It takes slower GnRH pulses from the hypothalamus at all stages of one's development.

The use of "faster and stronger" and "slower and weaker" is not a sexist difference. These adjectives may sound "politically incorrect" to some, but they are an accurate expression of the realities of how GnRH pulses and the HPG axis function in real life. These terms should not be taken to imply any value judgment or hierarchy.

The interaction of hormones we mentioned above, coupled with other hormones and neuropeptides, in the HPG Axis reaches every cell in our bodies. It affects neuron regeneration, food intake, temperature regulation, addictive behaviors, learning, memory, motivation, arousal, mood, aggression, as well as our social, courtship, mating,[31] and maternal behaviors.

This chapter is not meant to impress the reader with the complexity of psychoneuroendocrinology. We have tried to keep this sketch as elementary as possible by leaving out details about the roles of other neurotransmitters, like noradrenaline, dopamine, serotonin, and the natural amphetamines and opioids. We have also avoided mentioning the neurotransmitters that inhibit nerve impulse transmission, amino acids that excite these messages, and other brain peptides like the pineal secretion melatonin and corticotropin-releasing hormone. Only psychoneuroendocrinologists find these kinds of details interesting. They certainly are beyond our needs, although we do need the sketch of the HPG axis and its hormones in this chapter to understand and appreciate how pheromones are tied into our sexual development and behavior. Our next chapter will provide some lighter and intriguing examples of the extent to which GnRH neurons and GnRH are involved in guiding and regulating our sexual development and behavior.

TRACKING THE YELLOW HORMONE

Our exploration of the connections between odors and sexual behavior has linked together several very important facts, starting with the many examples we have of physiological and behavioral responses that are clearly related to and triggered by odors and pheromones. Obviously we are referring mainly to examples in which pheromones clearly affect the ovulatory cycle in mammals and the corresponding menstrual cycle in women. When we looked behind menstrual synchronization and other examples, we found the HPG axis that controls responses like menstruation, courtship and mating behaviors, aggression, and ovulation. We know that this axis is dependent on GnRH neurons and GnRH production, both of which are affected by pheromones. We also know that the second stage in the HPG axis involves the level and pulse of LH, the luteinizing or "yellow hormone," which regulates the levels of the two crucial sex hormones, testosterone and estrogen, in all mammals including humans.[32]

Because our pulses of GnRH are so minute, so short lived, and originate so deep inside the brain, researchers cannot measure them directly as they sometimes do in other mammals. The only way to detect and to measure human GnRH pulses is indirectly, by measuring the levels of LH, the "yellow hormone," in the blood or urine. A good example of this indirect approach is the discovery that estradiol increases the number of neurons that respond to odor stimulation while testosterone seems to have the opposite effect. Because estradial and testosterone levels depend on LH levels, and LH levels depend on GnRH levels, we can link GnRH levels with sensitivity to odors, and speculate on the possible effects of odors on our sexual behaviors mediated by shifts in the balance of estrogens and testosterone.

It seems obvious—and many scientists agree—that the human examples we have discussed are consistent with and in fact human equivalents of the connections scientists have uncovered between pheromones, hormones, neurotransmission, and odor sensitivity in the complex factors underlying the sexual behaviors of other species.[33] If this appraisal is correct, then pheromones may very well have a powerful impact on human behavior.[34]

To complete our sketch of odors and sex, there are a few additional examples that strengthen the connection between genes, hormones, and behavior in humans and other animals. These examples will fit in with our sketch of the HPG axis in this chapter and with our examples of pheromone action in earlier chapters.

8

FROM GENES TO
BEHAVIOR AND BACK

One of the most enduring and, until recently, most perplexing questions to challenge the human mind has been to explain how males and females manage to produce offspring very much like themselves generation after generation. Offspring look and act like their parents, grandparents, and great grandparents. But why? How?[1] Modern genetics has shown the answer lies in the information passed from parents to offspring in the elegantly coded amino acids in the deoxyribonucleic acid (DNA) that combine when an egg and sperm join to produce an offspring that reflects the biological and psychological heritage of its parents.

Unfortunately, the public image of DNA, and its functional units which we call genes is too often grossly simplistic and distorted. Genes, we often hear, control all our traits. Genes for eye color determine whether we have brown, hazel, or blue eyes. A child inherits recessive genes for cystic fibrosis from his or her father and mother, and inevitably develops this chronic, debilitating condition. Genes determine every aspect of our biological future. Or so it seems.

This popular view of genes operating on their own to control all aspects of a living organism is supported by a picture that genes are just little beads of DNA information, strung together along spiral coiled strands. Each gene magically, omnipotently it seems, controls some single trait. News stories of genetic engineers inserting normal healthy genes into plants and animals to overcome the harmful effects of a faulty gene, or improve on nature only enhance this simplistic picture.

For many scientists and certainly for many more lay persons in the first half of this century, Nature—our genes—and Nurture—our social environment—were viewed as two parallel, independent influences on our lives. Genes controlled our development before birth, while the social environment dominated from birth to death. But this dualistic view has dangerous political and social implications, especially when it is claimed that either genes or the environment are the dominant, perhaps sole force in our lives.[2]

Those who believe that omnipotent genes are the crucial factor in our development and that they clearly overshadow the social environment have concluded that society has a moral responsibility to keep the mentally retarded, social misfits, and other undesirables from passing on their defective genes to their too-many offspring. The omnipotent gene theory reinforced class divisions, discouraged upward social mobility through education, and encouraged ideas about limiting the gene pool through forced sterilization and other measures promoted by Nazi social theorists and others seeking an easy solution to complex human problems.[3]

In the same era, other theorists denied that genes imposed any limit on human development. All we had to do was focus our efforts on improving our social environment, reducing poverty, and eliminating social inequities. For over fifty years, Communist agriculture experts rejected modern genetics and concentrated on creating the best environment to improve their crops and animal husbandry. For humans, a totally egalitarian society was possible because all inequities are the result of a social class system. Sexist and class inequities can be eliminated if only we provide equal opportunity and reject all alleged differences between males and females to raise our children in a totally gender-free environment. The only "real difference" between males and females is their sexual anatomy, and that is irrelevant except for mating and reproduction. Genes may rule our development in the womb, but the important scripts for our lives and relationships have been inscribed on our brain's blank slate by society only after we were born.[4]

For the partisans of nurture and social engineering, "it has been fashionable to insist that [gender] differences are minimal, the consequence of variations in experience during development." The influence of our genes and hormones on the organization of the male and female brain early in pregnancy is essentially irrelevant when it comes to what we can accomplish by improving learning and the environment.[5]

Today, the idea of genes as beads on a string automatically controlling our biology and environment as an independent force influencing our personality and mental functions is nonsense. As Alice Rossi pointed out in her 1984 Presidential Address to the American Sociological Society, attempts to explain human behavior and efforts to change behavior that neglect the fundamental biological and neural differences between the sexes "carry a high risk of eventual irrelevance against the mounting evidence of sexual dimorphism from the biological and neural sciences . . . [Human diversity] is a biological fact, while equality is a political, ethical, and social precept."[6]

The model of Nature versus Nurture has now been replaced by an interactive model in which genes and the biological factors they control interact with environmental factors throughout life. At some critical times in our lives, especially during early pregnancy, genes do play the lead role. But they always function in the unique, ever-changing internal environment of the developing organism. After birth, the external environment may move front stage, but its effects are always colored by our genes. During pregnancy and after birth, our genes, proteins, hormones, and neurotransmitters interact to guide our developing sexual anatomy, lay down the neural pathways, and concentrate neural and hormonal receptors in different regions of the brain in ways that mold our Hypothalamic-Pituitary-Gonadal (HPG) axis and influence our sexual behavior. In this process, our sense of smell and response to pheromones, our sensitivity to daylight, seasonal cycles, temperature, and stress are woven into the interactive web as they feed into and affect the neurotransmitters, hormones, and receptors of the HPG axis. In each cell, 100,000 genes are constantly being influenced by and reacting to stimuli inside and outside the cell. True, each gene codes for a specific protein such as those that make up our enzymes, hormones and receptors but this code is influenced by other genes, the cell, the organism, and its whole environment.[7]

If you are still tempted to view genes as a predetermined information packet that automatically defines how an animal develops, consider the worried reaction of an audience leaving a movie theater after watching the 1993 film *Jurassic Park*. Yes, scientists have recovered intact genes from a 550-year-old human bone, a 2,000,000-year-old woolly mammoth frozen in Siberian ice, a 32,000,000-year-old termite, and a 120,000,000-year-old weevil. Many who read or watch *Jurassic Park* firmly believe that scientists will soon put such prehistoric DNA into an egg with the kind of amino acids the genes need to make a whole organism and produce a living clone of these prehistoric animals.

Even if we recovered all the genes from a cell of some extinct animal, it could not function properly or replicate itself, let alone produce a whole human, prehistoric mammoth, termite, or weevil. Human genes can only function and produce a human when they interact with the living environment of a human egg cell. Woolly mammoth genes will not function properly, unless they are in an egg cell with the amino acids that form the protein structures of a woolly mammoth. If we put defrosted woolly mammoth DNA into the egg of a closely related modern elephant whose modern genes we previously removed, the proteins and cell material of the modern elephant egg would not provide the same environment as the woolly mammoth egg protein, no matter how closely related they are. No one knows what woolly mammoth genes in an elephant egg, carried in the womb of a modern elephant, would produce. It just would not be a woolly mammoth, nor a modern elephant.[8]

This new understanding of how genes and environment interact is nowhere more significant, neuroendocrinologist Bruce McEwen points out, than in understanding how our brain develops and works. "Long regarded as a complex electrical control box or a biological computer, the brain is now recognized more and more for its plasticity to respond to and withstand environmental challenges, to change with use and experience, and to respond to internal hormone signals."[9]

This flexibility is rooted in the many different ways our genes produce specific enzymes, specific receptors for hormones and neurotransmitters, and specific hormones. Since variations in enzymes, receptors, and hormones in turn affect our personalities and sexual behavior, we need to examine a few examples that will help us appreciate this lifelong interaction of genes and their environment. We start with two examples of how genes affect our experience of being sexual persons by altering a specific enzyme.

A DON JUAN GENE AND GIRLS WHO BECOME MEN

Our first example involves a behavior commonly associated with Don Juan, a legendary Spanish nobleman with insatiable sexual urges. Or if you prefer an Italian version, with Giovanni Casanova, a well-known diplomat, colleague of Benjamin Franklin, Voltaire, and Frederick the Great, and a compulsive seducer of women. Whatever his ethnic roots, the libidinous, promiscuous male has provided a powerful leitmotif for classic poems, plays, novels, operas, and other musical works by the likes of Moliere, Mozart, Lord Byron, Richard Strauss, and George Bernard Shaw. Only recently have we learned that, in some cases, this behavior is linked with a defective gene that results in a shortage of a key brain enzyme that breaks down the hormone adrenalin and a neurotransmitter known as PEA.

Adrenalin, widely known as "the emergency hormone," increases heart activity, improves the power and prolongs muscle action, and increases the rate and depth of breathing. Adrenalin acts like a natural kind of "speed," increasing one's energy and preparing the body for "fright, flight, or fight." Like "speed," it also improves one's mood.[10]

While emergencies are fortunately rare and seldom everyday occurrences, our adrenal glands are constantly producing small amounts of adrenalin. So the body needs an enzyme that can keep the adrenalin level under control all the time, not just after an adrenalin surge helps us cope with an emergency. That enzyme is monoamine oxidase (MAO), which not only keeps our adrenalin under control but also breaks down phenylethylamine (PEA), a natural amphetamine-like neurotransmitter in the brain.

Persons with a normal level of MAO also have a normal level of adrenalin and PEA. They can get high watching grass grow and listening to music. Some people, however, have a genetic defect that prevents them from producing a normal amount of MAO. With low MAO and constant high levels of adrenaline and PEA, these people are hyperactive. Because they feel euphoric and invincible all the time, life is a constant routine of ecstasy and euphoria with no edge or newness. But, like everyone else, they enjoy and need the thrill and euphoric feeling of the novel and unusual experience. For someone with a low MAO level, the only excitement in life is an addiction to daring, risky behavior. Their highs come from skydiving, wind-surfing in the clouds, driving at high speeds, bungee-jumping, and the like. In some way, their brains then convert the experience of terror into an ecstatic euphoria.[11]

In the sexual arena, the gene for low MAO results in hypersexuality, a modern Casanova, Don Juan, or nymphomaniac. Low MAO also makes it difficult or impossible for a person to develop long-term attachments in childhood or pairbond as adults normally do.[12]

Our second example of a gene producing an enzyme that affects our sexual experience and behavior involves the 5-alpha-reductase (5AR) enzyme.[13] In this case, a child inherits a recessive gene from each parent that cannot produce the enzyme needed to convert testosterone to dihydrotestosterone (DHT). In the first three months of pregnancy, this embryo starts off on the male track. It has a male chromosome pattern of XY. It also develops testes, lots of testosterone, and internal male sexual anatomy. Meanwhile its MIH eliminates the potential for a uterus, vagina, and fallopian tubes. The only problem, a lack of the enzyme 5AR, shows up in the third month of pregnancy. Since DHT is the hormone that causes the external sexual anatomy to develop into a penis and scrotum, an embryo without 5AR and DHT develops external sexual anatomy that more or less resembles a clitoris and labia rather than penis and scrotum. (The anatomical effects of a lack of DHT are fairly clear. What a lack of DHT does in the pathways of the brain is anyone's guess at this point.)[14]

When an infant is born with no 5AR enzyme and DHT, it appears to be a normal little girl. Because this condition is so rare, the parents and midwife or attending physician would not be inclined to check carefully the clitoris and labia to make certathe infant really is a girl. A simple chromosome test would reveal the "girl" is a genetic male, but this test would not be performed unless there was some reason to suspect a problem. Because the infant with no 5AR or DHT appears to be a healthy, normal little girl, the parents will raise it as such. Even though she may have some doubts as she grows up, a child with 5AR-DHT deficiency will usually conform to her parents' expectations. She is not likely to argue with her own external anatomy and everyone who tells her she is a girl, even though somehow she feels now and then that maybe she is not like all the other girls.

This situation changes drastically with the onset of puberty. Even though the lack of 5AR and DHT continues through adolescence and adult life, the surge of androgens at puberty appears to be sufficient to turn the clitoral-like phallus into a small penis and fuse the labia more or less to form a scrotum. The testes may then descend into the new scrotum.[15] As secondary characteristics of a male develop, so does a sexual attraction to women as this girl becomes a man.

In three rural villages of the Dominican Republic, where Julianne Imperato-McGuinley and her colleagues first studied this condition, the "conversion" of a daughter into a son at puberty was acceptable because of the strong patriarchal tradition. Even so, affected children were subject to some ridicule, with taunts like *quevote* ("penis at 12") and *machihembra* ("first woman, then man"). Once researchers understood the genetic defect behind 5AR-DHT deficiency, they started examining newborns more carefully and checking their chromosomes when family histories suggested a risk of this gender problem. Most of the more than three dozen Dominican Republic children with 5AR-DHT deficiency managed to adopt a male gender role and later married, although the extent of their adjustment is still hotly debated.[16] Still, all of the Dominican Republic children who were born with this defect before the 1970s and were reared as girls eventually rebelled against being female and assumed male identities and life patterns as adults. After the 1970s, such children were properly identified and reared as males, even though their external sexual anatomy was not what it should be in childhood.

The message is clear: genes code for enzymes that in turn affect sexual behavior.

FOUR-YEAR-OLD MEN AND GENETIC MALE GIRLS

Moving on to other ways genes alter our sexual behavior, we have two good illustrations of how a defective gene can alter the activity of a hormone receptor and how this in turn clearly affects an individual's sexual behavior.

Normally, the GnRH gene helps to code for the function of neurons that secrete gonadotropin-releasing hormone (GnRH) in the hypothalamus and in scattered centers of the limbic and olfactory systems. GnRH then interacts with its receptors in the pituitary to trigger production of LH. When LH is picked up by LH receptors in the testes, it triggers testosterone production and secondary sex characteristics. Testosterone influences the structure and function of many different neurons and controls sex drive. After testosterone enters the brain, enzymes transform it into other hormones that influence the development of brain neurons and pathways. When androgens surge at puberty and are picked up by their receptors throughout the body, all the anatomical and psychological changes males experience as they go through puberty follow naturally.

In some boys, however, a mutated gene produces an abnormal receptor for LH that jams in the "ON" position.[17] The result is known as familial precocious male puberty. (Familial in this context means the gene occurs in certain family lines.) Before a boy with this genetic defect is four years old, he will show signs of a very early sexual maturation. The growth spurt that normally occurs in the teen years will occur between ages two and four years, with adult-like muscle development, a deepened voice, pubic hair, and sexual interest. While other boys have years to learn the skills they need to handle their budding sexual drive and avoid inappropriate sexual behavior, these four-year-olds have no idea of what is appropriate or inappropriate behavior. Sexually, they are men. But then, at age four, any sexual behavior is considered inappropriate in our culture!

The sense of smell relies on the same kind of receptors that are involved in premature puberty. In addition, the pheromones of other mammals can activate genes in neurons that control the HPG Axis and puberty whether it comes in the teen years or early childhood.[18] The LH receptor is a G-protein coupled receptor, which normally is activated by GnRH. Since pheromones stimulate the production of GnRH and of LH by acting on G-protein coupled receptors in olfactory neurons, it seems likely that pheromones may also be involved in the onset of puberty.[19]

Much more common than familial precocious male puberty is another condition in which a faulty gene creates a defect in an androgen receptor that alters sexual experience. You can see the results of this genetic mutation in some female fashion models who conform to our common male ideal of feminine beauty, tall with well developed breasts and long, graceful legs, a flawless, baby-like complexion with no hint of acne.[20] But behind the clear appearance of a female and the unquestioned psyche of a female gender identity may be a genetic male with XY chromosomes, testes in the abdomen, and a normal male high level of androgens and low level of estrogens in the blood.

What makes these women different from other women is a recessive gene on their X chromosome that leaves them with a defective androgen receptor. None of their body cells can bring testosterone into the cells where it can interact with the genes to masculinize the sexual anatomy and brain pathways. Because their body cells cannot respond to the masculinizing message of testosterone, their external sexual anatomy and gender identity are perfectly normal for a female. Their secondary sex traits are classic even ultra feminine because of estrogens from the testes and adrenal glands. Yet, because they have testes and MIH, they have no internal female sexual anatomy. They have no menstrual cycle and are obviously infertile.

At birth, infants with androgen insensitivity or testicular feminization, appear to be normal little girls and are so reared by their parents. Years later, during a pelvic examination, her gynecologist may tell her that her vagina is short, dead-ended, and not deep enough to allow for coitus unless dilated or surgically lengthened. Because this condition is well documented, a simple chromosome test will alert the doctor to the full extent of the woman's condition. Since there is nothing to be gained from telling her she is a genetic male with no receptors for the testosterone her testes and adrenal glands produce, the doctor will recommend "minor surgery" without telling her that her testes need to be removed before they develop a malignancy. Most likely the physician will simply tell her she is a perfectly normal, healthy woman although she cannot bear any children. Of course, the fact that she is insensitive to testosterone also means she has little or no sex drive.

There are other examples of how genes alter the receptors for specific hormones and neurotransmitters in ways that eventually affect our sexual behavior, but familial precocious male puberty and androgen insensitivity are particularly useful for our purposes here.

HORMONES, PHEROMONES, AND GENDER ORIENTATION?

When it comes to the genes that code for the hormones and their receptors which affect our sexual behavior, we have good evidence in both humans and non-humans, although interpreting this evidence is often hotly debated. Evidence that high or low levels of androgens in the womb may result in different structural developments and pathways in the corpus callosum, massa intermedia, and other brain areas of males and females stirs little debate until one asks questions about what these differences may mean for learning and math/language skills, or in the emotional lives of men and women.[21] While no one can dispute the fact that girls and women produce much lower levels of gonadal androgens than boys and men, or that this may make the adrenal androgen production of women a more important factor in the maturation of their sebaceous and apocrine glands, the mere hint that this difference may affect the lifelong production of pheromones based on androgen metabolism triggers heated debate.

Some of our strongest and most accurate evidence of gender differences in androgen production and metabolism can be found in various components of our urine. Properly analyzed, the end products of hormone metabolism in our urine may tell us a great deal about the current status of many different hormones, about our sex, and perhaps even about our sexual orientation.

Most of the androgen produced by males results from pituitary LH stimulating testosterone production in the testes, though other androgens are also produced by the adrenal glands. The liver converts testosterone and these other androgens to androsterone and etiocholanolone, both of which are excreted in the urine.

Twenty-five years ago, Margolese analyzed urine samples collected over a twenty-four-hour period from a group of healthy men and found that the ratio of androsterone to etiocholanolone can be used to discriminate between heterosexuals and homosexuals. Specifically, Margolese found that females and homosexual males excreted less androsterone than etiocholanolone (A<E), while heterosexual males secreted more androsterone than etiocholanolone (A>E). This association is perhaps one of the earliest examples of a hypothesis about a biological origin of sexual orientation.[22]

Not unexpectedly, given the social atmosphere twenty-five years ago, Margolese's suggestion was immediately challenged by a psychiatrist, who like most psychologists in his time, doubted that sexual orientation had any biological component. The challenge was met when urine samples from a mixed group of homosexuals and heterosexuals were analyzed and the results correctly identified the sexual orientation of every subject.[23] A few years later, Margolese and Janiger proposed "that the metabolic pathway which results in a relatively high androsterone value is associated with sexual preference for females by either sex, whereas a relatively low androsterone value is associated with sexual preference for males by either sex."[24] This same study may have provided the first evidence of a genetic basis for homosexuality. Of twenty-four heterosexuals, two reported having homosexual relatives.

Of twenty-eight homosexuals, seventeen reported having homosexual relatives, five of whom had two each.[25]

In 1977, this evidence, along with the statistical significance of confirmed findings that the androsterone to etiocholanolone (A/E) ratio discriminates between homosexual and heterosexual males, was dismissed mainly because there still were no standards available for male or female A/E ratios.[26]

In 1981, after interviewing 1500 men and women, Alan Bell, Martin Weinberg, and Sue Hammersmith admitted they could find no social factor or experience that could be consistently linked with homosexual orientation. They did, however, find "a powerful link" between the development of homosexuality and gender nonconformity, children who regularly adopted behavior patterns commonly associated with the other gender. In their sample, roughly half of the gay men and three-quarters of the heterosexual men were typically "masculine." Half of the gay men and a quarter of the heterosexual men showed some "effeminate" behavior. Two-thirds of the heterosexual women and one in five of the lesbian women were typically "feminine." One-third of the heterosexual women and one in five lesbians showed some "masculine" expressions in personal identity, interests, and activities. While expressing some behavior patterns commonly associated with the other gender may be linked with prenatal hormones and homosexual orientation, it is obvious that gender nonconformity is hardly a solid and consistent indication of a homosexual destiny.[27]

Sexual orientation is never as simple as the gender of one's sexual partner(s). Our orientation contains at least three gender-related factors: that of the persons we are sexually attracted to, that of the persons we fantasize being erotically involved with, and that of those we fall in love with. For some men and women the gender of the partners in these three categories do not match. Some men, for example, deeply love their wives but fantasize about having sex with a man when they have intercourse with their wives. This complex sexual orientation is closely linked with our *gender identity*, our unwavering personal conviction that we are male or female, and our *gender role behavior*, the behaviors we adopt to tell others we are male or female.[28]

At the same time, the link Margolese suggested twenty-five years ago between genes, hormones, and sexual orientation meshes nicely with several recent studies of genetic factors and family tendencies among the siblings and twins of homosexual men and women.

At Harvard University, Richard Pillard and James Weinrich interviewed fiftyone predominantly homosexual and fifty predominantly heterosexual men, all unmarried, asking about the sexual orientation of all their brothers and sisters over twenty years old. Then 115 sisters and 123 brothers were interviewed by a direct mailing. Four percent of the brothers of the heterosexual index subjects reported being homosexual. This matches the best estimates of how many American men are exclusively or predominantly homosexual. However, 22 percent of the brothers of homosexual index subjects were homosexual, suggesting a strong familial or hereditary influence.[29]

In 1991, Michael Bailey at Northwestern University joined Richard Pillard in a follow-up study of the 56 gay identical twins and 54 gay fraternal twins, and the adoptive brothers of 57 gay men. Fifty-two percent of the identical twin brothers, 22 percent of the fraternal twin brothers, and 11 percent of the adoptive, genetically unrelated brothers were also homosexual. We would expect results like this if sexual orientation is strongly influenced by some genetic factor(s).[30]

When Pillard, Bailey, and colleagues looked at the sisters of lesbian women, they came up with similar results. Close to half of the identical twins, 48 percent, 16 percent of the fraternal twins, 14 percent of the biological sisters, and only 6 percent of the adoptive sisters were lesbian.[31]

In a fourth study, Whitam, Diamond and Martin examined twin pairs in which one or both of the twins is homosexual. In two-thirds of the 34 male and four female pairs of identical twins, both twins were homosexual. Among the 23 pairs of fraternal twins, both were homosexual in a third of the pairs. Three sets of triplets showed a similar pattern.[32]

It is far too early to draw a definitive conclusion from these studies of genetic patterns in families. However, "Depending on one's assumptions about the prevalence of homosexuality in the general population and how well these small samples are typical of twins in the general population, these results suggest a hereditary influence somewhere between 30 percent and 70 percent."[33]

In the early 1990s these genetic studies were reinforced by two complementary discoveries.

In July 1993, the *Wall Street Journal, New York Times,* and other media picked up on a report in the prestigious journal *Science* of a breakthrough study of a "gay gene" carried on the X chromosome males inherit from the maternal side. Biochemist-geneticist Dean Hamer and colleagues at the National Institutes of Health, used gene markers, family pedigrees, and very sophisticated DNA replication techniques to identify a small group of genes (Xq28) at the end of the long arm of the X chromosome in gay men as the cause of homosexuality in some men. Their cautious conclusion was "that at least one subtype of male sexual orientation is genetically influenced."[34]

One possible clue to what this genetic factor might do in terms of setting up neural circuits and pathways that may be connected with homosexual behavior came from Simon LeVay at the Salk Institute in San Diego. Working with a small number of autopsied brains, LeVay has identified a neural circuit in the brain that he suggests may trigger sexual attraction to women. The INAH-3 center in the hypothalamus appears well developed in heterosexual men and relatively absent in heterosexual women. Moreover, the INAH-3 in gay men and assumed heterosexual women are similarly undeveloped.[35]

The possible associations and links between family pedigrees, genes, neural tendencies that affect the production of various hormones in the HPG Axis before and after birth, and the possible effects of these on sexual behavior will undoubtedly produce interesting debates. Much research remains to be done, first to confirm Hamer and LeVay's initial findings and then to find out how these neural pathways and circuit might be affected by genes and how they in turn direct behavior.[36] Yet we are compelled to note that the INAH-3 is located in an area of the hypothalamus known to contain GnRH neurons, more of which migrate to the hypothalamus of males than to the hypothalamus of females during prenatal development.

Jump-cut back to our starting point and ask what the link between genes, hormones excreted in urine, and sexual behavior might have to do with human pheromones, and perhaps with sexual orientation.

To start with, Moore suggests that "it is possible that the difference between the sexes is a difference in concentration of the same attractive odor, rather than qualitatively different odors." Similar findings in rats suggest that odors in the urine provide reliable stimuli for sex identification.[37] As we mentioned earlier, the presence of two

androgen metabolites in urine, androstenol and androstenone, correlate well with maleness and with characteristic male odors detected in
urine and from the underarm area. These "pheromones" also correlate
well with the hormone functions of the HPG axis.[38]

FROM WIMP TO MACHO BULLY AND BACK

If all this leaves you strongly inclined to believe that somehow genes,
hormones, neurotransmitters, and receptors all interact within the
brain to affect sexual behavior, you are not alone. That is also our conclusion, even though we have not yet mentioned two additional important discoveries.

In the first of these discoveries we find evidence that behavior can
alter gene activity and change hormone production. This discovery
came out of the research of Russell Fernald, a Stanford University neurobiologist, with African cichlids, a tropical fish and favorite of behavioral researchers.

Fernald found that the hypothalamic cells that trigger mating in
cichlid fish are six to eight times larger in a male who commands a
large territory with a harem of females with a macho attitude that keeps
other males at bay, than the same cells are in mild-mannered males
with no social clout. If a domineering male is confronted by a bigger
bully, its hypothalamic cells shrink and slow down production of
GnRH. This causes the testes of the outranked male to shrink and he
loses his desire and ability to mate.

Dominant male cichlids are larger and more brightly colored than
either drab females or wimpy males with no drive or ability to mate.
Unfortunately, the extremely aggressive attitude and rainbow hues of
the dominant males also attract the attention of predators looking for a
meal. When this happens, nearby meek males rush in to fight over suc-
cession rights and access to the females. When a victor emerges, his
behavior changes dramatically. More important for our interests, the
victor's new assertive and dominant behavior triggers an equally dramatic growth in the hypothalamic cells responsible for making GnRH.
GnRH in turn tweaks the pituitary gland to produce more LH and
growth hormone with anatomical consequences you can easily predict
based on our discussion of the HPG Axis in the previous chapter.
Stimulated by a surge in its hormones, the newly dominant male grows

bigger. His color changes from drab to rainbow hues. His testes enlarge and start making sperm so he can service his harem.[39]

For the first time we have solid evidence that social behavior and the environment can cause a specific change in the brain's anatomy and that this neural change in turn can cause a change in the testes that triggers a specific behavioral change regulated by the HPG axis. The sexual behavior of the male cichlid is far from that of humans, but the consistency and repeated patterns of genes, proteins, hormones, the limbic system, and the HPG axis certainly suggest important new questions about the much less obvious and more subtle influence of the social environment and contact with other humans may have on human sexual behavior.

Tantalizing hints of human parallels have already turned up in research showing that the testosterone level drops when a male monkey is challenged by a more dominant male and when a male wrestler or tennis player loses a match or tournament. The testosterone level rises when they win and stays up through the next match until they lose.[40] So human behavior can influence gene activity and alter hormone production! And pheromones are, so far as is known, the only social environmental influence that affects hormone levels.

THE ONES WHO GUIDE

We began the previous chapter by looking at chemical messengers, the gamones, that play a key role in fertilization, the very start of an individual's life. We also examined briefly the role of hedgehog and HOX genes that direct the migration and differentiation of cells in the first month of human pregnancy. At the time we indicated that the development of the brain and olfactory system was pivotal in this very early development.

Fortunately, just as we were finishing this book, two research teams announced a major breakthrough in their efforts to find the elusive factors that help wire up the brain by guiding GnRH and other individual neurons in their migration and in developing hundreds, even thousands of connections with other neurons. Their breakthrough research provides a perfect conclusion to this and the previous chapter and our examination of the HPG axis and the sequence from genes to enzymes, receptors, hormones, sexual differentiation, and behavior.

At three weeks, before the human embryo is the size of a pencil eraser, certain cells are producing scores, if not hundreds of chemical messengers that jointly serve as a kind of Department of Transportation for the neurons. These chemical messengers steer, instruct, heighten, and subdue the traffic flow of millions of axons as they migrate within the fetal brain. In the two paragraph description of this research in the Science section of the *New York Times* quoted here, we have italicized some key phrases that are crucial to our thesis about the role of odors in human development and sexual behavior.

> The researchers have christened the factors netrin-1 and netrin-2, after the Sanskrit word for "one who guides." Their work confirms predictions made [a hundred years ago] in 1892, when the legendary neurobiologist Santiago Ramón y Cajal proposed that axons [nerve branches] find their way to their destinations like *bloodhounds on a leash, sniffing chemicals in their environment and proceeding accordingly*. The netrins are like *scent markers* that tell the axons, "Yes, you're on the right path," or "Now it's time to veer sharply to the right and head north." They are called *chemotropic factors: they are chemicals that persuade axons to turn and bend. They are also growth stimulants, prompting the axons to elongate as they migrate*.
>
> The new studies also evoke the image of the developing brain as *a kind of Parisian parfumerie, where chemistry reigns and entices. And just as a particular perfume may attract one nose and repel another, so the netrins, and other chemotropic factors in the brain seem to lure some axons to move forward, while causing the axonal extensions of other neurons to rear back in distaste*. In this way, a single factor can perform multiple guidance tasks.[41]

After pulverizing and examining extracts of about twenty-five thousand embryonic chick brains in their quest for the Holy Grail long sought by neurobiologists, Marc Tessier-Lavigne, Tito Serafini, and their colleagues at the University of California at San Francisco were surprised to find that roughly 50 percent of the gene for the netrin scent factor of the vertebrate embryo matched a similar gene in the primitive round worm or nematode.

Nature is lazy. Once the genes for netrins appeared in the round worm or in some more primitive animal, these genes changed very little as they passed on to new and much more complex animals, including humans. From round worms to humans, these scent factor genes guide brain development and lay the groundwork for the sense of smell and its key role in sexual development and behavior.[42]

The consistency of netrin scents, GnRH neurons, the HPG axis, the VNO, and other olfactory elements across many animal species, from primitive animals to humans, provides strong support for our thesis that odors and pheromones play a major role in human sexual development and behavior just as they do in other animals.

9

THE EMOTIONAL MIND

Our nose and VNO are merely the entrance gates through which odors first must pass on their way to triggering the appropriate reactions in the mind-body complex that help make us the individuals we are. Receptors in the dendrites of nasal nerve cells and slightly different receptors in the VNO convert chemical messengers to electrical impulses and begin decoding them. Since the final decoding, translating, and processing of odors occurs in various circuits and switchboards in our central nervous system, we definitely will need to add some new details about how various neural circuits work to understand how odors influence our sexual development and behavior in the complex web of genes, hormones, and the HPG axis.

The brains of early fish, the first animals with backbones, first appeared long ago as three primitive swellings at the head of the spinal cord. There was a forebrain, a midbrain, and a hindbrain, very much like we find today in the brain of a human fetus at four weeks. Over the course of time, different sections of the primitive brain system have expanded to an incredible variety and complexity. Despite the variety and wide complexity of animal brains in today's world, brains share much of the same basic architecture and many of the same basic functions.

The most important development by far has been the growth of the "enchanted loom," Nobel-laureate Charles Sherrington's term for the conscious, thinking part of the forebrain, the cerebral hemispheres. The cerebral hemispheres fill the inside of the human skull like a giant mushroom, dominating all else in the central nervous system. Nestled inside the expanding forebrain, in the floor of its mushroom cap, are the olfactory bulbs, the dominant structure in the forebrain. Over the ages, the forebrain's olfactory bulbs that triggered much of the behavior of fish and reptiles eons ago, have lost ground as the conscious circuitry expanded. Nevertheless, these neural centers retain a strong and vital connection with the expanding limbic mind, creating a seething tropical world of learning and memories still powerfully affected by odors and pheromones.

The hindbrain or brain stem has remained essentially unchanged through millions of years. Many of its hard-wired, automatic switchboards for body functions, eating, breathing, and mating are still strongly affected by odor messengers in all animals from reptiles to humans.[1]

Life and survival on land made harsher demands than life in the ocean. Instead of oxygen-laden water flowing effortlessly over gills, the first amphibians and reptiles had to pull air into their lungs and expel it several times a minute to meet a higher demand for oxygen. Four legs had to be coordinated for walking within minutes of hatching. Some developed forelimbs to grasp and hold food. Finding a mate, nest building, establishing a territory and defending it with ritual postures and threats, mating, and fighting off predators were also crucial abilities. In many respects, the reptilian brain is a classic embodiment of Freud's "Id," with an oral-genital fixation and hard-wired behavioral pathways poorly equipped for learning to cope with new situations but marvelously robotic in survival behaviors.[2]

We can survive without the brain's conscious, thinking circuits, but a newborn without a smoothly functioning reptilian brain or brain stem dies within minutes because she or he cannot even breath. That is because we humans should really have a two-year pregnancy. That cannot be because the cerebral cortex is growing so rapidly that if the fetus is not born at nine months, the head will become too large to pass through the birth canal. This means we are born with nerve pathways in the conscious brain still undeveloped. Unlike the newborn mammal with four legs, we cannot walk when we are born. Unable to crawl or feed ourselves, we can breath and suckle and carry on other basic life functions because of reflexes hard-wired in the brain stem. In the months after birth, the hard-wired behavioral patterns of the reptilian brain control behavior and life functions while the neurons in the more sophisticated, conscious neural circuits of our cerebral hemispheres develop and gradually take over many, but certainly not all, functions of the brain stem.[3]

The reflex smile of newborn infants is one of the more important behavioral patterns controlled by the reptilian brain, because it seduces adults into taking care of the helpless infant. In a few weeks, the infant's developing memory circuits connect the mother's breast odor and the body odor of caregivers with the experience that a smile is rewarded with cuddling, rocking, and being fed. As the infant's reflex smile invites care and love from a parent, the infant quickly learns that smiling results in more tender care. Soft-wired, conscious neural pathways, mediated by odors and learning, take over from the hard-wired reptilian brain circuits.[4]

Similarly, a hard-wired reflexive need for the infant to raise and turn its head to clear its nasal passages and mouth for breathing as it sleeps in the crib is essential for survival. A breakdown in the brain stem control of this reflex may sometimes result in death from Sudden-Infant-Death Syndrome (SIDS) when the infant sleeps on its stomach and face down. Lewis Lipsit, a developmental psychologist, has suggested that lethargic and unresponsive infants are more susceptible to SIDS because the voluntary centers of their brains do not develop to take over this coping mechanism from the reflexive reptilian brain, leaving them at risk for suffocation.[5]

"Except for altruistic behavior and most aspects of parental behavior, it is remarkable how many *patterns of behavior* seen in reptiles are also found in human beings."[6] Even though we may be able to moderate or partially control some of the hard-wired behaviors in the reptilian brain with yogic concentration, we can never eliminate them. Nor would we want to.

THE EMOTIONAL-VISCERAL MIND

Nestled in the floor and walls between the cerebral hemispheres are the neural circuits of the emotional-visceral limbic mind which includes the paired thalamus, amygdala, hippocampus, and nine or so tiny circuits known as the hypothalamus. Because these circuits or nuclei contain clumps of specialized nerve cells that secrete many different types of hormones, the limbic mind opens the door to a world of emotions, unavailable to the reptilian brain. Deeply affected by smells, the limbic mind can add a range of feelings, emotions, and hot passions to the emotionless "Four F's" initially controlled by the brain stem. Limbic pathways and circuits also add sensitivity and a feeling of individuality and personal identity to the behaviors originally controlled by the reptilian brain.

Not long ago, neuroscientists believed the limbic mind and hypothalamus only processed information from the olfactory and digestive systems. Now we know they also handle information from the eyes, ears, and the sensory systems involved in taste, touch, pressure, heat, and cold. Two of our three limbic subdivisions are closely related to odor and pheromone detecting systems. One takes care of feeding, nursing, and kissing. The other is involved in various sexual behaviors. Both regulate aggressive and violent behavior. The fact that the main pathway to the third limbic subdivision bypasses the olfactory system reflects a shift from smell to other influences on our social and sexual behaviors.[7]

At the heart of the limbic mind, different areas of the hypothalamus serve as major bridges between the reptilian brain and limbic system. This sets the stage for the hypothalamus to play a major role in controlling sexual behavior. The steady release or pulsing cycle of GnRH we described earlier is handled by the hypothalamus. And GnRH is directly or indirectly responsible for all the hormones produced by the pituitary, ovaries, testes, adrenal glands, and the neurosecretory cells in the brain. All animals with an internal skeleton and central nervous system are continually processing odor and pheromone clues from the outside world that set the GnRH circuits in the hypothalamus into action.[8]

Several areas of the hypothalamus influence sexual behavior. Damage in the preoptic area of a male rat wipes out all its sexual behavior. When this same area is stimulated electrically or with testosterone, the male becomes compulsive and obsessed with sex, a veritable sex-maniac.[9] This area is also vital to maternal behavior. On the other hand, damage to the preoptic area of a female rat makes her much more receptive to mating.[10] Another tiny area of this switchboard is three to seven times larger in normal males than in females and twice the size of the same area in castrated males. As with many recent discoveries of differences in the male and female brain, we have no idea what this difference might mean for our sexual behavior.[11]

Natural or induced lesions in a center just behind the preoptic area wipes out all sexual behavior in female rats. Female hormones cannot reverse this effect unless the hormone is injected directly into this area. Again we do not understand what is actually going on here.[12]

And then there is the INAH-3 circuit mentioned in chapter 8. LeVay and others believe that this nerve circuit, about the size of a grain of sand in heterosexual men and almost non-existent in heterosexual woman and gay men, somehow affects sexual attraction to women.[13] Additionally, Dean Hamer suspects that a "gay gene" might fit into this hypothesis. "The most simple hypothesis would be that the Xq28 makes a protein that is directly involved in the growth or death of neurons in the INAH-3. Alternatively, the gene could encode a protein that influences the regulation of this region by hormones."[14]

Other limbic regions serve as relay stations for sensory information traveling from the reptilian brain stem to the thinking brain. These relays link odors with memories especially when they are associated with sex, punishment, and pleasure. Limbic pleasure centers also produce natural amphetamines and opioids which, as we will see in our next chapter, play an important role in altruism, sexual attraction, bonding, and love.[15]

All told, the limbic mind and hypothalamus are major players in human sexual behavior, triggering emotions of all sorts including sex drive and attraction, aggression, anger, fear, the pleasures of eating and mating, nursing, and bonding. Despite its considerable genetic hardwiring, our limbic mind can learn from experience and from the softwired thoughts of our cerebral hemispheres.[16]

THE TRIUNE BRAIN

The cerebral hemispheres crown our reptilian and limbic brains. A hundred billion neurons, with neurotransmitters and neuromodulators, create an "enchanted loom," a fluid, sparkling electronic screen that somehow is self-conscious and is somehow capable of describing the world outside and inside in symbolic language. Somehow, this "loom" can read, write, and do arithmetic. It converts visual images, sounds, and sensations of touch, pain, pleasure, taste, and heat from outside into a unique consciousness of self and other.

"Mother of invention and father of abstract thought, [the mushrooming cerebral hemispheres] promote preservation and procreation of ideas," Paul MacLean tells us.[17] Each of the hundred billion neurons is capable of making thousands of chemical connections with other neurons, and capable of communicating electrically with other neurons even when not physically connected by a chemical synapse. In a flash of time, these neurons manage, decode, and interpret a thousand trillion "bits" of information. In the process, they add a new dimension to the seething tropics of limbic emotions, opening the door to a cooler, more rational, soft-wired climate of abstract analysis, deduction, reasoning, logic, planning for the future, moral discrimination, and love.[18]

Another gender difference in the thinking brain occurs in the prefrontal areas, which influence the parental care and bonding circuits of the limbic mind. These areas are more richly developed in women than in men, suggesting that emotional and bonding messages from the limbic mind may retain more of their power in women than in men. This same area gives women a greater ability to integrate sensual pleasure and orgasm. Several researchers have reported that women enjoy a greater capacity than men to integrate pleasurable experiences and orgasmic highs. For most men, James Prescott suggests, the orgasmic experience is reflexive-automatic, genital-focused, and handled primarily in the reptilian and limbic minds and in the old cerebellum. Women, on the other hand, can experience a much more integrated, whole-body, and transcendent orgasm involving the frontal and temporal regions of the thinking brain as well as the brain stem and limbic systems.[19]

Oddly, no one gets upset when we suggest that much of what we know about how specific genes function in humans comes from our study of those same genes in animals. Everyone is delighted when scientists discover how a particular gene operates in rats that will help us control or cure a disease in humans. No one is upset when we use animal hormones, enzymes, or other proteins to treat human diseases. Nor do people object when we use animal tests of medications to decide how to use these medicines with humans.[20]

Our reaction is often the exact opposite when it comes to suggesting ways the reptilian and limbic minds are still involved in human behavior and emotions. For many, research on animal behavior and brain functions has no relevance for understanding similar brain functions and behaviors in humans. And yet it is undeniable that in addition to sharing genes, hormones, proteins, and enzymes with animals, we also share some important brain structures and resultant behaviors with other mammals and primates. Many of our basic "circuits," "switchboards," and "mainline cables" are very similar, if not identical, and react to similar stimuli, including odors and pheromones, in similar ways.

We have several examples of how pheromones influence production of GnRH from the hypothalamus, and how GnRH regulates production of pituitary hormones that, in turn, regulate production of testosterone and estrogen in the ovaries and testes. We have also seen how pheromones are derived from the various sex hormones our bodies produce, and how, depending on the animal species involved, pheromones can induce or delay the onset of puberty, synchronize menstrual cycles or suppress ovulation, and directly or indirectly influence sexual development and all sorts of sexual behaviors.

Considering the research of Linda Buck at Harvard University, Stuart Firestein at Yale University, and others (chapter 4), it is apparent that in different animal species including humans, aromatic chemical messages function in very similar ways, sometimes even producing similar developmental or behavioral effects. Regardless of the animal species, it is G proteins in smell neurons that convert aromatic chemical messages into electrical impulses the brain can react to and decode.[21] And regardless of the animal species, particular pheromones and their G proteins they activate trigger GnRH production. Beyond the link between odors, G proteins, and premature puberty in four-year-old boys (chapter 8), we have only a few scattered anecdotal suggestions of other pheromone effects on GnRH and sexual behavior that parallel other pheromone effects reported in nonhuman primates and other mammals.

Some fascinating pheromone effects in mice, for instance, would be even more arresting if researchers were to find a related human effect. In the Lee-Boot Effect, for example, female mice housed together in small groups of four or more with no males around experience a kind of ongoing pseudopregnancy and do not ovulate. The cause is a urinary pheromone that causes the corpora lutea, ruptured egg follicles left in the ovaries after release of eggs, to remain active for extended periods of time, producing hormones that inhibit further ovulation.[22] In the Whitten Effect, urinary pheromones of female mice crowded in large groups cause extended estrous cycles and eventually suppress the production of eggs altogether.[23]

In the Bruce Effect, a recently impregnated mouse placed in a cage with a normal male other than the one who induced the pregnancy will likely miscarry.[24] Except for convents of strictly cloistered nuns and possibly women's prisons, we have no human populations that match the environmental uniqueness of the mice that exhibit the Lee-Boot or Whitten effects.

Still, Cutler has reported that the irregular menstrual cycles of women exposed to male pheromones become more regular. We also know that pregnant cosmetologists who are continually exposed to the aromatic chemicals in cosmetics, especially formaldehyde-based disinfectants, experience an almost two-fold increase in spontaneous abortions.[25]

Despite the sparsity of documented parallels, many scientists are convinced that research on the evolution of brain functions can provide vital insights into the possible effects of pheromones on human sexual behavior. In pursuing this research, we will likely find that some, perhaps a good number of behaviors widely assumed to be purely learned actually start off as genetic or unlearned neural encoded patterns inherited from the survival strategies of our ancestors, responses that are in many cases activated by pheromones.[26]

In Paul MacLean's well-documented and widely accepted model of a triune brain, we are like a giant neural network with a peripheral nervous system and our senses guided simultaneously by "three drivers, all of different minds and all vying for control." In popular terms, the human brain amounts to three biological computers interacting in a network. Each central processing unit has "its own special intelligence, its own subjectivity, its own sense of time and space, and its own memory, motor and other functions."[27]

Yet within this triune brain, between the three minds, there are no hard and fast boundaries. True, each has its own "driver, its own distinct chemistry and structure." And each brain can operate somewhat independently. There is however one crucial exception: the two lower minds have no neural machinery to express their experiences in words and share them consciously. For MacLean, the reptilian mind provides the basic plots and actions, the limbic mind adds emotional sensitivities to the developments of the plots. Meanwhile, the new mammalian brain has the capacity to develop these plots and emotions in almost any way the individual author wants to see the plot expressed:[28]

> In an evolutionary sense, they are eons apart. And yet they are very much interconnected, forming a triune human brain in which "the "whole" is greater than the sum of its parts, because with the exchange of information among the three formations each derives a greater amount of information than if it were operating alone.[29]

LIMBIC LEARNING

Despite the hard-wiring of behaviors in the reptilian and limbic brains, we have considerable evidence that some of these behaviors can be influenced by learning, especially from the equally ancient sensory systems of smell and touch.

Nurturing touch can soothe a fast-beating heart, enhance the immune system, speed the healing of a wound, lower blood pressure, and even enhance intelligence. The cold, heat, and pressure messages of touch are initially processed by the reptilian and limbic brains, decoded and interpreted as pleasurable or painful. Pleasurable messages trigger production of natural opiates, endorphins, which tell the thinking brain something nice is happening. The sheer sensual pleasures of smell and touch an infant experiences suckling at the breast not only trigger production of oxytocin, "the hormone of bonding and love," but also stimulate nerve cell growth in the pleasure centers of the limbic system that influence social behavior and bonding later in life.[30]

Neuropsychologist James Prescott has also documented the powerful, long-term effects cuddling, rocking, and massaging a baby have on its brain circuits. The powerful combination of smell and touch, enhanced by sight and sound, stimulates development of the wiring between the cerebellum or "little brain" at the rear of the brain and the emotional centers of the limbic system directly in front of it. When an infant is deprived of smell, touch, and motion messages, the connections between the limbic system and cerebellum are poorly developed. According to Prescott, poor connections between the limbic system and cerebellum reduce or inhibit the inability to experience pleasure and love latter in life.[31] We also know that every organ system including our immune defense system appears to be influenced by these interactions.

In one area we have had some intriguing breakthroughs. Pavlov's turn-of-the-century experiments pioneered our knowledge of how limbic memories can be reprogrammed to link the stimulus of a bell or the smell of food with eating and the need for saliva. In a more recent experiment, a mouse was picked up for only two minutes a day in the two weeks before it was immunized. The stress this mouse experienced in being picked up by a hand big enough to squeeze it to death clearly reduced the ability of its immune system to react to the immunization.[32]

If the stress of being picked up can reduce the effectiveness of an immunization, could other sensory input enhance the immune response? Researchers pursuing this possibility have used odor and taste messages to retrain the limbic memories that affect the immune system. Doctors began by combining a strong odor and taste with a very toxic immune suppressing drug. When they gave this combination to an animal with a defective immune system that was attacking and destroying the animal's whole body, its immune system was slowed down and the destruction of cells stopped. After the limbic mind learned to link the immune suppressing message of the toxic drug with the strong smell and disgusting taste, the smell and taste could be used alone without the toxic drug to tone down the immune system.[33]

The first human use of this knowledge saved the life of a young women suffering from an autoimmune disease that threatened to destroy her body as if it were transplanted foreign tissue. She could only take an extremely toxic drug once a month, and then only for a few months, not nearly long enough to save her life. When the young woman took her first dose of cyclophosphamide, she took it with a strong dose of cod liver oil and rose perfume. Stimulated by the disgusting cod liver oil and the strong odor of rose perfume, her limbic memory connected these sensations with her body's strong response to the immune-suppressing drug. With this link established in the limbic brain, the stimulus of rose perfume and cod liver oil with a much reduced drug dose proved just as effective as a full drug dose in suppressing her body's immune attacks on her red blood cells. Five years later, the young woman was doing well, thanks to her reprogrammed limbic smell and taste memories.[34]

Odors and pheromones stimulate a variety of neurons in the limbic system, cerebral hemispheres and other parts of the body to make GnRH, the key hormone in the system of sex hormones that influence all kinds of sexual responses and behaviors. Associations between pheromones and hormone levels indicate that pheromones may alter the speed or strength of the GnRH pulse and levels of LH. These effects, in turn, alter the levels of testosterone and estrogen, which then appear to alter the number, structure, and function of nerve cell connections that influence both learning and memory. Odors and pheromones also influence many ways in which males and females differ in their production of serotonin, dopamine, and other neurotransmitters.[35]

MacLean reminds us that the earliest limbic brains were primarily devoted to processing odor messages from the outside world and controlling feeding, fighting, fleeing, and mating behaviors. Although the limbic brains of today's mammals are much more sophisticated because they decode and integrate many other messages besides the olfactory, the limbic brain remains true to its ancient emotional bias. For eons, these messages have triggered two elemental behavioral patterns, aggressive-dominance and courtship-mating behaviors.

To close our excursion into the limbic mind and its place in the triune brain we can offer Paul MacLean's provocative interpretation of a custom found in tribal cultures around the world where men use houseguards—stone monuments representing or showing an erect phallus—to mark their territory or home for other men and women. Unlike the males of other species, men do not mark their territories and assert their dominance with urinary pheromones. For MacLean, this behavior suggests a question. Could the phallic markers at the entrance to an aboriginal village or hut tap into deep-rooted limbic memories of the threat of aggression and dominance nonhuman males have signaled from ancient times with their urinary pheromones and genital display?[36] Might the phallus-like houseguards awake some kind of Jungian archetypal memory of pheromones in all mammals? "It is as though a visual urogenital symbol is used as a substitute or subliminal reinforcement for [the] olfactory, urinary territorial markings of animals."[37]

Marcel Proust was much more poetic in uncovering the heart of the limbic mind when he wrote in Remembrance of Things Past, "When from a long-distant past nothing subsists, taste and smell alone . . . remain poised a long time, like souls, remembering, waiting, hoping, amid the ruins of all the rest, and bear unflinchingly, . . . the vast structure of recollection."[38]

10

NATURAL OPIATES, INFATUATIONS, AND BONDING

Instinctively a mother rat licks her nipples, unknowingly applying a salivary scent that guides her blind, hungry newborn to her breast and milk. Wash the nipples and the newborn pups lose their way and die of starvation.

After a ewe gives birth and nuzzles its newborn lamb, a chemical reward, a bonding hormone known as oxytocin, released in the mother's brain tells her, "This particular lamb's odor is important. Pay attention to it." Inspired by this pleasure reward, mother wildebeest and their newborn calves rely on scent to find each other in an annual migration of hundreds of thousands of other wildebeest mothers, fathers, and calves.

Odors help nonhuman and human mothers bond to and identify their own infants. Human mothers, for example, regularly brush their noses in their baby's hair to inhale its sweet odor as they cuddle it. As we have seen, mothers can also identify their own infant by smell as well as they can by the sound of its cry, while infants can discriminate between the breast odor of their mother and other women.[1]

Despite similarities, there are important differences in the outcome of aromatic clues and hormones that inspire mating and parenting across the animal species. Driven to mate by odors and the effect that odors have on hormones, reptiles have little if any concern for pairbonding or parenting behavior. This mating ritual ended, snakes and crocodiles leave mates and offspring to fend for themselves without the slightest twinge of emotion.[2] Beyond the emotionless reptilian world, mating and reproducing heats up in the lower mammals as the circuits of the limbic system expand to add passion and pleasure to courtship, mating, and parenting. In the higher primates, mating and parenting become ever more complex, flexible, and conscious behaviors. Young mammals learn by watching their elders and then mimic them in their own sexual rehearsal play. Programmed reactions to pheromones and body odors still encoded in the primate's brain stem and limbic mind are now enriched by new pleasure-related behaviors of touch, nuzzling, and cuddling that trigger infant/mother bonding, nursing, and parenting programs.[3]

Humans retain these efficient, hard-wired circuits to assure survival of the species, no matter how often or how much we manage to submerge or sublimate these drives with the artistic, linguistic, altruistic, creative, and spiritual output our soft-wired, programmable and reprogrammable cerebral cortex makes possible. While humans are not driven as billy goats and rams are by the aromatic aliphatic acids of females, our brain stem and limbic mind constantly remind us we are still animals, not disembodied spirits. Genes and hormones direct and color our behaviors, influenced more often than we expect or are willing to admit by aromatic messages from the world around us.

With our near relatives, the chimps and great apes, the role of odors and pheromones has decreased significantly. Yet male primates still sniff the air for the scent of those vaginal odors and females still react to male pheromones. But the bonobos or pigmy chimps, our closest relatives, certainly have escaped the robot-like programs of bonding and mating that totally dominate lower mammals. With surprising frequency their sexual play mimics that of humans.[4]

In the *Anatomy of Love*, anthropologist Helen Fisher offers a snapshot of the "love life" of the bonobos:

> Sex is almost a daily pastime. Female bonobos have an extended monthly period of heat, stretching through almost three-quarters of their menstrual cycle. But sex . . . is not confined to estrus. Females copulate during most of their menstrual cycles—a pattern of coitus more similar to women's than any other creature.
>
> And females bribe their male friends with sex quite regularly. A female will walk up to a male who is eating sugarcane, sit beside

him, beg palm up, as people do, and then look plaintively at the delicacy and back at him. He feels her gaze. When he gives her the treat, she tips her buttocks and copulates; then she ambles off with the cane in hand. A female is not beyond soliciting another female either, sauntering up to a comrade, climbing into her arms face-to-face, wrapping her legs around her waist, and rubbing her genitals on those of her partner before accepting sticks of cane. Male-male homosexuality, fellatio, also occurs.

Bonobos engage in sex to ease tension, to stimulate sharing during meals, to reduce stress while traveling, and to reaffirm friendships during anxious reunions. "Make love, not war" is clearly a bonobo scheme.

Did our ancestors do the same?

Bonobos, in fact, display many of the sexual habits people exhibit on the streets, in the bars and restaurants, and behind apartment doors in New York, Paris, Moscow, and Hong Kong. Prior to coitus bonobos often stare deep into each other's eyes. And bonobos, like human beings, walk arm in arm, kiss each other's hands and feet, and embrace with long deep, tongue-intruding French kisses.[5]

A question about these spontaneous, erotically playful cousins: Might the bonobos indulge in French-kissing because it brings the subliminal stimulation of salivary pheromones being pumped into their VNOs while they consciously tease each other's sensitive erogenous lips and oral cavities? Might this be a factor in the popularity of kissing among men and women around the world?

Bonobos enjoy variety in their erotic play. Females sit on a male's lap to have vaginal intercourse, crouch while their partner stands, have intercourse while both are standing up, and playfully reverse the missionary position with the female on top facing him. They even enjoy intercourse while hanging in a tree. They engage now and then in mutual genital play. And always they gaze intently at each other as they "make love."[6]

Female chimps learn to mother by watching and imitating older females in the troop. While smell still plays a role in the bonobos' mother-infant pairbonding and adult sex, its role is very much diminished as the thinking part of the brain expands. We humans probably depend even less on pheromones and odors for mother-infant and adult pairbonding, but smell has not disappeared entirely as a factor in human sexual interactions and parenting interactions. Quite the contrary is the case. As in other species, it can be shown that humans depend just as much on chemical signals as do other species.[7]

THE REWARDS OF NATURAL AMPHETAMINES

In Sherrington's "enchanted loom, millions of flashing shuttles weave a dissolving pattern, always a meaningful pattern, though never an abiding one." Electrical impulses ride neurotransmitters from one neuron to another, guided by neurohormones and neuromodulators. Without this sparkling electrochemical web, we could not carry on any of the mental processes we humans enjoy so much.[8] Nor could we experience the spontaneity and self-awareness that makes us unique individuals.

What makes human life so enjoyable is being energetic, alert, happy as often as we can be and free of pain as much as possible. Being human means being motivated and inspired to transcend our narrow bounded world of self, to get out, to do things, to interact with other humans. The first meaning of the verb *inspire* in *Webster's Dictionary* is "to infuse an animating, quickening, or exalting influence." That implies an active role, someone or something inspires someone to act. But behind the active inspiration might there be something deeper, something more basic and passive that goes back to the primal experience of nursing at the breast and *breathing in* the scent of mother's breast? Especially if that experience of *breathing in* results in the release of a neurostimulant in our triune brain that leaves us with incredibly satisfying and pleasurable feelings of euphoria and ecstasy?

Neuroscientists have isolated, identified, and experimented with one such neurostimulant, a kind of natural amphetamine called phenylethylamine or PEA. PEA is found at the end of some nerve cells where it helps the electrical impulse jump from one neuron to the next. It has also been found inside the circuits of the brain stem, limbic system, and cerebral cortex. PEA seems to act indirectly on the central nervous system by increasing the levels of norepinephrine, a hormone that acts as a neurotransmitter, and dopamine, which among other functions serves as a short-term sexual activator.

According to Michael Liebowitz, a research psychiatrist at the New York State Psychiatric Institute, our brain's PEA acts like cocaine and speed, revving up the brain circuits, making our senses more awake and sensitive, producing euphoria, and generally making us feel good. PEA is also a key factor in our "falling in love," creating that euphoric, "blown away" experience we humans so value and romanticize. Falling in love means we can't sleep or eat. We are giddy and do silly things. Thoughts of the beloved occupy every cranny of our mind and memory. Ordinary pleasures pale in our euphoria.

So is falling in love just a matter of a flood of PEA?

Neuropsychologists tell us the scent of a loved one, seeing or touching him or her, and making love send a storm of messages to the limbic brain. The memory, emotion, and pleasure centers of the limbic system integrate these fragmented messages which we describe as desire, passion, and love, and passes them on to the hypothalamus. The hypothalamus produces an adrenocorticotropic hormone (ACTH) releaser that causes the nearby pituitary gland to produce ACTH itself. When ACTH is picked up from the blood by adrenal gland receptors, the adrenal cortical cells produce corticosterone that increases the breakdown of glucose. This, combined with PEA, is somehow translated by the "enchanted loom" into the classic symptoms of being sexually turned on and in love.

These chemical reactions, Liebowitz tells us, are "nature's way of insuring that we seek out and form relationships that last at least long enough to reproduce the next generation." But it is also good to remember that the natural highs of being in love, cuddling, making love, and having orgasms, like the "runner's high," push human experience to their limits and beyond.[9] These are positive highs, nature's way of giving us pleasure and joy. Only when circumstances deprive people of natural highs do some turn to cocaine, synthesized amphetamines, and street drugs that briefly mimic euphoric pleasure, but in the end, result in a physical addiction.[10]

If, as psychologist Anthony Walsh suggests, "each time we see or anticipate seeing our lover, the whistle blows at the PEA [and ACTH] factory and we get another fix," why do we not become addicted and spend all our time pumping up PEA and ACTH production?[11]

Living organisms cannot operate continually at peak load; they require time to rest and recuperate. Our brain circuits become acclimated to "high messages" triggered by the pleasant things of life if they happen too often. Automatic replay of a favorite piece of music, or a daily menu of filet mignon or lobster dinners, or working in a candy store surrounded by chocolate can leave us indifferent to what was once a lovely peak experience.[12]

How long can the glorious exhilaration of being in love last? Dorothy Tennov, whose 1979 book on Love and Limerence is a classic, and John Money in his 1980 study of Love and Love-Sickness both agree that PEA and whatever other neurostimulants are involved in the high of being in love can only rev up the limbic brain for somewhere between eighteen months and three years before the system becomes exhausted.

When Helen Fisher, a research anthropologist at the American Museum of Natural History in New York City, compared United Nations data on the incidence and patterns of divorce in sixty-two societies and extramarital sex in forty-two cultures, she discovered a "four-year itch" pattern that meshes nicely with the three or four-year amphetamine-driven bonding of infatuation and lusty, romantic sex Money and Tennov noted.[13]

One factor that can keep a relationship going as the euphoria of being "in love" wears thin is a shift from stimulating amphetamines to the brain's calming natural opiates. "When the magnetic effects of pure attraction dissipate, something else must occur if the pair-bond is to endure. Lovers must become attached to one another after the delights of sheer attraction are only sporadically or dimly felt."[14]

These natural opiates or endorphins promote a more relaxed bonding between lovers, the bonding of friendship and long-term intimacy. Endorphins affect a region of the brain that controls feelings of panic that arise when the euphoria and obsession begins to fade and one wonders what is next.[15] Will I survive without all that wonder-filled passion?

Some men and women cannot make the transition from passionate attraction to long-term bonding. They continually fall in and out of love. Liebowitz calls them "love junkies," or "romance junkies." Hastily picked, unsuitable lovers are quickly rejected. An irresistible attraction is quickly followed by a painful crash, and a frantic search for another passionate love. The quest turns into an endless, destructive cycle as the exhilaration of the chase and being in love is followed by despair.

When scientists injected some mice with PEA, they jumped about and squealed with a kind of mouse exuberance and exhilaration animal behaviorists call "popcorn behavior." When rhesus monkeys are injected with PEA they smack their lips and make pleasure calls, much as they do when they are courting another monkey. Baboons injected with PEA will press a lever in their cage more than 160 times in three hours when pressing that lever gives them PEA-laced food that maintains their high PEA level of euphoria.[16]

Fortunately, like every biological system, the brain circuits have their own built-in checks and balances, with defensive feedback loops. The brake on this PEA pleasure system is MAO, an enzyme that breaks down PEA and other neurotransmitters. After a few months, a year or two, the brain gets worn out from the infatuation highs of PEA. Production of MAO increases and the passion fades.[17]

In a love addict, it seems, the brain is producing too much MAO from the very beginning. This wipes out the PEA effect falling in love gives the normal person. This leaves the love addict constantly looking to new lovers for that wonderful high being "in love" brings. One possible treatment for this kind of love addiction would be to use a medication that blocks MAO and reduces its breakdown of amphetamines. Psychiatrists have long used such MAO blockers to help chronically depressed persons. Some antidepressant drugs work very well to block excess MAO, allowing PEA and other natural amphetamines to work on the brain and let the person experience natural happiness and psychological highs.

When Liebowitz and Klein gave a love junkie a MAO blocker for a few weeks, this long-term love-sick male became more relaxed, less panicky. He began choosing his partners more carefully. For the first time he was able to apply the lessons he learned in long-term but unsuccessful psychotherapy. Treating "love addicts" with MAO blockers is now quite common and successful.[18]

Other researchers have found that some people who suffer from a malfunctioning hypothalamus and a poorly functioning pituitary cannot fall in love, although they do marry for companionship. Could a lack of PEA or overproduction of MAO from the limbic system contribute to their "love blindness," as Money suggests.[19]

The role PEA plays in falling in love, love addiction, and love blindness brings us full circle to our earlier question about the origin of human *inspiration*. To what extent can we trace the "lust for life" or what the French call *joie de vivre* back to infancy when the infant first breathes in the mother's scent while being breast or bottle fed. Limbic memories of mother's scent are connected with the PEA euphoria of being cuddled, warm, safe, and fed. What more could an infant want? So, how likely is it that this euphoric experience in infancy may become somehow the foundation for our euphoric reaction when we encounter the scent of a lover later in life? To what extent does the euphoria of childhood nurturance and its effects on the brain prepare us for bonding with a lover later in life?

NATURAL OPIATES AND THE CUDDLING HORMONE

If PEA and other natural amphetamines are at the root of our sexual attraction and falling in love, might there also be some other neurostimulants in the limbic brain that are at the root of our long-term bonding?

Neuropsychologists suggest the answer to this question can be found in endorphins (natural or endogenous morphines), which calm the mind and reduce anxiety. Like morphine, endorphins are very powerful painkillers, stimulating the limbic pleasure-processing areas and tranquilizing the pain/aggression-processing areas.[20]

The brain secretes endorphins when we feel comfortable and secure. Infant brains release endorphins when they are cuddled, rocked, and nursed. Maternal brains react in a similar way, producing their own endorphins in response to the scent of the infant and the stimulation provided by the infant squeezing mother's breast and suckling on her nipple. For the mother this stimulation may even result in an orgasm. This perfectly natural and not uncommon experience, like any other orgasm, has a powerful effect on secretory cells of the brain, triggering production of the "cuddling or satisfaction hormone," oxytocin.

Endorphins and oxytocin taken together are very effective in reinforcing the mother-infant bonding, just as the oxytocin produced by the limbic system during love play and the endorphins released during orgasm reinforce the bonding between two lovers.

Since 1991, when the first scientific conference was held on oxytocin, researchers have been excited about this hormone because it gives us a good example of how the brain's anatomy and a specific neurohormone can be linked with a variety of behaviors, how behavior can affect the brain and how the brain can affect behavior. Hidden in this excitement is the definite but still unspecified involvement of odors and pheromones in the production of oxytocin and other hormones and neurotransmitters.[21]

For many years, obstetricians have used oxytocin to spur uterine contractions during labor and facilitate breast feeding. Now oxytocin appears to be one of the more importance hormones in the HPG axis.

Once the body has been primed by estrogen and testosterone at puberty, oxytocin triggers the search for a partner.[22] Oxytocin also spurs maternal feelings as birth approaches. An oxytocin-treated female rat will pick up and nuzzle its pups much more than an untreated rat mother does. Given additional oxytocin, a male rat is more likely to build a nest and zealously guard its pups. When the same males are injected with an oxytocin blocker, they not only neglect their pups, they may even turn them into a convenient meal.

The parenting behavior of ewes is easily upset and eliminated. If a lamb is separated from its mother by accident or design for six hours after birth, the mother ewe will totally ignore it. Since ancient times, sheep breeders have known that if they vaginally stimulate the mother ewe for five minutes, her lost nursing urge returns. Today, reproductive physiologists like Anne Perkins and James Fitzgerald, who work in Montana with the U.S. Sheep Experiment Station across the state line in Dubois, Idaho, tell us that the vaginal stimulation releases a burst of oxytocin that is probably responsible for restoring the ewe's nursing and maternal drive.

Oxytocin receptors have already been identified in the brain region associated with the sensation of sexual fulfillment that follows climax. More important for research on links between sex and smell is the discovery of oxytocin receptors in limbic areas that are associated with smell, sight, the endocrine system, and ovulation control. This gives scientists firm ground for boosting oxytocin's role in mating and reproductive behaviors and pursuing questions about the possible role of smell in this web of interacting causes and effects.

FRIENDSHIP VERSUS SEXUAL LOVE

The effects of natural amphetamines, opiates, and oxytocin, added to our understanding of how odors, pheromones, genes, brain anatomy, neurotransmitters, and hormones affect human and animal behavior, suggests a couple of provocative questions.

The first involves a jump cut to some observations from Israeli kibbutzim. Twenty years ago, Lionel Tiger and Robin Fox, two prominent sociologists, reported that the widely respected "Law of Propinquity" does not hold in the Israel kibbutz. "The Law of Propinquity" expresses common sense backed up by research evidence—namely, that we usually find our mates near where we live.[23]

For over eighty years, the left-wing kibbutz movement *Hashomer Hatzair* has provided a lifestyle and culture all its own for a small minority of the Israeli population. In the kibbutz, children eat and play together. They compete and cooperate like children anywhere, but they also share a self-contained life within the world of individual families. Children from many different kibbutz families live not with their parents but in children's houses where they sleep together in the same dormitories.[24]

If "The Law of Propinquity" is universally valid, then most of the kibbutz children should grow up, fall in love with, and marry spouses from their own kibbutz. Unexpectedly, Tiger and Fox found a kind of "antibonding effect" in three major Israeli kibbutzim federations. Not one couple of 2769 married couples raised in the kibbutzim had spent their first five years together in the same infants' house. Tiger and Fox suggest that the kind of bonding and friendship children develop with peers in a kibbutz seems to preclude their being sexually attracted to each other and marrying.

Another example of this "antibond effect" turned up in a study of marriages in two Pakistani villages. The two villages were identical in every way, including the custom of arranging marriages for their children as soon as they were born. There was one difference, however. In one village, infant brides remained with their parents until after puberty when they left home to live with their husbands. In the other village, the newborn bride was taken immediately after birth to her new husband's home where she was raised with him from infancy. Most of the couples raised together found it difficult to relate to each other sexually.[25]

Do children who grow up together in an Israeli kibbutz or live with their future spouses during childhood react to the unique body odors of the other children in a way that makes these peers unattractive, even unacceptable as sexual partners? Do unfamiliar body odors and pheromones promote falling in love and having sex?

Remember the research of Yamazaki, Yamaguchi, and Gilbert who found that humans and mice can identify siblings or litter mates by body odor and that mice avoid mating with closely related mice (chapter 1). This ability to distinguish closely related individuals from strangers and its link with mating patterns may shed some light on the marriage patterns in the Israeli kibbutz.

This connection becomes more logical when we look at Carole Ober's provocative ten-year research of marriage patterns among the Hutterites, an isolated religious group in North America. The thirty-five thousand Hutterites scattered in communities across Canada and the northern United States are all descended from a group of about one hundred Russian immigrants who came here in the 1870s, so individuals often share similar genes. In exploring their fertility patterns, Ober found that men and women with similar immune systems were much less likely to marry one another than chance would have suggested. Among the 852 adults Ober tested, she expected that 68 would have the same five key immune system genes as their spouse. But she found only 24 shared the same key genes with their spouses, meaning that many Hutterites had avoided marrying someone with the same five immune system genes.

Faced with explaining how these people could detect differences in the immune system of others and avoid marrying someone with a similar set of genes, Ober claimed the most likely explanation was some kind of subtle, subconscious odor. "Sweat and breast milk could be odor cues governing behaviors," she said. Ober also suggested that Hutterite infants are sensitized to their mother's breast pheromones, and then later in life avoid marrying a person whose pheromones subliminally signal that the immune system genes each inherited from their mothers are the same. She admits that this hypothesis is somewhat daring, but no other explanation is apparent.[26] (We agree, and anxiously await publication of her findings in a peer-review scientific journal.)

Our second question also focuses on the role of pheromones in sexual attraction in research on what psychologists call the Coolidge Effect.

According to a popular legend, Calvin Coolidge, our thirtieth president, visited a farm in the 1920s. In the morning, his wife was impressed by the amorous energy of a bull in the pasture, and suggested that her guide point this out to the president with the suggestion she would like him to be equally amorous. In the afternoon, the guide passed along the First Lady's comment. The President, being an astute observer, asked whether the bull always visited the same cow. "Of course not," the guide replied. "Well, tell that to the First Lady." In simple terms, the Coolidge Effect states: "Variety is the spice of life."

After orgasm and ejaculation, a male mammal typically experiences a refractory period during which he cannot be sexually aroused for some time. If the same female is removed and reintroduced after each mating, the refractory period becomes longer and longer with each successive mating. However, if a different female in heat is introduced after each mating, the male's refractory period is brief.

In one typical study, rams had a refractory period of less than two minutes between ejaculations when different ewes were sequentially introduced into the pen. When the same ewe was reintroduced, the refractory period lengthened to almost eighteen minutes after five trials. Beamer and his colleagues tried to fool the ram by covering the familiar ewe with different skins and Halloween masks. That attempt failed, and the researchers had to conclude that "This phenomenon . . . is due to the unique odor of each female."[27]

Might men and women have a similar nonmonogamous response to new and unfamiliar body odors? We have no experimental evidence to support a positive answer, but we do have a few fascinating circumstantial clues.

In their classic study of *Patterns of Sexual Behavior*, for instance, Ford and Beach found that 84 percent or a 156 of a 185 contemporary cultures allow men more than one sexual partner. Less than 16 percent restrict men to one mate and only 5 percent completely disapprove of premarital and extramarital relations. More to the point, 72 of 185 culture actually approve of specific types of extramarital relations, although again women are more restricted than men. Eighteen of the 185 cultures, however, placed no restrictions on the extracurricular activities of their women.

Recent sex-therapy practices suggest another possible clue. From the 1960s through into the mid-1980s, some sex therapists worked with sexual surrogates to help men with erectile problems. After some sexual counseling and psychotherapy, the patient was introduced to a surrogate therapist. While the patient and surrogate worked through a series of sensual exercises with graduated intimacy, the patient refrained from all sexual intimacy with his wife. Considering what we know about the effect of a new sexual partner on other mammals, one might speculate that some men with erectile problems may respond to surrogate therapy because it revives the PEA(amphetamine)-mediated passion with the novel stimulation of the surrogate therapist that can then be transferred to the wife when he resumes sexual relations with her.[28]

In prehistoric times, when men and women had an average life expectancy of thirty or thirty-five years, our species could survive if each couple stayed together four or five years to give their first child a good chance of living. Neural tendencies in the triune brain, mediated by pheromones, PEA, and endorphins, increased the prevalence of this pattern. Those same tendencies persist today, but with one major change, a dramatic doubling of our average life expectancy. That factor alone has created major stress for our concept of marriage being "until death do us part" and "forsaking all others."

One common adaptation to the interaction of these two realities of life is the pattern of serial monogamy, in which husbands and wives become dissatisfied as the passion fades and greener, more passionate pastures appear on the horizon. Somewhere around half of all American marriages end in divorce and remarriage to a stimulating new partner. The other half survive the transition into calmer, less romantically intense, less passionate, perhaps much less sexy long-term friendships. Some long-term relationships survive despite the prevalence of extramarital affairs, or because the couple renegotiate their commitment to allow each other some freedom to have emotional, perhaps sexually intimate co-marital relationships.

The implications of the connections we suggest here between pheromones, hormones, neurostimulants, and sexual bonding provoke a flood of unanswerable but certainly controversial questions for one to ponder and debate.

"Permanent togetherness," according to Gerhard Neubeck in an anthology on *Extramarital Relations*, "results in quantitative and qualitative exposure that may lead to satiation." But then as Erich Fromm said, "Love is not the same as making love."[29]

11

MAKING HUMAN PHEROMONES

Given the important role pheromones play in activating the genes in hormone-secreting nerve cells that control sexual development and behavior in other mammals, we should not be surprised that we share with them several rather elaborate systems for producing and distributing pheromones. Nor should we disregard the possibility that what we know about how other animals make and distribute pheromones may well help us with gaps in our research and knowledge about human pheromones.

Among humans, and other mammals at least, the most important source of pheromones is the skin, and three different types of glands, eccrine, sebaceous, and apocrine, that secrete chemicals onto the surface of our skin.[1]

We have more eccrine glands than any other type of gland. Evaporation of watery sweat from eccrine glands all over the body helps to keep us cool, even when we build up excess body heat from a work out at the gym, adapt to the dogs days of summer, or experience an intense release after orgasm.[2] Sebaceous glands are also found over most of the body, but we have fewer sebaceous than eccrine glands. Our forehead, scalp, and face have the largest and most active sebaceous glands; our palms and soles none. The secretions of sebaceous glands are oily and contain substances that the bacteria on our skin thrive on. These bacteria, along with the secretions of eccrine and sebaceous glands, play a vital role in pheromone production.[3]

Secretions of both the eccrine and sebaceous glands contribute to our body odor, but it is the milky secretions from the apocrine glands that are mainly associated with pheromone production in other mammals. The human fetus develops an abundance of apocrine glands along with the hair follicles that cover its body while in the womb.[4] At birth, however, we have fewer apocrine glands than either sebaceous or eccrine glands.

Sometime before birth, before the hair follicles are fully developed, the apocrine portion of the hair-gland complex is reabsorbed, except in the hair follicles located around our nipples, in our genital area, our armpits, and the area of our navel.[5] Conflicting reports on the number and the location of apocrine glands nearly defy analysis. Some claim that apocrine glands may also be found in our scalp, on our forehead and cheeks, under our nose, and at the base of our eyelashes. They probably also occur in several other areas, particularly in the bearded portion of the face.[6]

The apocrine and sebaceous glands associated with hair follicles are extremely sensitive to sex hormones.[7] Androgens increase the size of apocrine and sebaceous glands, the number of these glands formed, and the amount of secretions they produce.[8] Estrogens decrease gland size and the amount of secretion, but they do not decrease the number of glands that are formed.[9]

During pregnancy, the mother's androgen levels ensure that the sebaceous and apocrine glands of the fetus will develop fully and that both types of glands function briefly right after birth. After birth, bacteria on the infant's skin convert the adrenal androgens from the sebaceous and apocrine secretions into the characteristic body odor of newborns.[10] Unlike the eccrine sweat glands, sebaceous and apocrine glands then regress and remain inactive until puberty when the androgen levels rise to stimulate them once more.

Puberty begins several years before teenagers show the obvious signs of sprouting to adult height, developing muscle mass or breasts and curvy hips, and genital growth. When the person is between the ages of eight and ten, his or her adrenal glands start to increase the amounts of androgens they produce, which activates the growth of hair around the genitals and in the underarms.[11] This surge of adrenal androgens, led by dehydroepiandrosterone (DHEA), causes the apocrine and sebaceous glands associated with the pubic and underarm hair follicles to enlarge and begin producing their secretions.[12] This early effect of adrenal androgens on pheromone production is enhanced when androgen production from the testes and ovaries begins to increase. This activates secretion from apocrine and sebaceous glands all over the body.[13]

Apocrine gland secretions have no odor until bacterial growth enhanced by sebaceous gland secretions start decomposing them. There is, however, a major sex difference in the character of the pheromones produced by the teenager. While infant boys and girls produce similar body odors, teenage boys and girls definitely show sex differences in their body odors because their adrenal glands and testes or ovaries produce different levels and ratios of sex hormones. The intensity of detectable body odor varies with the number of apocrine and sebaceous glands, with their size, with personal hygiene, with diet, with the levels of the various sex hormones, and with sex differences in the predominant type of bacteria found on the skin surface.[14]

Men produce more and stronger body odor than women because androgens are the predominant sex hormone in males. Also, most males have a particular type of odor-producing bacteria on their skin. Some women have this same bacteria, but their lower levels of androgens combine with levels of estrogens and progesterone dominate in different phases of their menstrual cycle, so even the women with the skin bacteria characteristic of males do not have a strong male body odor. The shifting balance of estrogens and progesterone during the menstrual cycle is also responsible for cyclic changes in a woman's odor.[15]

From adolescence through adulthood the development and activity of the apocrine and sebaceous glands remain fairly stable. Pheromone production, however, begins to decline for women at about age fifty and for men about age seventy.[16] From puberty to old age, the activities of the glands involved in pheromone production depend on both the individual's sex and age. That is because the activities of the eccrine, sebaceous, and apocrine glands are so strongly influenced by the production of androgens in the ovaries, testes, and adrenal glands.[17]

A well-known genetic defect gives us an interesting insight into this connection. In the human adrenal glands, cholesterol is channeled through three main metabolic pathways. Some of us unfortunately inherit a defective gene for an enzyme deficiency that blocks the conversion of cholesterol to cortisol. The body needs cortisol and when it does not get enough, feedback loops get the message to the adrenal glands which then increases cholesterol production. That overproduction coupled with a shifting of the cholesterol products from the blocked path into one of the other paths results in an increased androgen production in that other pathway. Children with this condition, known as CAH or congenital adrenal hyperplasia, experience some serious symptoms from the surplus androgen, masculinizing of their bodies. A minor, but interesting from our viewpoint, result is an increased activity of the sebaceous and apocrine glands caused by the surplus androgens. Likewise, a deficiency in androgen production in either sex is associated with a decreased activity of the apocrine and sebaceous glands, and their resulting pheromone production.

Allowing for the differences in our body sizes, humans have proportionately more and larger apocrine glands than any other animal.[18] As recently as 1986, however, scientists reported that apocrine glands had no known function in humans although they knew they were associated with pheromonal activity in other animals.[19] Now that we know humans have a pair of VNOs, which function as pheromone detectors,[20] it seems fairly reasonable to suggest that the structure and function of our apocrine and sebaceous glands are part of a pheromone production system, just as they are in other mammals.

SKIN PHEROMONES

In addition to the variety of sweat pheromones we produce with the help of our hormones and skin bacteria, we also produce a rich complex of other chemical signals in our skin cells, urine, and saliva.

The skin is, by far, the largest of our body's organs.[21] An adult's skin covers up to a hundred thousand square centimeters; roughly the area of a nine-by-twelve-foot rug. It provides us with a wrapping that protects us from the effects of wind and rain, prevents toxic chemicals and deadly bacteria from entering our body, and helps to ensure against excess loss of body fluids. In addition, our skin cells also contain more enzymes than any other organ, and this diversity allows for considerable versatility in converting sex hormones like androgens, estrogens, and progesterone into pheromones. DHEA may be converted into testosterone, the primary androgen, at sites such as the hair follicles, which contain our sebaceous and apocrine glands. Testosterone, in turn, may be converted to androstenol and/or androstenone.[22] This conversion allows the by-products of hormone break down to become airborne as we constantly shed skin cells.[23] Moreover, estrogens, progesterone, and other hormones are converted to other active chemical substances that may function as pheromones.

Our skin also makes fatty acids. So many different types of fatty acids are made that there is little doubt that no two individuals make exactly the same fatty acids or exactly the same amounts of them. Among other things, slight variations in enzymes and in body temperature cause changes in fatty acid production, which, along with eccrine, sebaceous, and apocrine secretions, help provide each of us with a distinctive chemical signature. This unique combination of odors enables many other animals to recognize each other, just as it allows a dog to recognize the scent of its master or a friend.[24] Fatty acids produced by the skin help to give us an equally distinctive chemical print or pheromone signature.[25]

Mammals produce pheromones as part of the many metabolic processes that go on in the cells and organs of the body. These end products, including the breakdown of sex hormones, are filtered out of the blood circulating in the kidneys and excreted in the urine. At least two of the chemically active substances found in our underarms and in our skin are also found in urine. Because they are found in the urine of both sexes only after puberty, and because concentrations of both androstenol and androstenone are greater in the male, many scientists believe that these and similar chemicals in the urine may also function as human sex pheromones.[26]

Pheromones in our sweat? Pheromones in our skin cells? Pheromones in our urine? What about pheromones in our saliva? Although it is more than 99 percent water, saliva, like urine and blood, accurately reflects many results of our body's processes, including the breakdown of sex hormones.[27] Since testosterone is present in our saliva, it should come as no surprise that androstenone, and many other chemicals that are considered pheromones in other animals, are also found in our saliva as well as in our blood and urine.[28] From our saliva, these aromatic messengers pass easily into our breath.

SPREADING THE MESSAGES

Whether they come from our skin, the hair on our head, our underarms, our genitals, or saliva, pheromones must find a way to get to another member of the same species before they can influence that individual's sexual development or behavior.[29] Pheromone distribution then is just as important to chemical communication as pheromone production. It is no surprise, then, that our elaborate pheromone production systems go hand in hand with equally elaborate systems for their distribution.

While eccrine sweat glands are never associated with hair follicles, sebaceous glands sometimes are, and apocrine glands always are, although not all hair follicles are associated with apocrine glands. In other more furry mammals, hair seemingly plays a major role in the distribution of pheromones. This might lead you to the suspicion that human hair plays a much smaller role in distributing pheromones than it does in other much more furry mammals. That is not true. The flaw in this conclusion is that numerically at least, we have as many or more hairs per body surface than some very hairy primates. The difference is our body hairs are much finer and nearly invisible.[30]

The growth of body hair, like the number, the structure, and function of apocrine and sebaceous glands, depends on androgens. In terms of human pheromone distribution, our androgen-dependent abundance of body hair in particular areas is significant for several reasons.

First, the underarms, chest, genitals and lower abdomen contain an abundance of gender-specific body hair and large numbers of apocrine glands. Each of these areas responds to sexual stimulation with vasocongestion, which means that blood cells pool beneath the surface of the skin and produce warmth.[31] Warmer skin temperature makes these particularly hairy areas conducive to evaporation. Warm skin also makes apocrine and sebaceous secretions more volatile, increasing the distribution of our pheromones in response to sexual stimulation. Added to this, the hair in these areas traps odorless secretions and allows bacteria to change them into odorous pheromones.

Secondly, our skin cells, like our regenerating olfactory neurons, are constantly being replaced.[32] The loss of our fur—but not our hair—may in fact enhance the distribution of the pheromones found in our skin cells. We no longer have the fur that would trap our skin cells and keep them close to our body.

The protection our skin provides costs dearly in terms of the number of skin cells that die and are shed from our body. So, in the process of protecting us from the environment, our skin makes us part of our environment as we continuously shed dead skin cells into the air around us. Estimates suggest that every hour we lose about a thousand skin cells per square centimeter of exposed body parts.[33] A person of average size sheds nearly forty million cells a day in an invisible airborne cloud of particles that contains sex hormones and their pheromone metabolites. The constant loss and replacement of our skin cells is an effective way to constantly update others on our hormone status.

The ability of trained dogs to follow a trail of dead skin cells supports the claim that human skin cells contain pheromones. Unlike volatile, gaseous pheromones produced from the breakdown of glandular secretions, the pheromones in skin cells are relatively stable and easily tracked by persistent bloodhounds.[34]

In real life, the messages of gaseous pheromones blend with more solid pheromones in the cloud of microscopic skin cells we inhale when we encounter a person. These messages make contact with the mucous lining of the VNO, and in some cases with the main olfactory system receptors, just as they do in the bloodhound. From the olfactory receptors, the resulting electrochemical messages find their way to the subliminal circuits of the limbic mind, to GnRH neurons that trigger hormone production in the HPG axis, and which affect our sexual development and behavior.[35]

There are times, however, when the subliminal messages of pheromones are so strong they break through to our consciousness. Other animals may regularly sniff the pheromones left behind in the urine of other animals to locate a mate or find out who has been wandering through their turf. Humans, on the contrary, have been socialized to ignore the scent of urine, or to be repulsed when we unavoidably encounter it in some not so civilized urban setting. But in the clinical laboratory, the scent of urine may be a valuable diagnostic tool. Urine, as noted above, contains aromatic by-products derived from the breakdown of hormones and other substances. These aromatic by-products often contain clues to the person's specific state of health.

Anyone who has performed clinical tests on urine will attest to the unique odor of different urine samples. The various components of an individual's urine reflect a great deal about the current status of their many different hormones. The various components also provide clues to the sex and sexual orientation of the individual.[36]

When a physician requests an urinalysis, the odor of that person's urine is not written down on the lab report the physician reviews.

However, given the opportunity to speak with the physician, a good laboratory technologist will comment if the odor provides any diagnostic implications. When, for instance, a patient has a urinary tract infection, the particular type of bacteria causing the infection may be tentatively identified by the odor it produces. Also, if the patient's body chemistry is grossly dysfunctional, as in the case of a diabetic whose sugar level is out of control, the odor will give the condition away. When a diabetic's sugar level is dangerous, the aromatic message in the urine will be reinforced by a similar odor of acetone on the person's breath. That is because the aromatic ketone that shows up in the diabetic's urine also shows up in the saliva, whence it passes into the person's breath. Once the diagnostic implications are relatively clear, treatment can begin immediately without waiting for the laboratory tests to ascertain the patient's blood sugar level and confirm the diagnosis of diabetic ketoacidosis.

The odor of androstenone, the ketone form of a sex hormone present in saliva, probably serves a similar purpose, providing equally good evidence of reproductive fitness and overall health of the persons we encounter, whether or not we consciously recognize the message. In the near future, depending on more advanced technology or perhaps just more advanced training in odor recognition, health care professionals may diagnose heart attack victims on the spot by detecting in their breath the high level of pentane and other odors associated with this deadly condition. A simple breath-testing machine might allow persons with various chronic conditions to check their status several times a day at home or work.[37]

THE MOST INTIMATE OF PHEROMONES

In addition to finding pheromones in skin glands and cells, urine, blood, saliva, and breath, researchers have found evidence of pheromones in the vaginal secretions of many other species of mammals for whom they serve as powerful sex attractants.[38] Extracts of vaginal secretions from rhesus monkeys, for instance, increase male grooming behavior, mounting activity, and ejaculations. These effects are evident even when the female shows no other physical or behavioral signs that she is sexually receptive or "in heat." When researchers tested these extracts by blocking the male's pheromone-detecting system, these substances have no effect on his behavior, clearly indicating that they qualify as true pheromones.[39]

Production of vaginal pheromones varies with the female's sex hormone levels, especially her estrogen level.[40] A midcycle rise in the female's estrogen signals high sexual attractiveness in rhesus females with a marked increase in vaginal pheromones. An interesting aspect of this phenomenon is that rhesus females have a monthly menstrual cycle that is more similar to the human female's fertility pattern than it is to the fertility cycle of other primates.[41]

Researchers have isolated and identified several aromatic short-chain fatty acids in the vaginal secretions of both rhesus monkey females and women.[42] Production of these vaginal fatty acids, like the production of androstenol, androstenone, and fatty acids in the skin, depends on the level of the sex hormones,[43] but with a major difference. The links between androgens and the production of androstenone and androstenol are relatively simple. Production of vaginal aliphatic acids, in contrast, is much more complex and varied, depending as it does on variations in the monthly cycle of estrogens and progesterone and on the types and numbers of bacteria in or around the vagina. Because of this complexity, no single aromatic chemical has been shown to be a major contributor to vaginal odor in either monkeys or humans.[44] Still, scientists have discovered that the response of male rhesus monkeys to vaginal odors often depends on the specific situation and in some cases on the male's past experience.

The variability in the composition of vaginal odors suggests that the male's response may also vary from a strong attraction to aversion and even disgust, depending on the balance of hormones in the course of the menstrual cycle.[45] Preliminary research suggests that human vaginal odors change slightly in both pleasantness and intensity during the menstrual cycle. More pleasant odors are associated with ovulation and the concurrent peak in fertility. These results, however, were obtained from a clinical study in which males smelled used tampons kept in jars. This completely artificial approach may well have affected the male's rating of the pleasantness of the various samples of vaginal odor. A more natural setting may have yielded different results that more accurately represent the real reactions of men to vaginal odors.[46]

On a less clinical note, the popularity of male-female oral-genital sex suggests that many men may find vaginal odors pleasant.

Unfortunately, no human study has yet been designed to properly test whether men's interest in performing oral sex shows any consistent link with different stages in the woman's menstrual cycle and whether the sex appeal of human vaginal odors changes in parallel with this interest. If such a study could be carried out in a natural setting, the results might tell us more about the true nature of male responses, if any, to vaginal pheromones, than the tampon sniff test described above.

Particular vaginal odors, like specific breath and urine odors, may indicate the presence of abnormal conditions. A yeast infection, for instance, causes a characteristic musty vaginal odor, while an overgrowth of the bacteria *Gardnerella vaginalis* is marked by a fishy-smelling, amine-type odor. The one-celled parasite *Trichomonas* likewise produces its own characteristic odor in vaginal discharges. These conditions and others can easily be detected when a physician requests examination of a patient's vaginal discharge. Typically, a laboratory technologist will confirm this olfactory diagnosis with microscopic examination of the specimen, but the original clue comes from the nose.[47]

All told, warm-blooded animals, including humans, take great care to produce strong and clear aromatic messages, even if we are unaware of our reactions to them. Whatever the source of these aromatic messengers, the evidence is clear that they do affect and influence the sexual development and behavior of other animals. Whether or not they have similar important effects on humans remains to be determined, but if they do not, then scientists will have to figure out why we produce these aromatic messengers from many different sources.

Meanwhile, there is no denying that there are many different odor clues that indicate a person's health and reproductive status. Whether or not we detect these clues consciously or unconsciously, these odors do provide the same pheromonal messages.

12

A KISS ISN'T
JUST A KISS

Among the few pieces still missing from our exploration of the
mysteries of odors and sex are some details about how
pheromones manage to get from one person to another.

In looking for answers to our earlier questions about animal
pheromones, the history and anatomy of smell, pheromone effects, and
connections between odors, genes, hormones, our triune brain, and
behavior, we found many bits of research and insights about animal
pheromones that gave us clues into the role these chemical messengers
may play in human sexual development, physiology, and behavior.
Allowing for important differences between humans and other animals,
we could still rely on the thread of biological consistency to lead us to a
better understanding of the scent of eros in human life. Sometimes the
pieces that fit into our puzzle were based on solid scientific research. At
other times, the insights were tantalizingly incomplete or inconclusive.
Still, we could rely on the thread of consistency.

Our question in this chapter poses a new problem for which the
thread of consistency is not as helpful. If scientific research on other
aspects of human pheromones has been scant until recently, even less is
known about how people manage to communicate chemically with each
other, especially when pheromones operate below the level of consciousness. This question plunges us into the variability of cultures which regulate, often very informally, how men and women connect and interact,
how we move from superficial encounters to erotic intimacy.

What we know about the production and nature of pheromones
in other species clearly indicates that sex pheromones most likely serve
more or less similar functions in humans as they do in other species.

But signaling and priming pheromones cannot tell us who is a stranger, friend, or lover; they cannot bond mother and child, inspire oral sex, or convey any other information, unless they can get from one person to another. So, despite the vagaries of culture and human social interactions, we need to explore this piece of our puzzle.

Fortunately, despite the fact that no "specific" human behavior has been directly linked to chemical communication via pheromones, there are a number of nonspecific human behaviors that can be indirectly linked to the distribution of pheromones. As you might expect, since animal pheromones often involve courtship and mating, most of our clues will come from patterns in human courtship behavior that are shared by many different cultures.

Dancing is probably the most common of these threads. In many cultures, "fast" dancing often precedes "slow" dancing in our courtship behavior. The link between pheromone production and distribution may not be immediately evident in this courtship "strategy," but consider what we know about the distribution of pheromones in other animals and the connection may be easier to see.

In fast dancing, friction between uncovered skin and the air releases a cloud of airborne pheromone-containing skin particles around each dancer, which they share particularly if they are dancing close to each other. Fast dancing also produces body heat and the need to cool the body. Skin bacteria quickly turn hormone elements in the increased secretions of apocrine and sebaceous glands into pheromones. This combination of airborne skin cell pheromones and the more volatile gaseous pheromones from glandular secretions during fast dancing is often followed by a more intimate slow dance that increases our exposure to the subliminal chemical messages of our dance partner.

Other mammals have a fur coat that protects and insulates them from their environment as well as trapping their pheromones. The obvious body hair of humans has no other function than ornament and sexual lure.[1] Still, as in other animals, secretions from our apocrine and sebaceous glands that are trapped in our hair may serve as a subliminal sexual lure regardless of cultural variations.

Picture dance partners who are engaged in a romantic close dance. Within the confines of this dance, it is common for men and women to partially raise their arms to embrace. Men also commonly raise their arms much higher than women do when they turn their partner in a circle, as they do in ballroom, country, square, or western dancing.

Remove the romance from the picture and you are left with the biological fact that underarm hair and warmth are particularly effective means to ensure that pheromones evaporate and are distributed. But only when the arm is raised. When the arm is held beside the body, the underarm apocrine scent organs are nearly closed off and not exposed to the air.[2]

An important step in male courtship behavior comes when the male tentatively slips his arm around his partner's shoulders and she snuggles against his chest. All the casual observer may see in this is a tender, romantic escalation of intimacy. The behavioral biologist looking for ways humans might exchange their pheromones sees something more subtle—another way males unconsciously maximize release of their underarm scent near the female's VNO. That is not a very romantic interpretation, but if this behavior subliminally reinforces the physical tenderness and escalates the attraction, should romantics object?

In different eras and cultures, the small couch commonly known as a "love seat" has provided men with a ready opening to getting an arm around a woman. Furniture designers may only have been playing to the romantic interests and expectations of the buyer, but behind the "love seat" may be another aid to sharing the subtle influence of pheromones.

Kissing, rubbing noses, and other variations that involve exchange of saliva and sharing breath are also a popular courtship behavior throughout human cultures. We do know that the concentration of at least one human pheromone found in our saliva is higher in men than in women.[3] Does this mean that kissing is merely another covert means for males to slip their sex pheromones to their partner?[4]

The answer to that question, and other related issues of kissing, may lie in a pragmatic, unromantic scientific analogy of that all-American sport of "baseball." The game starts when the two players step to the plate together and first encounter each other's pheromonal cloud. "First base" is achieved when the male puts his arm around the female and she lets it stay there to savor his scent. The first and subsequent kisses might be considered "second base," with the male reaching "third base" when he fondles, kisses, and sucks on her breasts. By the time an unromantic, game-playing boy gets to "third base," he and his partner have shared a fair amount of their unique pheromonal clouds and salivary messengers. He has enticed her with his apocrine, sebaceous, and eccrine scents, and she lured him with her breast scent. In a world of cause and effect, any apparent coincidences are likely to arouse suspicion. How coincidental do you think the link is between human pheromones and progressive intimacy?

Pursuing the baseball metaphor to bring our point of "scoring" home, consider the progression of the runner from "third base" to "home base" in what not so long ago was considered the ultimate intimacy: sexual intercourse. However, the growing emphasis on Safer Sex in the 1990s and attempts by feminists to move males from their narrow phallic-coital obsessed definitions to a broader experience of sexual pleasure, intimacy, and satisfaction, may be giving "scoring" a new meaning. Emphasis on the "home run" or "balling" may be changing with the emphasis on the added dimension of oral-genital sex, especially cunnilingus.[5]

We have already explored the effects of vaginal aliphatic acids on male monkeys and other mammals, and how production of particularly attractive vaginal pheromones increases with the rise of estrogen levels associated with a woman's fertility. Could it be that oral-genital contact, the new "ultimate intimacy," might be a means of assessing the reproductive fitness of a woman whose vaginal secretions provide odorous cues? On the other hand, if a woman enjoys female-male oral-genital sex, could she be responding to the subliminal invitation of the pheromonally active glandular secretions behind the ridge of the penile glans? Are the straight male and lesbian devotees of cunnilingus unknowingly pursuing an age-old quest for pheromones under the hood of the clitoris and in vaginal aliphatic acids? Are heterosexual women and gay male devotees of fellatio similarly pursuing the age-old mammalian quest for male pheromones trapped under the foreskin of the uncircumcised male or in the pubic hair of a circumcised male?[6]

We do not offer these interpretations and suggestions to ignore the loving intentions of the giver, or to deny the pleasure reflexes and wonder-filled relaxing endorphin release that oral-genital sex normally produces for the recipient. We are simply suggesting the strong possibility of an added dimension based on our scientific curiosity.

Romance and scientific curiosity are not incompatible. In fact, to support our claim that these two views of oral-genital sex are quite congenial, we would cite a fiery encounter in Sandra Brown's bestselling romance novel, *French Silk*.

> "This is dangerous as hell, but. . . Ah, God, I can smell you." He
> leaned forward and burrowed his face in the cleft of her thighs,

nuzzling, gnawing, kissing her madly through the giving fabric of her dress. "Too bad you can't bottle this."[7]

Humans pheromones *have* been bottled, or at least that is what some fragrance companies have recently claimed. But eighty years ago, long before the concept of human pheromones began to develop, Havelock Ellis noted that the attraction of oral-genital sex might well be based in our attraction to genital odors.[8]

SUPPRESSING THE PHEROMONAL EFEFCT

Whether or not one accepts this scientific interpretation of alleged interactions between pheromones and human behavior in the courtship dance does not prove anything. So, to further support our claim, we suggest another approach using a different kind of circumstantial evidence. Many cultures have endorsed behavioral patterns and customs that, knowingly or not, effectively squelch pheromone production and distribution. We would suggest that this type of suppression is linked to an attempt to restrain or repress the progressive nature of escalating intimacy linked to sharing pheromones.

Some religions, for example, limit pheromone distribution that might lead to a sexual consequence by forbidding dancing altogether or limiting it to same-sex couples. Similarly, shaving the underarms and/or legs may be a cultural remnant of antisexual Victorian mores designed to reduce the amount of pheromones retained on the female body. Considering that during most of our history, bathing was infrequent and that underarm deodorants were unheard of, there may well have been a genuine need to suppress the distribution of stimulating human pheromones from the underarm area of women.[9]

Completely covering the hair with a veil or *chador* as women do in some Muslim cultures prevents pheromone distribution from the hair.[10] Covering the whole body, from head to toe, in a *burka* with a only a slit for the woman to see through, as fundamentalist Muslim women do, creates a full barrier to distribution of all female pheromones.

In his first letter to his disciples in Corinth, St. Paul reminded the Christians that

> if a man refuses to remove his hat while praying or preaching, he
> dishonors Christ. And that is why a woman who publicly prays or
> prophesies without a covering on her head dishonors her husband.

Yes, if she refuses to wear a head covering, then she should cut off
all her hair. And if it is shameful for a woman to have her head
shaved, then she should wear a covering. But a man should not
wear anything on his head.[11]

Why was Paul only concerned about women covering their hair, and
then only in public? The context of his remarks make it obvious that
Paul was convinced that men should show their respect for Christ's
authority when praying in public by removing their head covering as
they would for a civil official. And that woman should show their def-
erence and submission to their husbands by keeping their heads covered while praying or prophesying in public.

That obvious motivation does not, however, eliminate the possibility of something more behind this custom than maintaining male
dominance over women. Paul obviously knew nothing about the chemistry of women's pheromones, but perhaps he and other men of his time
knew about their real effect from folklore and everyday observations.
Were the early Christians perhaps concerned about pheromones
trapped in women's hair distracting men from their religious pursuits
and diverting them into the pursuit of sexual pleasure? The presence of
head coverings for women in many different cultures and times suggest
this is not an unreasonable possibility.

And then there is that quaint and ancient Western custom of the
groom lifting the bride's veil to give her a "first kiss." If the bride walks
down the aisle on a white runner designed to protect her from evil spirits coming up through the floor of the church, and if she wears her veil
down to protect her from other men until her husband lifts the veil and
publicly declares with a kiss that she belongs to him, is it too unreasonable to suggest that the bride's veil might also have been borrowed and
adapted from the Muslim tradition of veiling women, both single and
married? Of course, one could counter that when Western brides
replaced the wool veil with a lace veil, they eliminated its function as a
pheromone barrier. "On the other hand, one could argue," as Charles
Wysocki does, "that in the course of evolution human beings are shed-
ding control by pheromones and leading more of an independent life. If
one takes that view, then the kiss is nothing more than a vestigial
behavior for transmitting pheromones."[12]

Far less sexist than women's veils is our age-old use of breath
deodorants, and antiperspirants and deodorants for the underarm. For

centuries men and women chewed parsley and mint to release their deodorizing chlorophyll and pleasant herbal scents. In our century, chemists replaced parsley and mint from the garden with mint-flavored alcohol-based mouthwashes and breath sprays that may, in effect, substitute their alcohol base for the alcohol-based pheromone androstenol. Alongside the longstanding gender equality of breath and mouth deodorants, most cultures have consistently put more emphasis on customs that limit distribution of women's pheromones more than men's pheromones.

When it comes to pheromone distribution from the breasts or chest, the sexist bias in Western, especially American, cultures reflects the gender bias in shaving the underarm. In most Western cultures women are required to cover their breasts. Men are not. But female fashions reveal an interesting cycle. An era of puritanical uptightness with neck-clutching high collars and long sleeves with wrist-tight cuffs is sooner or later followed by an era reflecting more comfortable attitudes toward sexual mores in plunging necklines and sexy cleavages that enhance pheromone distribution, especially from women's sexy eveningwear.

Now it seems unlikely that breast pheromones would have a greater effect on men than the chest pheromones of men would have on women, especially considering that women generally have a much greater ability to detect and identify various odors, and males produce stronger body odors than women. Why then can men go almost anywhere bare-chested and women are arrested for going topless on the beach?

While we are on the subject of women's breasts, why is there so much focus on women keeping their nipples and areola covered at topless and go-go performances? Behind this obsessive interpretation of "indecent exposure" might there not be lurking a fear of female breast pheromones and an effort to limit their distribution? Or is this gender disparity just another aspect of a male-dominated culture?

Since we are pushing into relatively virgin territory in this chapter, we might play devil's advocate with the sexist biases mentioned above and suggest that perhaps the women have gotten off easier when it comes to penile-clitoral pheromones because far more males are circumcised than are females.

Among prehistoric farmers, males ensured the fertility of their fields by offering their foreskins to the gods in the fields. Early Egyptians believed humans were created with both a masculine and a feminine soul. Since the male's feminine soul was thought to be located in the foreskin and the woman's masculine soul in her clitoris, circumcision at puberty made the boy or girl fully male or fully female. African and Arabic cultures adopted circumcision from the Egyptians as a religious rite for both males and females.[13]

Male circumcision passed into the Jewish world with Abraham, who had his sons circumcised. Joshua required it for all Jewish males as a sign of the covenant between the Jews and God. Although popularly regarded as one of the essentials of a true believer, neither male nor female circumcision has any warrant in the Qu'ran. Muslims usually circumcise boys after age eight or nine and before puberty.[14] Again, we are offering a rhetorical question, for which we have no answer, just a strong curiosity about whether the presence of pheromones in the smegma of the clitoris and penis might have played some role in the origins of circumcision in prehistoric times, and its popularity through the ages, especially in our puritanic American culture.[15]

THE SCENT OF A LOVER

> . . . she brushed her hair and put on jeans and an old sweater of Steven's. It was a way of staying close to him. She could wear his clothes if she couldn't have him.[16]

When one of us mentioned this quote from Danielle Steel's novel *Heartbeat* to a friend, she smiled and immediately provided us with an unexpected anecdotal confirmation in a story about her mother. For years, her mother always kept a white towel on the headrest of her husband's favorite lounge chair to protect the upholstery from his hair oil. After his death, the mother saved the last such towel in a zip-lock plastic bag and brought it out to smell when she felt alone and wanted to remember her lover.

Recent hair styles also suggest some questions about the changing scent of a lover. Both the feminist and men's movements encourage women to be more assertive, competitive, and even aggressive at the same time men are urged to be more sensitive and in tune with their emotions and express their feelings more openly. As socially imposed gender roles are less sharply drawn and become more androgynous, it is curious that women's increasing "masculine" traits are reflected in their "masculine" short hair styles, while men's longer hair styles reflect their greater willingness to express the feminine side of their personalities.

Shorter hair on the head traps less pheromones and lessens the difference in the distribution of odors that are characteristically male or
female. Thus, a woman with short hair might smell more masculine,
and a long-haired man more feminine. Being that more and more
women are looking for the sensitive, emotional male and more and
more men becoming comfortable with assertive women, this gender
cross-coding in hair styles may in fact be helpful.

The classic Western stereotypes of the petite, long-haired, blonde
who has more fun and the tall, dark, and handsome man she wants to
have fun with raises some intriguing and as yet unresearched questions.[17] A tall man, for example, has up to one and a half times more
pheromone-producing skin than a short man has.[18] A dark-skinned man
has more apocrine glands, and therefore produces more pheromones
than light-skinned males. A man with a beard traps more apocrine
secretions than one who shaves his facial hair. And while some women
knowingly prefer the "distinguished" or more "manly" look of men with
neat mustaches or beards, for other women the clean-shaven "look" is a
turn on. But is what women see what they hope to get, or is it what they
smell that they hope to get? And does this hold true equally for men?

In many mammals, the levels of androgens and dominance go
hand in hand. For upright bipeds like men, taller signals bigger and better. Hormonally, taller means more androgen, and more androgen
means more aggressive, a greater reproductive fitness, and stronger sex
drive. Information about androgen levels conveyed on the breath or
through other body odors may serve to warn others not to pick a fight,
or perhaps to entice a potential mate with a subliminal advertisement
of his virility, and his ability and readiness to mate.

In all races, adult women are, on the average, about four inches
shorter than men.[19] This disparity means that intimate contact in an
upright posture provides exposure to pheromones from different areas of
the body. When dancing "cheek to cheek," for example, a man is most
exposed to pheromones from the hair on top a woman's head. She, on
the other hand, is most exposed to pheromones from his face and chest.

Curiously, men often knowingly prefer women with a particular
hair color. Sixty years ago, Iwan Bloch, a highly respected pioneering
sexologist, reported that in his research women who naturally exuded
the odor of amber were "much less frequent, and more sought after" by
men. Women with ash-blond hair, he noted, "are wont to exude a very
delicate amber odor" which men generally prefer to a musky scent.

Sometimes women with chestnut brown hair have this odor [of amber], but more often they have a sort of violety odor which appears to be connected with the excretions of the sebaceous glands. Brunettes not infrequently have an odor of ebony wood which, during their periods, combines with a light but not unpleasant musk odor. Galopin goes so far as to think that he can divide even the lovers of these women according to these different categories. Men who love the violet and amber odor are more tender and more faithful. Yet blond women are able to hold their lovers longer than their swarthier sisters, who, though they are loved more passionately and despotically, are loved less deeply and permanently.[20]

Back in 1914 Havelock Ellis commented on the link between a woman's hair color and the odor of her armpit.

Its gamut covers the whole keyboard of odors, reaching the obstinate scents of syringa and elder, and sometimes recalling the sweet perfume of the rubbed fingers that have held a cigarette. Audacious and sometimes fatiguing in the brunette and the black woman, sharp and fierce in the red woman, the armpit is heady as some sugared wines in the blondes.[21]

One readily apparent racial difference in human anatomy is hair color. But the link between anatomical racial differences and physiological differences is often ignored or denied. This subject is so emotionally charged that few scientists dare study it for fear they will be branded racists just for being interested in the subject.[22] Similar perils are even more evident when someone tries to take the next step and suggests a link between racial differences and differences in sexual behavior. Despite this sensitivity, a few comments on these differences are necessary to shed some further light on the mysteries of odors and sex.

An observation from Boyd Gibbons extensive review of "The Intimate Sense" for National Geographic offers a good springboard for our brief discussion:

During the World Wars, German soldiers claimed they knew the whiff of the English, and the English said likewise. More recently, North Vietnamese soldiers reported that they often smelled Americans before seeing them. Jack Holly, a Marine Corps officer who led reconnaissance patrols deep into the triple-canopy jungles of Vietnam, told me, "I am alive today because of my nose. You couldn't see a camo bunker if it was right in front of you. But you can't camouflage smell. I could smell the North Vietnamese before hearing or seeing them. Their smell was not like yours or mine, not Filipino, not South Vietnamese either. If I smelled that smell again, I would know it."[23]

Anecdotal? Yes, but these experiences are real and supported by research stretching back to Ellis's fine summary of what was known eighty years ago about racial differences in body odors. Ellis, for instance, reported that many, though not all blacks have a stronger body odor than other races, which is made even stronger by cleanliness, which opens the pores of the skin.[24] Europeans, he reported, are "considerably more odorous than are many other races—for instance, the Japanese—and there is doubtless some association between the greater hairiness of Europeans and their marked odor, since the sebaceous glands are part of the hair apparatus."[25]

These differences correlate well with racial differences in the development of apocrine glands.[26] Blacks have more apocrine glands than whites, and whites more than Asians. Some blacks have apocrine glands on the chest and abdomen, both above and below the navel. In contrast, whites rarely have apocrine glands on the abdomen, and when they do the glands only occur below the navel.[27] Japanese rarely have apocrine glands on the pubic mound or labia majora. They also have no apocrine glands on the chest, other than those around the nipples. While men have larger apocrine glands than women, the experts disagree on whether men or women have more apocrine glands.[28]

Racially, the most striking fact about apocrine glands is their weak development in the underarm area of orientals. Approximately half of the Korean population have no apocrine glands under their arms. Similarly, underarm apocrine glands are sparse and do not touch one another in the Japanese.

The underarm skin of men and women of most races has a visible flat, oval structure consisting of many separate but adjoining apocrine glands.[29] The axillary organ is designed specifically to produce and disperse odor-producing substances. When secretions from the apocrine and sebaceous glands mix with the watery sweat of the nearby eccrine glands, the diluted secretion flows over the surface of the axillary skin and hairs. Bacteria then break down this relatively odorless material into aromatic substances.[30] In all races, differences in development of the axillary apocrine glands correlate with the odor of their secretions.

All whites and blacks produce axillary odor, but only 10 percent of Japanese and only 2 or 3 percent of Chinese have any axillary odor.[31]

Since both black and Asian men and women have little body hair compared to whites, racial differences in apocrine gland development do not appear to correlate with the amount of body hair. However, development of the apocrine glands and the production of odors may vary with racial differences and with sex differences in levels of testosterone or with the production and metabolism of other androgens.[32] Since levels of testosterone are higher in men than women and higher in black women than Caucasian or Oriental women, both gender and racial differences in odor production appear to correlate with testosterone levels.

Besides relationships between apocrine gland number and distribution, the pigment of skin, hair, and eyes, androgen concentrations, climate of origin, and scent, there are marked differences in structure between the races, and to a lesser extent between the subraces of humans. For example, the relative breadth of the nose in various groups in different parts of the world correlates with average annual temperatures, relative humidity, and atmospheric pressure.[33] Higher temperature and higher atmospheric pressure increase the volatility of pheromones. Higher relative humidity also increases human odor production. A short, wide nose with flat nostrils, well adapted to a hot, moist climate or high altitude, maximizes transfer of odor molecules to the olfactory bulb and assists in scent detection.[34] So the climate, the volatility of odors, and shape and structure of the nose also play a role in pheromone distribution.

Do these differences in odor production have any cultural significance?[35] Consider the number of times women have exclaimed, "Men stink" or, "Men are pigs." It is worth noting that the same pheromone produced by the male pig is found in the underarm sweat of men, and in quantities much higher than occur in women. A man will seldom exclaim, "Women stink."

"Stinking" often precedes a racial or ethnic epithet. Do racial and ethnic differences in odor and pheromone production contribute to racial prejudice? Familiarity with the odors of different cultures can improve communication and reduce interpersonal space between people of different nationalities.

Which brings us back to our main theme: the often ignored importance of olfactory communication important in human interpersonal relations not just in sexual relations.

13

THE JOY OF ODOR

A few years ago, the National Advisory on Neurological and Communicative Disorders estimated that over two million Americans live in a world with some problem that seriously hampers their ability to enjoy the odors and tastes of everyday life. Every year approximately a quarter of a million Americans show up in a physician's office complaining that they have lost their sense of taste or smell. Yet doctors receive little or no training in how to evaluate or treat these complaints. Despite the prevalence of olfactory disorders and their links with other health problems, physicians seldom ask their patients about their ability to smell and even more rarely test this special sense as a part of their diagnosis.[1] Even if a doctor does take a patient's complaint seriously, his examination for odor sensitivity is likely to be very crude when compared with examinations for impaired hearing or vision.[2]

When our ability to see, hear, feel, or taste is reduced or lost, we quickly recognize that something serious has happened. We know a blind or deaf person could easily be unaware of a life-threatening situation. Or that a person with an impaired touch sensation might not recognize when the water in the shower is scalding or the soup too hot. But an impaired ability to smell? "An inconvenience, yes, and it does reduce some of the pleasures of eating. But you can live without it." We have an allergy attack, a cold, or the flu, and can't smell anything. "Oh, it'll come back. Why be concerned? Why complain?"

Only recently have psychophysicists, neurobiologists, embryologists, and medical specialists become aware that an impaired sense of smell, known as anosmia, may indeed be a symptom of something seriously wrong. Absence of a response to smell in a newborn infant, for example, may indicate some major problems and malfunctions in the brain, a variety of abnormal chromosomal and genetic conditions, or diabetes. Within hours after birth, odors will elicit reflex responses in a newborn with increased saliva and strong breathing. When that response is not normal, there may be a problem.[3]

Natural selection has made the normal development and function of our olfactory system a major factor in the normal development of the thinking part of our brain, in our memory and learning functions, and especially our sexual development and behavior. An awareness of that reality suggests a few questions about the two million Americans who have little or no sense of smell.

Before we deal with those questions, we need to get our terminology clear. In any frontier science, researchers frequently get into heated debate as they struggle to develop a clear set of terms to describe their sketchy data and emerging hypotheses. Because attempts to understand the human sense of smell and its consequences have been so limited until recently, you cannot find much consistency in the operational terms and definitions we have used over the years. That situation, fortunately, is rapidly changing.

Early researchers, for instance, at first favored "ecto-hormone" before agreeing on "pheromone." They had trouble agreeing on what was a "primary" odor. Coming to a consensus on how to control the purity and measure the strength of the odors they used to test the ability to smell consumed considerable energy.

Witness the implied ambiguities in some of the early reports. In 1918, Blakeslee reported on a single family of Russians in which some members could only smell pink verbena flowers while others could only smell red verbenas.[4] But there are different species of verbena. McWhirter, in 1969, reported that five to eight percent of the undergraduates at Oxford University could not smell freesia flowers.[5] But what strain or variety of freesia? Some freesia strains are quite fragrant; others not so.

A 1916 classification based on clinical tests came up with more than four hundred different scents, but settled for six main odors: fruity, flowery, resinous, spicy, foul, and burned or scorched. Amoore included sweaty, spermous, fishy, urinous, and musky odors in his list of more than thirty primary odors.[6]

In the late 1980s, a herculean stride was made when biopsychologists at the Monell Chemical Senses Center in Philadelphia joined forces with the National Geographic Society. In less than a year, 1.5 million men, women, and children on six continents responded to a carefully designed questionnaire and reported on their abilities to detect and identify six very carefully measured primary odors: rose, banana, cloves, musk, sweat, and mercaptan, the smell of rotten meat. Because of its unequaled size and international character, the results of this study are a major resource for this chapter.[7]

The term *anosmia* literally means "lack of the ability to smell." But the inability to smell what? Many men and women think they have an excellent sense of smell and would reject being labeled anosmic, but about half of us cannot smell androsterone, a pheromone in boar's saliva and a major aromatic element in human sweat. Should we really use the term anosmia for the one in ten Oxford undergraduates who could not smell freesia but who had no trouble recognizing other odors? Or for the Russians who could not smell pink or red verbenas?

Some researchers today prefer the terms "selective or specific hyposmia," "hypo" being the Greek prefix for "reduced, inhibited, or impaired" and "osmo," the Greek for "smell." Increasingly, the term *anosmia* is being reserved for persons who totally lack any sense of smell, although some continue to talk about "selective or specific anosmia."

In 1982, Trygg Engen estimated that only about two out of a thousand Americans were totally anosmic. That appears to be a serious underestimation in view of more recent studies, starting with an estimate of two million anosmic Americans offered by the National Advisory on Neurological and Communicative Disorders. Two million is about 1 percent of the American population, an estimate that is close to the *National Geographic* survey data in which 1.2 percent of the 1.4 million American respondents reported they experienced permanent anosmia. Two out of three in the *National Geographic* survey also reported at least one temporary experience with anosmia, usually associated with an allergy attack, a cold, the flu, or a pregnancy.

Hyperosmia, an abnormal heightened sensitivity to odor, is the opposite of hyposmia. One of our friends, a healthy woman, can identify the various ingredients in a recipe or complex fragrance. An unusual odor in the house, cigarette smoke, or cooking smells, will wake her from a deep sleep. She also reports that her sensitivity has decreased with age and attributes this to reduced hormone production.

People with faulty hormone production in the cortex of their adrenal glands, a condition known as Addison's syndrome, are extremely sensitive to odors. In terms of thresholds, they may be as much as a hundred thousand times as sensitive as persons without this disease. Fortunately, treatment with adrenal cortex hormones, gluco-corticoids like prednisone, can usually bring the smell threshold of these persons down to the normal range. [8]

A similar exaggerated sense of smell has been reported in young people with cystic fibrosis of the pancreas, although later researchers turned up conflicting results.[9]

Forty years ago, LeMagnen first reported that the sensitivity of women to certain musk-like odors varies with the menstrual cycle. Schneider calls this phenomenon a "relative hyperosmia."[10]

Anosmia has many expressions in the human population. It can be impaired or heightened, total or partial, more or less temporary or per-manent. Relatively few of us are olfactory champions, and those who are often take advantage of their sensitivity as gourmet chefs and soumiers, connoisseurs of gourmet foods and fine wines, teas, and coffees. Or in the fragrance industry, creating fine perfumes or engineering flavors and aromas to enhance the sales appeal of any product you can imagine.

Most of us operate on a somewhat less sophisticated plane, in a rather pleasant world where our olfactory systems function somewhere below the 100 percent level.

WHAT CAUSES ANOSMIA?

From what we have already seen about the evolution, anatomy, and functions of our olfactory system, we can quickly come up with some ideas about what causes the various forms of anosmia. A genetic or chromosomal origin is certainly possible. Something may also have gone wrong with the migration of GnRH neurons during fetal development, creating some problem in the hypothalamus, or in the processing circuits of the main or accessory olfactory bulbs. The toxic effects of various environmental challenges is certainly worth mentioning: the nicotine in cigarettes, prescription medications that have unexpected side effects on olfactory neurons, and a wide spectrum of infections of the olfactory and respiratory systems. We certainly do not want to pass over the possible effects of surgery, head injuries, and even trauma to the olfactory system that occurs during cosmetic and therapeutic surgery on the nose.

At present, we are far from having satisfactory explanations for the many expressions of anosmia and hyposmia, but we do have some good insights and leads.

Start with genes. The strongest case for a genetic cause of anosmia is found in adults with a malfunctioning hypothalamus that causes underdeveloped ovaries or testes and the body build and physical characteristics of a juvenile. This condition, known as Kallmann's syndrome, has been studied in patients ranging from age ten to fifty years. Men with Kallmann's tend to have no beard and poorly developed genitals. Kallmann's is rarer in women, where it causes poorly developed breasts, scant pubic hair, a small pelvis, and absence of any menses.

Individuals with Kallmann's typically experience anosmia due to a missing gene. This gene (Kalig-1) produces a protein vital to the migration of GnRH neurons into the brain, and to the connections the GnRH neurons make in the hypothalamus and in the olfactory system. When the gene is missing, structural abnormalities affect both the sense of smell and sexual development. In addition, boys and men who have Kallmann's syndrome show almost no sexual interest. They are unlikely to be sexually aroused whether alone or with a partner.[11]

One of the more common conditions involving an extra or missing chromosome, known as Turner's syndrome, affects an estimated one in three thousand newborns. This is not as common as Down's syndrome, which involves an extra copy of the number 21 chromosome. Girls with Turner's syndrome have only one X chromosome, instead of the usual two XXs.

The lack of a second X chromosome (45,XO) has many different consequences for the newborn infant and its future. The most obvious effects are physical. Since a second X chromosome is needed for functioning ovaries to develop, girls with only one X do not develop functioning ovaries. Without estrogen and progesterone from functioning ovaries, these girls do not develop the secondary sex characteristics of breasts, pubic hair, and feminine fat deposits girls usually experience at puberty. They also have no menstrual cycles. Girls with Turner's syndrome are usually given estrogen replacement to trigger development of the appropriate secondary sex characteristics.

Because they have no ovaries, these girls also fail to produce the normal small amount of testosterone that gives women their sexual drive or libido. The common theory is that the lack of any sexual interest or libido in women with Turner's syndrome is due to this missing ovarian testosterone.

But another explanation is possible. Girls with Turner's syndrome often experience language, motor, and learning deficiencies as a result of that missing second X chromosome. Might the missing second X chromosome, or the lack of ovaries and their hormones before birth, also somehow interfere with the normal development of the hypothalamus, olfactory bulbs, and/or olfactory neurons? If so, might this anosmia contribute to the lack of libido in women with Turner's syndrome?

We do know that some men with undeveloped testes have no sense of smell at all, and that women with menstrual problems often have an impaired sense of smell. Robert Henkin, at Georgetown University, has found that about a quarter of the men and women with anosmia he studied reported a loss of libido, and some of the men complained of shrinking testes and reduced beard growth. It would certainly be helpful to know how normal or deficient the olfactory sensitivity is in women with Turner's syndrome, and whether their anosmia is linked with their lack of libido.[12]

Mutant genes inherited from parents or a gene mutation early in embryonic development suggest another hypothesis. Non-smellers may lack the gene needed to make the receptors for androstenone, the key odor in human sweat. On the other hand, some people may have inactive receptors that can be awakened when challenged by exposure to this scent.[13]

In his thorough review of The Perception of Odors Trygg Engen reported that "the most common cause of anosmia is apparently head injury."[14] Sudden blows to the head can shear olfactory axons where they pass through openings in the bony plate at the base of the skull to reach the olfactory bulbs. Severed axons may grow back, but the damage may also be permanent. This type of damage is not uncommon, nor is its effect on human sexual behavior. Anecdotal evidence of the importance of the link between sex and the sense of smell may even be used as legal evidence in the form of expert testimony. At least one attorney we encountered is aware of the link between head injury, the loss of the sense of smell, and the loss of libido. We know of this attorney because he contacted Kohl after reading in the Chicago Tribune the title of his presentation at an annual meeting of the Society for the Scientific Study of Sex. "Are olfactory-hormonal relationships primary determinants of human sexual behavior?" was the presentation's title; the same question this attorney sought to answer in court. It seems a client suffered a head injury and had lost his sense of smell along with his sex drive. Although Kohl sent the attorney information from several areas of related research, he was not able to find out the outcome of this case, or whether it was settled out of court.

Douek notes that plastic surgery of the nose is also sometimes a cause of anosmia, but the data regarding such incidents is poor.[15] Recent discoveries about the ultrastructure of the VNO and the effect alleged pheromones have on the electrical activity in the human VNO makes it imperative that those doing surgery to correct a deviated nasal septum or other problem consider ways of reducing the risk of damage to the VNO.[16] Robert Henkin, former director of the Center for Sensory Disorders, Georgetown University, warns that "Sex without smells is not quite the same." Moreover, one in four people with little or no smelling ability experience a decrease in their sex drive.[17]

We do have some evidence of links between anosmia and multiple sclerosis, Parkinson's disease, chronic renal failure, consistent lack of menses, cirrhosis of the liver, vitamin B12 deficiency, and diabetes mellitus. Nasal passage polyps, overgrown adenoids, and other growths that block the access of air to the upper nasal passages have also been linked with anosmia.

Nasal and sinus infections, influenza, acute viral hepatitis, and allergic infections of the nasal passage (rhinitis) and sinuses (sinusitis) frequently lead to temporary anosmia. Smoking and some prescription medications may damage the olfactory nerves or inhibit their normal functioning.

AN INTERNATIONAL SMELL SURVEY

In 1986 and 1987, the National Geographic Society joined with Avery N. Gilbert and Charles J. Wysocki, biopsychologists at the Monell Chemical Senses Center in Philadelphia, to design a survey of our ability to detect and identify the scent of roses, cloves, bananas, a sulphur-containing gas, musk, and human sweat. The questionnaire and test samples reached members of the society in the September 1986 issue of *National Geographic* magazine as part of an article on "The Intimate Sense of Smell." On the questionnaire, readers were asked to provide the usual demographic information and to answer a series of questions about their experiences with smell. After scratching each odor sample, they could check whether or not they could detect each odor and whether or not they could identify each odor using a list of possible descriptive terms.

Even though a minuscule amount of each odor was used in each test sample, making up the tests that went to approximately a million respondents consumed a lot of test odors. A single ounce of androstenone donated for this survey would cost $200,000 on the commercial market. Each minute sample of these expensive odors was enclosed in a microscopic bubble safeguarded by a chain of polymer molecules until the spot was scratched.

The response to the survey was overwhelming and totally unexpected. A phenomenal 1.5 million men, women, boys, and girls sent their test results to the National Geographic Society. One hundred thousand results came from outside the United States. Many readers photocopied the survey and shared the odor samples with family members. Whole classes of students from the elementary school level through college responded. It will take someone working forty hours a week, fifty weeks a year, ten full years just to key the results of the surveys into a computer. Only when the data is entered can any kind of in-depth analysis be undertaken.

Meanwhile, 26,200 survey responses were randomly selected for a preliminary analysis. The results of that analysis produced some intriguing and sometimes unexpected insights into the extent and kinds of specific anosmia or hyposmia women and men experience.

To begin, nearly two out of three men and women reported having suffered a temporary loss of smell one or more times. Some 17 percent reported two or more episodes, and 2.3 percent claimed three or more episodes. Slightly over 1 percent reported a permanent loss of smell. Colds and the flu were linked with three out of four of the reported cases of temporary anosmia. Allergies were linked with 17.7 percent, and prescription medications and exposure to other chemicals with 6.2 percent of the reported incidents of partial anosmia. Head injuries and pregnancy were both associated with less than 1 percent of the temporary anosmia reports.

Pregnancy appears to reduce American women's sensitivity to odors. Pregnant American women also rated the smells of banana, sweat, and musk less intense than nonpregnant women of the same age. In other countries, pregnancy seemed to have fewer effects on women's ability to detect specific odors, and on the way they rated these odors, from weak to intense and unpleasant to pleasant. Why there was such a difference is an intriguing, unanswered question.

While past studies by other researchers typically compared the ability of smokers and nonsmokers to detect extremely low levels of odors, the National Geographic/Monell survey asked about smoking habits and measured response to odors well above the threshold level. Only a quarter of the smokers identified themselves as having an "excellent" sense of smell. Smokers reported a weaker response to sweat, cloves, and gas, a stronger response to banana and musk, and no difference from nonsmokers in their rating of rose. In general, smokers rated unpleasant odors less unpleasant and pleasant odors less pleasant than did nonsmokers.

The sense of smell also decreases with age. Men and women reach their greatest sensitivity at about age twenty, and slowly decline thereafter. At age eighty the decline for women slows; for men the rate of decline increases.

The general results of the preliminary analysis for the six odors contains some further surprises.

CLOVES (Eugenol): The warm, spicy, pungent odor of cloves had the highest rating of the six odors for both detection and identification in both men and women.

ROSE: This fragrance also achieved near universal detection, although one in five men and women could not identify it correctly.

BANANA: Like cloves and rose, the essence of banana was also easily detected by almost all the respondents, although only half of the men and women could identify it correctly.

SULPHUR-CONTAINING GAS: A mixture of mercaptans is an unpleasant odor added to natural gas as a warning. Over 97 percent of those surveyed could detect this odor, but only three out of five could identify it. A little over half of those over age sixty and only one in four persons over age eighty described the mercaptan mix as unpleasant, meaning that they are definitely at risk of not detecting a dangerous gas leak in their home or apartment.

MUSK: One in four women and one in three men could not detect the musk sample, despite its strong odor. Two out of three women and three out of four men could not identify the specific odor of musk.

SWEAT: While men have more androstenone in their armpit sweat, women are better at detecting this odor. Still, three out of ten women and one out of three men could not detect this odor. Only one in four, male and female alike, could correctly identify it. Curiously, some of those who were able to detect androstenone said it smelled musky or like urine. Others described it as a floral-like scent!

Percentages of respondents who could detect a particular odor and identify it correctly.

Eugenol	Isoamyl acetate		
Could smell it	CLOVES	ROSE	BANANA
Women	99.5%	99.5%	99.3%
Men	98.9%	99.0%	99.0%
Identified it correctly			
Women	89.6%	84.5%	52.8%
Men	83.2%	81.6%	49.4%

	Mercaptans	Galaxolide	Androstenone
Could smell it	SULPHURED GAS	MUSK	SWEAT
Women	97.8%	74.6%	70.5%
Men	97.0%	62.8%	66.7%
Identified it correctly			
Women	59.3%	34.8%	26.0%
Men	58.1%	22.9%	24.2%

When the results for androstenone from New York, Chicago, Denver, and Los Angeles were analyzed, researchers found almost identical results. When they looked at the responses from outside the United States, significant variations were evident from region to region.

Percentages of respondents in different areas of the world who could not smell androstenone.

	United States	United Kingdom	Caribbean	Asia	Latin America	Australia	Europe	Africa
Men	37.2%	30.0	29.2	25.5	24.6	24.2	24.1	21.6
Women	29.5%	20.9	17.5	17.2	17.7	17.9	15.8	14.7

Why is this specific anosmia 7 to 9 percent more common in the United States overall? And 16 percent higher than in Africa? Why is insensitivity to androstenone 6 percent higher among British men and women than it is in their counterparts on the other side of the Channel? Could genetic differences among the dominant races in the eight regions explain these results? Most of the respondents in this survey described themselves as Caucasian. So a racial theory may not hold up to scrutiny.

Reacting to these preliminary data, Gilbert and Wysocki point out that many variables might account for these results.

Perhaps people in certain regions who had difficulty detecting the scents were less likely to return the survey. Or there may have been environmental effects on the different populations. We know, for example, that repeated exposure to androstenone can improve the ability to detect it.[18]

Might Americans have greater difficulty than others in detecting androstenone because our Puritan ethic of "cleanliness is next to godliness" promotes our obsession with underarm deodorants, antiperspirants, and women shaving their underarms? Might these practices leave Americans less exposed to androstenone, and consequently less able to detect this odor?

Before we enter the twenty-first century, we can expect the data from the 1.5 million respondents will yield many more important discoveries about our sense of smell, published most likely in the *National Geographic* and a variety of papers in technical and professional journals.

FROM GRAPE JUICE TO CHATEAU YQUEM

Every time Robert Francoeur pours a glass of grape juice, clear or darkest purple, the mild fragrance reminds him of an intense, emotional experience from ten years ago. Invited to a dinner at Dick and Eva's apartment, he was ready for a wonderful experience, including pungent Hungarian paprikash chicken and the walnut, cinnamon, and apple strudel created and baked by Eva.

What no one was prepared for that evening was the aperitif Dick took without thinking from the wine rack. He was around the corner, in the already aroma-packed kitchen when without warning an overwhelming, wonderful bouquet swept through the apartment. Dick had uncorked a bottle of sauterne, a Chateau Yquem, vintage 1959.

All conversation stopped as the bouquet flooded our olfactory systems and overpowered their higher faculties. In silence, everyone savored the incredible vintage aroma.

From our birth to the grave, the joys of odors enrich and mold our days and our loves with powerful limbic memories.

14

THE HEALING POWER
OF AROMATIC OILS

Modern aromatherapy uses aromatic oils to add zest to food, to perfume the air we breath, to influence our moods, to help us lose weight, and even to cure illnesses. Its origins extend back at least thirty thousand years to when our ancestors first learned to use fire to cook food.

It is not hard to picture a cave somewhere in Europe or Asia, or perhaps an open African savannah, long before recorded history. Some unheralded women are sharing casual chit-chat as the evening meal cooks on a carefully tended fire. Extrapolating from what we know of nomadic hunter-gatherer cultures today, it is easy to imagine one of the Cro-Magnon women mentioning to her friends that her favorite recipe for roast leg of bear used cypress wood and dried leaves from a thyme bush to give the meat a special woody, nutty quality. Another woman may have admitted her preference for adding basil leaves to hickory wood to get a pepperminty but hotter flavor with a hint of thyme and licorice.

Equally plausible would be another woman in the circle commenting that her husband breathed easier when he inhaled the pleasant smoke of burning cedar wood. And another woman remarking that sick animals often got better after eating the leaves of certain plants. Her dogs, she may have reported, ate juniper berries when they had skin problems and geranium leaves when they had diarrhea.

In all likelihood, however, aromatherapy started thousands of years before Cro-Magnon women and men began to cook their food. One theory is that the medicinal use of herbs and other plants started when early nomadic hunter-gather people learned from watching animals that some plants were poisonous, some could induce or cure vomiting or diarrhea, and others could cure headaches or help digestion. Once on the track of a beneficial plant, they used four senses—sight, touch, taste, and smell—to sort out the different plants and herbs for different uses.

Another undocumented milestone in aromatherapy occurred sometime in the New Stone Age, six to nine thousand years ago, when humans discovered they could get an oily liquid by pressing olives, nuts, or the seeds from sesame, castor, and other plants. These oils added zest to cooking. They were also soothing when massaged into the skin or hair.

Known to chemists today as "fatty oils," these oils have one problem. With time, they turn rancid and develop an extremely foul smell. That problem was solved by soaking aromatic herbs in oils being stored for later use. Along the way, Neolithic man discovered that massaging herb-scented fatty oils into the skin often produced the same beneficial effect those herbs had when chewed, inhaled as smoke, or taken as a tea.

Not surprisingly, our earliest human records (Sumerian cuneiform tablets and ancient Egyptian hieroglyphics) contain references to the powerful effects of aromas. The early Sumerians celebrated the sensual and healing delights of aromatic oils from plants, herbs, and trees, and burned resinous gums like myrrh and frankincense from desert plants. Temple friezes at Karnak show Egyptian pharaohs burning incense to please their gods.

Even earlier is Shen Nung's *Herbal*, the oldest surviving medical text written in China about 4,700 years ago. With detailed information on 305 plants, the *Herbal* clearly proves that the ancient Chinese were well versed in aromatherapy. *Ayurveda* or "the knowledge of longevity," the oldest form of Indian medicine, is at least three thousand years old. This healing system, using herbs and essential oils, is still widely practiced in India as part of different massage techniques and acupressure therapy.

Glass perfume bottles in the tombs of noble men and women, ancient Chinese, Etruscans, Jews, and others, tell us they valued the charm of fragrances, whether they came from everyday herbs or were imported from distant exotic lands.

Fragrant oils were popular all over the ancient world as remedies for a variety of physical, mental, and emotional complaints. At a time when people commonly thought that bad odors were a clue to diseases, some ancients even believed that bad odors caused diseases. If this was so, then it seemed logical to assume that pleasant odors could chase away diseases in this life and after death. Embalming with fragrant spices, mainly cumin, marjoram, and cinnamon, could protect dead loved ones and prepare them for life in the next world.

Our ancestors also celebrated the immense pleasures to be gained by using fragrant essential oils to stimulate the primitive emotional centers and memories in the brain stem and limbic system. The Egyptians believed aromatic oils had almost divine power because they had been created by the gods. King Tut was buried surrounded by alabaster vessels filled with essential oils that still had their original fragrances more than three thousand years later when his tomb was opened. Ordinary Egyptian women, along with Cleopatra, enjoyed perfumes and used them to snare men.

Ancient myths traced the power of rose water and rose oil to the divine origins of the rose itself, which they said came from the blood of Adonis, the blood of Venus, or the sweat of Mohammed. Rose water is easy to make; just add rose petals to water or alcohol. Rose oil, legend says, was discovered accidentally at the wedding of a Persian princess and the Emperor Djihanguyr. A canal around the palace gardens was filled with rose petals for the pleasure of the wedding guests. As the sun heated the water, the oils in the petals separated and floated to the surface where it appeared like a scum. Once the powerful fragrance of this "scum" was discovered, it was not long before the Persians were mass producing and marketing Persian rose oil. Today, the best rose oil comes from Bulgaria, where the damask rose is grown in a mountainous area of only 240 square miles. It takes thirty roses to make one drop of Bulgarian rose oil and sixty thousand roses to make one ounce!

The early Jews bought frankincense and myrrh from Egypt or their Persian neighbors for ceremonies in the Temple of King Solomon in Jerusalem. Legendary wise men brought these same spices from the East to celebrate the birth of Jesus. Frankincense to evoke a sense of faith, inspiration, inner strength, and the spiritual. Myrrh to evoke a sense of strength, stability, confidence, and meditation.

At Roman banquets, the wings of perfumed white doves circling overhead fanned sensual air on banquet guests. After the banquet, the guests could sleep off their hangovers on saffron-stuffed pillows, or recuperate at the public baths where relaxing, therapeutic rose water scented the steam and Persian rose oil and therapeutic herbs were used for massages.

As the Roman Empire disintegrated and outsiders raided the countryside, the great cities and infrastructure of Europe disintegrated. Europeans descended into the Dark Ages. Even the touted glories of the Middle Ages palled against the rising cultures of Byzantium, the Middle East, and Asia. "A thousand years without a bath" is the way Ruth Winter sums up the European atmosphere between the fall of Rome and the Renaissance, which

> gives you an idea of how people and places smelled. Europeans had no drains, little soap, and a marked distaste for bathing. They lived in a stinking environment, where the odors from the castle drains were used to keep the moths from the lord's clothes hanging in the garderobe, which was also a lavatory. There was no refrigeration, and most cattle had to be slaughtered before the onset of winter and their meat crudely preserved; so off-tastes were added to off-odors leading to a great demand for costly spices.[1]

A thousand years ago, after Constantinople had replaced Rome and provided a bridge from India and Asia for traders bringing spices over the Silk Road from the Far East to Europe, the Muslims celebrated aroma engineering. Their paradise, Mohammed said, would contain three pleasures: women, children, and perfume. Sandalwood, musk, incense, rose water, and other scents were treasured in the harems. They even mixed a little musk in their cement to enhance the spiritual, otherworldly atmosphere of their mosques with a sensual power.[2]

During the Christian Crusades to liberate the Holy Land from the Moslems in the eleventh, twelfth, and thirteenth centuries, Christian princes found profit in licensing traders to import spices and perfumes from the Middle East, especially when they sacked Constantinople between 1204 and 1261. Of course, only the rich few in Europe could afford these luxuries; the vast majority of Europeans were serfs and suffered in a world of stenches.

Still, the Crusades sporadically opened trade with India and the Orient, permitting herbalists and perfumers to expand their knowledge of aromatherapy and make it a major element of medieval medicine and culture. When the Black Death swept across Europe, killing millions, physicians of the time protected themselves head to toe with black leather garments. A long beak on their hood was packed with a potent combination of incense, mace, wormwood, myrrh, aloes wood, musk, ambergris from whales, nutmegs, myrtle, bay, rosemary, sage, roses, elder, cloves, juniper, rue, and pitch to ward off the plague and its stench.

In 1261 this temporary door to the spices of the East closed when Byzantine rule was restored to Constantinople, and the Muslim Ottoman Turks renamed the city Istanbul. With the overland route to spice-rich China, India, and Ceylon blocked, Columbus sailed west to open a new land of spice in the Americas. Portuguese explorers found a way around Africa to bypass the high cost of dealing with the Arab middlemen. New uses were discovered for spices that made them ever more desirable. With spices used to disguise rancid meats and liven up a bland diet, the Renaissance celebrated a fragrant world.

During the eighteenth century, the birth of chemistry opened the door to modern aromatherapy as inquisitive experimenters found ways to mimic the aromas of plant extracts with chemical compounds.

In our own century, the ancient wisdom of using essential oils for therapy began to reemerge when the French chemist Renée Gattefosse discovered the beneficial properties of lavender oil. Most people know lavender as a common component in potpourris, sachets, toilet waters, and dried bouquets. Few know that it has long been widely regarded as the most useful and versatile medicinal oil. In his book on *The Art of Aromatherapy*, Robert Tisserand reports that lavender oil is widely used by herbalists to treat abscesses, acne, asthma, boils, bronchitis, burns, carbuncles, colic, convulsions, depression, dermatitis, diarrhea, on to influenza, insomnia, and migraine headaches, and down to typhoid fever, vomiting, and whooping cough.

Until the Age of Aquarius burst forth in American youth of the 1960s, Americans were satisfied with a rather limited bouquet of aromas, potpourris and sachets: Chanel for some, White Shoulders or Evening in Paris for others. And of course, Old Spice for the men to splash on after a shave.

In the scent revolution that came with the sexual revolution, the flower children dumped Old Spice and White Shoulders when they embraced the natural muskiness of sex without guilt and soap. Soon musk fragrances were being advertised as the inescapable invitation to the bedroom. What followed was an unabashed explosion of personal scents for both men and women that seems likely to continue to grow with eighty new fragrances introduced each Christmas season. Meanwhile, the chemists continue their quest for that elusive pheromone that would draw men and women together as irresistibly as the pheromones of a boar or of a moth work their lusty lure.

MODERN AROMATHERAPY

It is a long way from these unrecorded milestones to the fragrance-deluged world in which American men and women spend five billion dollars a year on personal fragrances. The worldwide fragrance market reached $12.5 billion in 1991.[3] We swim in a world of synthesized scents created by chemists to hype the sale of everything from taco chips and fake "buttered" popcorn to kitty litter, lemon-scented garbage bags, watches, compact disc recordings, and dolls. In late 1994, a French petroleum refinery began adding a vanilla scent to their gasoline and lemon scent to their diesel fuel.

In recent years, chemists have been recruited by manufacturers of all kinds to help them exploit the primitive emotions and moods that spring to life when particular odors find their way to our limbic emotions. Today's world drowns the subtle aromas of nature in a kind of inescapable "Muzak for the nose." That is the blunt description Richard Dodd, founder of Coconut Grove, an environmental design firm in Miami, Florida, uses to describe our world of engineered odors.

Dodd's business logic is simple, and characteristic of both ancient and modern aroma engineers. We design the environments we work, play, eat, and sleep in to make them more pleasant and enjoyable. Every day American businesses spend billions of dollars to create the desired mood. Spaces are carefully and expensively sculptured with color, furnishings, carpets, drapes, and yes, Muzak.

Today's aromatherapy adds a new dimension to this environmental engineering. A few years ago, Richard Dodd convinced a Florida Marriott Hotel to let him bathe their lobby in a subliminal stress-relieving blend of jasmine, orange blossom, lemon, peppermint, and lavender in the hope of making their customers recall their pleasant time at Marriott.[4] Dr. Alan Hirsch, who set up his own Smell and Taste Treatment and Research Foundation in Chicago, has made news in Las Vegas when his aroma engineering at a Las Vegas casino increased the patrons' spending by 53 percent.[5]

Aroma engineering is already an exploding field, big business, and likely to get much bigger as the research breakthroughs described earlier are applied to practical commercial, medical, and educational uses. In ten years, aromatherapy has grown from ground zero to a quarter of a billion dollars in sales in 1994.[6] The range of applications seems unlimited. At the Monell Chemical Senses Center in Philadelphia Gisela Epple is studying the effects of specific odors on children in stressful situations. At Bowling Green State University in Ohio, psychologist Peter Badia is studying the effect of odors on sleep and the kind of dreams we have. At the University of Minnesota, psychologist Mark Snyder has found that a person cannot have a relationship with somebody whose smell she or he does not like.

We may also encounter scent-engineered environments when visiting a doctor, chiropractor, hair stylist, local hospital, at the office, work, or health club, or while shopping or flying overseas on some airlines. At the mall, we may detect a distinct potpourri scent outside Victoria's Secret, or a relaxing, spiritual mix of eucalyptus, spearmint, lavender, and geranium at the New Age bookstore. Essential oils are everywhere in our world.

Oils? Slippery, soothing, viscous, smelly liquids lubricate the moving pistons and cam shafts in our cars and motors. Oils heat our homes and provide light. Essential oils, those that aroma engineers and therapists use, are different.

Like our less aesthetic fatty oils, essential oils are made by plants and trees. Petroleum oils come from plant material decomposing under pressure inside the earth's crust over thousands of years. Essential oils, by contrast, are made in the chloroplasts of living leaves. Some of these colorless, volatile, water-insoluble molecules, like the oil of turpentine, are not pleasant to smell; others are pleasingly fragrant.

Essential oils come from a variety of plant parts—calamus oil from the aromatic roots of a flower called sweet flag, the oils of rosemary and thyme from leaves of those plants, and the oils of lavender, clove, and rose from flowers. Cinnamon oil is found in the bark of laurel-like trees in Ceylon and the East Indies, black pepper oil in dried berries, orange and lemon oils in the rinds of those fruits, and myrrh and amber in the sap or resin of plants.

The quality of a particular essential oil varies depending on what part of the plant it is extracted from and the season of year or time of day it is harvested. Climate, the way the plant is cultivated, and the kind of soil it grows in, also affect the quality of an essential oil, just as they affect the quality, flavor, and bouquet of coffee beans or teas. Rose oil from Bulgaria is exquisite, cinnamon from Sri Lanka the best.

Unlike more stable fatty oils, aromatic essential oils are highly volatile and quickly evaporate into the air. This characteristic makes the essential oils produced by flowers a key factor in attracting bees for pollination.

Essential oils are soluble in alcohol and ether, but not in water. When heated, however, individual molecules of essential oils quickly evaporate and mix temporarily with heated water molecules. Chemists call this simple process steam distillation. Put the leaves, bark, fruit, root, or sap in a vat; pass steam over it and the heated essential oils are released to mix with the steam. Cool the steam and the essential oils separate from the water so they can be skimmed off.

Chemists also extract essential oils with ether, or soak plant material in alcohol to dissolve them. When chilled to a precise temperature, the essential oil solidifies and can be separated out. This solid oil is known as an "absolute oil." Chemists also use the term "absolute oil" to refer to the particularly heavy and concentrated oils extracted from rose, jasmine, carnation, and tuberous begonias.

Mechanical extraction is also used for some essential oils. When an orange is peeled and the rind bent, tiny capsules of a fragrant essential oil burst into a mist. Squeeze that oil into a burning match and it burns momentarily. The essential oils of lemon, lime, tangerine, and orange, are squeezed or pressed from the rind or peel after it is separated from the fruit.

USING AROMAS

Japanese industrialists claim that scientific circulation of appropriate aromas through an office air-conditioning system improves the productivity, efficiency, and concentration of their clerical staffs. A whiff of lemon in the morning wakes the staff up to the challenges of the day. Just before lunch comes the soothing scent of rose, followed by a late-afternoon perk-up bouquet of "tree-trunk-oil." They say it works.[7]

At the world-famous Sloan-Kettering Cancer Center in New York City, anxious, nervous patients are relaxed for magnetic resonance imaging (MRI) scans with the fragrance of vanilla. Researchers at Case

Western Research University of Dentistry recently reported that a floral fragrance diffused throughout a dentist's office significantly reduced anxiety among patients waiting to undergo root canals. Diana McNab, a sports psychologist and professor at Seton Hall university in New Jersey, uses vanilla to relax her athletes for coaching and counseling, and lemon, peppermint, and evergreen to stimulate. At Duke University, Dr. Susan Schiffman, who has done extensive research on fragrance, says a whiff of peppermint, menthol, or eucalyptus can give a definite pick-up before a workout or game.[8] In 1993, Perfume Company of Newtown Connecticut marketed a new fragrance, Vanilla Fields, to play on the calming effect of vanilla.

A complementary aromatherapy kit helps first-class passengers on Virgin Atlantic Airways relax during their flight and arrive refreshed. To relieve residual anxiety and irritability from the drive to the airport, parking, and check-in, the kit provides lavender oil. Lavender dabbed on the temples, behind the ears, in the hollow of the neck, and on the back of the hands and the tops of the feet soothes the nerves and encourages a restful take-off. Later, just before landing, passengers are treated to a triple wake-up bouquet. Dabs of stimulating lemon-grass oil are absorbed into the blood stream and wake up the body and brain. Eucalyptus oil gives a jolt to the nasal sinuses and probably also to the emotional centers of the limbic system. And a peppermint mouth rinse prepares the traveler for a warm welcome at the gate or baggage claim area, or at least freshens the mind for the business ahead.

The fragrance of fresh-baked bread is a classic, often irresistible, turn-on for shoppers. One Connecticut supermarket chain has gained customer approval and enhanced its appeal by recycling the aroma of its bakery throughout the store. Many supermarkets have their bakeries in the front of the store so that shoppers are bathed with hunger-stirring aroma as soon as they walk into the store.

Ordinary restaurants use colorful, fresh, inexpensive carnations on their tables, forgetting that carnations have the smell of the dead because they are so often used in funeral displays. Roses provide a more congenial and relaxing floral accompaniment for a fine feast. Few things can spoil a carefully crafted gourmet bouquet like garlic residue on a kitchen knife used on a dish that should have no hint of garlic. Gourmets also warn about the residue smell of a detergent on glassware or of scented soap on the hands after a visit to the restroom.

Scents do more than improve productivity and enhance gourmet banquets. No one knows that better than Procter and Gamble, Lever Brothers, Colgate, and others who spend billions of dollars a year for hundreds of millions of pounds of fragrances to mix into their soaps, detergents, fabric softeners, disposable diapers, hair shampoos, and conditioners in the quest for more sales.

Yet even those who are ecologically minded and think they are immune to all the hype of enticing, irresistible smells are mistaken. Millions of years of odor exposure have conditioned us to spontaneously gravitate to and buy nicely scented products. Our environmentally sensitive search for all-natural products may pull us to the "unscented" toilet paper, but even there a *soft smell* hidden in the "unscented" paper reinforces our "squeeze test." We are hooked by our nose despite good intentions. Even Ivory Soap, which advertises that it is 99.44 percent pure has its own unique perfume, which also shows up in its dishwashing detergent.

Fifty years ago, as the Germans cleaned up the bombed-out areas of their country, they used a common, cheap, and easily available disinfectant, chlorine. The pungent odor of chlorine was linked with the painful memories of war's devastation in the memory circuits of German limbic systems. Even today, Germans prefer pine-fresh scented cleaning products and avoid any hint of chlorine.

"Pine-fresh" is by far the most popular scent for women in other lands besides Germany. American and Brazilian women love it. Venezuelan women love it so much they want ten times as much pine fragrance in their floor cleaners as American women get. In Venezuela family reputations can be enhanced by the strong "pine-fresh" scent that drifts out open windows twice a day to tell everyone, "this house has really clean floors."

"Pine-fresh" does not always win out, especially when it comes to body fragrances. Romance-inclined French women prefer fragrances with sophisticated, exotic, warm flowery notes. Jasmine-based scents are popular, perhaps because the most fragrant jasmine bushes in the world are very common in southern France. But this popularity raises an unanswered question that goes beyond French preferences: why is jasmine almost universally described as "seductive" and "romantic?"

In a similar vein, what about sandalwood? In Bali, famed for its sensual dance and erotic character, Indonesian women prefer fragrances that combine sandalwood with floral scents.

Japanese culture emphasizes simple and delicate beauty in which every detail has meaning, whether it be in its traditional sparsely furnished home, in the presentation of a meal, or in an exquisitely simple meditative Zen garden. Japanese women prefer delicate, fine fragrances, and avoid the blunt, obvious scents Americans often favor.

As for men and the fragrances they prefer for themselves and their women, that depends. Should it be an earthy fragrance with a contemporary twist, a bracing blend of citrus, herbs, and woods for the man of action, a distinctively assertive masculine scent, a warm sensuous musk, or easy-going cool nautical? Yet it is not really his choice because women generally select the fragrance they prefer on their men and give that aftershave lotion or body cologne to them as a present. After a man knows what turns on the woman he wants to attract, he naturally repeats with the scent she likes. As for men buying a perfume for a woman friend, forget it! The woman knows her moods best and whether her body chemistry goes well with light and ethereal or heavy and musky, rich floral or exotic woods warmed with amber, the harmony of fruits and flowers or the freshness of an ocean breeze, a sophisticated feminine or a seductive Oriental palette.

As for the home, a potpourri of rosemary perhaps with touches of eucalyptus, geranium, juniper berry, and bergamot in the morning can be stimulating. Many tea drinkers are drawn to Earl Gray tea, which is flavored with bergamot. Tangerine can bring cheer and light to the ordinary and mundane. At night, a bouquet of neroli, chamomile, lavender, and rose relaxes one for sleep. Ylang Ylang, a tropical Asian essential oil used in Bali as a scent for the wedding bed and in expensive massage oils, brings an appreciation of beauty.

Bottled "Peace of Mind" sleep inducers, energy boosters, and stress relievers. Sensuality, tranquility, exhilaration, and euphoria. Scented body splashes, soaps, and shower gels to beautify, soothe, cool, or heat.

TOMORROW'S FANTASY WORLD

In its early years after coming from Europe, the American flavor and fragrance industry was closely associated with the fashion industry and centered in New York City. Today fifty-two of the seventy-five American companies dealing in flavors and fragrances have their headquarters just west of the Hudson River, in New Jersey.

In its early years, the focus was on perfumes and toilet waters for women, a few aftershave lotions, fragrances for soaps and household cleaning products, and flavors for chewing gums, desserts, and beverages. Then, some fifty years ago, the industry took a quantum leap forward when flavor chemists decided to find out what it was that made raspberries smell and taste the way they do. They found the key chemical was a relatively small molecule called a ketone that could be easily duplicated by chemists. This discovery opened the door to modern flavor and fragrance engineering.

In the 1970s, consumers' advocacy groups forced the food industry to display the word "artificial" on the labels on all products containing nature's flavors duplicated in the laboratory. In American culture, the adjectives "synthetic" and "artificial" carry very strong negative overtones. They raise strong suspicions that such flavors and fragrances are "unnatural," meaning second-rate or, even worse, unhealthy—possibly dangerous, even poisonous.

The reality is that "synthetic," "artificial," "laboratory-created" raspberry flavor and other synthetic aroma/flavors are chemically identical with those found in nature. Natural and duplicated flavors and fragrances contain the same identical chemicals, arranged in the same structure so that they fit the receptors in our taste buds and nasal passages. Smell receptors in the upper nasal passages and in the VNO cannot tell the difference between natural odors and flavors and those duplicated in the laboratory.

There are, however, some real differences, though probably not the ones you might expect. The duplicated aromas and flavors are much more reliable and consistent than the variable flavors and aromas extracted from natural fruit and flowers. Since they can be produced by combining chemicals off the shelf, laboratory flavors and fragrances do not require the destruction of natural resources. Most important from a business viewpoint, they are much less expensive. It costs $35 to extract a pound of strawberry essence from a large number of fresh perishable strawberries that must be processed at their fragrance peak. A pound of the same essence can be duplicated in laboratory flasks for only $4. Small wonder our world is becoming more and more fragrant.

What about the future links between smell and sexuality?

In 1974, George Dodd, at Warwick University in England, isolated and identified alpha-androstenol, a hormone in male sweat, the "first direct-acting human sex pheromone." Ten years later this fragrance was incorporated into the world's first pheromone-containing perfume/cologne, Jovan's Andron for Men and Andron for Women, in 1983. Jovan White Musk for Women followed in 1990 and Jovan White Musk for Men in 1992.

In 1993, Quintessence took Jovan Musk another step by introducing Jovan Musk2, "a pheromone-based cologne designed to trigger a sensual reaction between the sexes." Laboratory duplicated alpha-androstenol is advertised as the "ultimate sensory ingredient" in Jovan Musk2. Combined with vetiver, vanilla, storax, sandalwood, amber, and African cedar, alpha-androstenol provides a "truly masculine yet irresistibly sexy, romantic fragrance."

Another company developing and marketing pheromone-containing perfumes is EROX, organized in 1992. Among the scientific consultants for EROX are many of the leading researchers whose work we have mentioned in this book. David Berliner, a former Professor of Anatomy at the University of Utah, has identified some twenty human pheromones and is the founder of EROX and president, CEO, and Director of its Pherin division. Jose Garcia-Velasco, Lawrence Stensaas, David Moran and Thomas Getchell, experts on the VNO; and Richard Michael and Luis Monti-Bloch, experts on human pheromones, also work with EROX.[9]

EROX claims that it has synthesized the first human pheromones that can alter people's moods by triggering feelings of self-confidence and relaxation. This company hopes to capture a 1 percent share of the $4.9 billion U.S. market within two years of its "fragrances-plus" approach. EROX doesn't claim its fragrances will turn the human wearer into an irresistible magnet for every person of the other sex within a mile or two, as the queen bee pheromone does with drones or the canine estrous pheromone does for males within a mile or two. "It's not a sex attractant," Pierre de Champfleury, president of EROX, says. Rather, "It's about feeling better about yourself. It's about creating a sense of well-being."[10]

The EROX fragrances combine synthesized pheromones with perfumery formulations that affect the brain through the olfactory system. Ann Gottlieb, a fragrance consultant for EROX, describes the women's scent as warm semioriental with a touch of brightness on top. "The men's also is a semioriental, but much more crisp."[11]

Of course, television talk show hosts are already having a field day with these new fragrances. Winifred Cutler told "The Montel Williams Show" audience that the fragrance additive she developed and is marketing as Athena Pheromone 10:13 contains a secret formula with human pheromones. Is her formula, containing the adrenal hormone DHEA, the love potion for women that she claims it is? Cutler says that a similar "love potion for men wouldn't work." According to her, "in biology . . . you don't have the male luring the female. You have the female, her role is to lure and to choose from among the ones that pursue which one she wants. And the male's role is to get it up and move toward the female."[12] Other evidence from EROX, and even some comments from the studio audience, suggests that, in biology, males do lure females—and that the pheromones of the male are part of the lure.

Marilyn Miglin describes her years of research in ancient Egyptian temples, uncovering "astonishingly complex and unforgettable formulas" that she translated into a Masterpiece Fragrance she has named Pheromone. Pheromone's "vibrant blend of ingredients" includes jasmine blossoms gathered in full bloom before dawn, Tonka extract from the Ambrette seeds of a rare tree in Venezuela soaked in rum, orange blossom oil, lotus blossoms from Marrakesh, sacred Egyptian Kypri, provocative Cyprinium, and mysterious Mendesium. "The incredible formula also includes Ylang-Ylang, Fo-ti-tieng, Aegyptium, Penny Royal, Iris, Rosemary, Sandlewood, Attar of Rose, Patchouli, Lotus Palm, and Oak Moss." None of her ingredients meets the criteria of a true human pheromone, but formulas like this and pheromones containing human pheromones are perfect for audience participants on television talk shows to test in the field and then report back to the nation on their wonderful effectiveness.[13]

Behind the television and media hype, however, is some very serious research on fragrances and their effects on human behavior and sexuality.

In the near future, we will enjoy convenience foods and snacks, as well as balanced full meals, that have all the fragrance and taste appeal of Mother Nature's best with the added advantage of fewer calories, less sugar, and less fat. The goal of Ungerer & Company, a 100-year-old New Jersey fragrance and flavor company, is to create a time-released microscopic container, a liposome, that can deliver a fatty scent/taste to restore the appeal of low fat prepared foods without adding calories and fat.[14]

In the near future, foods and other products will be designed with enhanced fragrances and flavors to compensate for the our declining sensitivity to odors and tastes.

In the near future, we will know whether a specially scented nasal inhaler will provide a safe and effective way to lose weight and keep it off. Alan Hirsch has already tested such an inhaler containing an odor faintly reminiscent of Fritos corn chips. The more his 3,193 overweight patients sniffed, the more weight they lost, an average of thirty pounds over six months.[15] A nasal inhaler will soon be available to suppress the cravings of chocoholics.[16]

In the near future, home gourmets deciding what to cook will be influenced by "scratch and sniff" cook books.

Aroma engineering will make our experience at the movies much more realistic with the authentic *Scent of a Woman* permeating the theater as we watch and listen to the film. In 1994, the Fox Television Network promoted a few days of sensory enhanced programming. The viewing audience could purchase both 3D glasses and "scratch and sniff" cards to be used "on cue" when the programs aired.

Meanwhile, Robert Moss and his team of researchers continue to add details to the complex relationships among pheromones, other social or sexual stimuli, the VNO, the main olfactory system, and the activation of genes in GnRH-secreting nerve cells in the hypothalamus and in other limbic structures.[17] They have already shown that pheromones and gene activation in GnRH neurons are linked both directly and indirectly (through other hormones—including neurotransmitters—and their receptors) to the mating behavior of rats. This cause and effect relationship between pheromones and behavior is paralleled in studies of many other species.[18]

Anne Perkins and her colleagues are also continuing to offer additional insight into the important influence GnRH has on levels of other hormones. These hormones and their receptors play a primary role in sexual differentiation of the brain, exerting especially powerful effects on structures of the limbic system that correlate well with the sexual orientation and the sexual behavior of sheep.[19]

We have alreay cited the works of Simon LeVay and of Dean Hamer whose studies of human neuroanatomy and of human genetics correlate well with what we know about human sexuality from the study of other animals.[20] The recent release of Bruce McEwen's book,

The Hostage Brain, extends the availability of easy-to-read information about genes, nerve cells, hormones, sexual differentiation of the brain, and behavior.[21]

The scientific research is ongoing, and what we have referred to as Ariadne's thread—the biological consistency among species—is ever more apparent. Yet, even our current knowledge tells us that the pheromones of other mammals are not the only social-environmental stimuli to infleunce genes. These genes are found in nerve cells that secrete GnRH. This hormone, GnRH, "the biological core of mammalian reproduction" is secreted from the hypothalamus and from structures of the limbic system. And the influence odors have on GnRH secretion is essential to the interface between the social environment, the brain, and the behavior of many other species.

Many of the studies we have cited show that pheromones influence our physiology and behavior in the same way that they influence the physiology and behavior of these other species. We have provided you with both scientific and anecdotal information about the influence of odors on human courtship behaviors, on many other human behaviors, and on the probable cause and effect relationships between pheromones and human sexual behavior. Now, we ask that you consider this question: Are human odors—the subliminal scents called pheromones—the scents of eros?

As you consider this question, keep in mind that the beginning of the twenty-first century and the start of a new millennium are only a scant five years away! This turning point is close enough for us to recall the analysis Havelock Ellis offered at the beginning of the twentieth century, when he wrote that:

> No sense has so strong a power of suggestion, the power of calling up ancient memories with a wider and deeper emotional reverberation, while at the same time no sense furnishes impressions which so easily change emotional color and tone, in harmony with the recipient's general attitude. Odors are thus specially apt both to control the emotional life and to become its slaves.[22]

It seems equally appropriate to parallel this turn-of-the-century appraisal of the connection between the sense of smell and our sexuality with a statement from another leading sexologist who has been at the forefront of research on the connections between genes, nerve cells, hormones, and human sexual behavior. Admittedly, we cited this fore-cast by John Money earlier in this book, but it provides an appropriate postscript and a prelude to speculation about what our continued research into the web of connections between odors, pheromones, genes, nerve cells, hormones, neurotransmitters, sexual development, and sexual behavior holds for us:

> This new knowledge will, in all probability, enforce a complete rewrite of the differentiation and development of human sexuality and eroticism early in the twenty-first century.[23]

NOTES AND
REFERENCES

INTRODUCTION:
RASPBERRIES AND THE BIRTH OF THIS BOOK

1. A. Karlen, *Sexuality and Homosexuality: The Complete Account of Male and Female Sexual Behaviour and Deviation—With Case Histories* (London: MacDonald, 1971), 402.

2. J. V. Kohl, "Luteinizing Hormone: The Link Between Sex and the Sense of Smell?" (paper presented at the annual meeting of the Society for the Scientific Study of Sex, San Diego, California, 1992).

3. R. T. Francoeur et al., "Hormones and Human Sexual Behavior," Symposium: annual meeting of the Society for the Scientific Study of Sex, Chicago, Illinois, 1993; J. V. Kohl, "Are Olfactory-Hormonal Relationships Primary Determinants of Human Sexual Behavior?" (poster session at the annual meeting of the Society for the Scientific Study of Sex, Chicago, Illinois, 1993); "Olfaction, the Endocrine System and Human Sexual Behavior?" (symposium presentation at the annual meeting of the Society for the Scientific Study of Sex, Chicago, Illinois, 1993).

4. A. Perkins, "Hormones and the Behavioral Response of Male-Oriented Rams to Rams or Estrous Ewes" (symposium presentation at the annual meeting of the Society for the Scientific Study of Sex, Chicago, Illinois, 1993); A. Perkins and J. A. Fitzgerald, "Luteinizing Hormone, Testosterone, and Behavioral Response of Male-Oriented Rams to Estrous Ewes and Rams," *Journal of Animal Sciences* 70 (1992): 1787–94; A. Perkins, J. A. Fitzgerald, and E. O. Price, "Luteinizing Hormone and Testosterone Response of Sexually Active and Inactive Rams," *Journal of Animal Sciences* 70 (1992): 2086–93.

5. E. Coleman, "Compulsive Sexual Behavior: New Concepts and Treatments," *Journal of Psychology and Human Sexuality* 4 (1991): 37–52; "The Role of Psychotropic Medications on Hormonal Pathways and in Human Sexual Behavior" (symposium presentation at the annual meeting of the Society for the Scientific Study of Sex, Chicago, Illinois, 1993); E. Coleman and J. Cesnik, "Skoptic Syndrome: The Treatment of an Obsessional Gender Dysphoria with Lithium Carbonate and Psychotherapy," *American Journal of Psychotherapy* 44 (1990): 204–17.

6. Kohl, "Olfaction, the Endocrine System and Human Sexual Behavior?"
7. Kohl, "Are Olfactory-Hormonal Relationships Primary Determinants of Human Sexual Behavior?"

CHAPTER 1: THE MYSTERY OF ODOR

1. J. Money, *The Destroying Angel* (New York: Prometheus Books, 1985), 195.
2. H. Ellis, *Studies in the Psychology of Sex: Sexual Selection in Man*, vol. 4 (Philadelphia: Davis, 1914), 46.
3. Cited in Irving Bieber, "Olfaction in Sexual Development and Adult Sexual Organization," *American Journal of Psychotherapy* 13 (1959): 852.
4. Bieber, 851.
5. L. Thomas, "Notes of a Biology-Watcher: On Smell," *New England Journal of Medicine* 302 (1980): 731–33.
6. J. V. Kohl, "Luteinizing Hormone: The Link Between Sex and the Sense of Smell?" (paper presented at the annual meeting of the Society for the Scientific Study of Sex, San Diego, Calif., 1992); R. T. Francouer, "On the Scent of a Lover," *Forum* (November 1993): 40–45.
7. M. Schleidt, "The Semiotic Relevance of Human Olfaction: A Biological Approach," in S. Van Toller and G. H. Dodd, eds., *Fragrance: The Psychology and Biology of Perfume* (Amsterdam: Elsevier Applied Science, 1992).
8. As we will see later, humans have a pair of vomeronasal organs (VNO), a key structure in the detection of pheromones in both humans and other mammals. As of 1994, other parts of the accessory olfactory system which have been documented and studied in other mammals have not been found in humans. Also, while the VNO in humans does respond to specific pheromones in clinical tests, the mechanism behind this response is not known at present.
9. Cited by Schleidt, 38.
10. P. MacLean, "The Brain's Generation Gap: Some Human Implications," *Zygon: Journal of Religion and Science* 8 (June 1973): 113–27; A. Walsh *The Sciece of Love: Understanding Love and Its Effects on Mind and Body* (New York: Prometheus Books, 1991).
11. A. Kohn and F. Fish, "Wasted Resources/Missed Opportunities," *Journal of Irreproducible Results* 38, no. 1 (1993): 15.
12. G. Brum, L. McKane, and G. Karp, *Biology: Exploring Life*, 2d ed. (New York: John Wiley and Sons, 1994), 518–38.
13. Geneticists say such genes have a pleiotropic effect.
14. J. Cohen and I. Stewart, *The Collapse of Chaos* (New York: Viking Penguin, 1994); "Our Genes Aren't Us," *Discover* 15 (April): 78–84.
15. "In addition to environmental factors, genetic differences have also been demonstrated to be important. In a series of studies, Yamazaki and his colleagues have convincingly shown that differences in the H-2 major histocompatibility locus of the mouse, *Mus musculus*, particularly in the H2-K and Qa: Tla regions of chromosome 17, result in individual odor differences." [Z. T. Halpin,

"Individual Odors Among Mammals," in J. S. Rosenblatt et al., eds., *Advances in the Study of Behavior*, vol. 16 (Orlando: Academic Press, 1986), 53]. Because the mice within an inbred strain are genetically so similar, sharing as they do the same MHC genes and 98 percent of the rest of their genes, they are very close to being identical twins. See also: K. Yamazaki et al., "Recognition Among Mice: Evidence From the Use of a Y-Maze Differentially Scented by Congenic Mice of Different Major Histocompatibility Types," *Journal of Experimental Medicine* 150 (1979): 755–60, and A. N. Gilbert et al., "Olfactory Discrimination of Mouse Strains (*Mus musculus*) and Major Histocompatibility Types by Humans (*Homo sapiens*)," *Journal of Comparative Psychology* 100 (1986): 262–65.

16. Halpin, 49.

17. Gilbert et al.

18. See also: L. Gedda, D. Casa, and M. Comparetti, "Twin Zygosity Diagnosis: Experiments with Bloodhounds," *Rivista Di Biologica* 73 (1980): 95–97; J. N. Labows and G. Preti, "Human Semiochemicals," in Van Toller and Dodd, *Fragrance*, 84.

19. We are not ignoring or denying the importance of creative, artistic, nonlinear knowledge and "lateral thinking." Our focus and interests here are on the scientific method and its limitations, in an effort to understand a specific question about how odors and the sense of smell might affect and influence animal and human behavior.

CHAPTER 2: IN THE DARKEST NIGHT

1. H. E. Fisher, *Anatomy of Love* (New York: W. W. Norton, 1992), 41.

2. L. Thomas, "Notes of a Biology-Watcher. A Fear of Pheromones," *New England Journal of Medicine* 285 (1971).

3. Bert Holldobler and Edward O. Wilson of Harvard University co-authored the Pulitzer-Prize winning book *The Ants* (Cambridge, Mass.: Harvard University Press, 1990). In 1994, two new studies show that two different species of male moths respond to the down-wind trails of female pheromones in much the same way as the ants deal with pheromone-based food trails laid down by previous ant explorers.

4. M. Jacobson, *Insect Sex Attractants* (New York: Interscience Publishers, 1965).

5. E. O. Wilson, *Sociology: The New Synthesis* (Cambridge, Mass.: Harvard University Press, 1975).

6. H. H. Shorey, *Animal Communication by Pheromones* (New York: Academic Press, 1976).

7. Our descriptive definition is based on several technical definitions proposed by P. Karlson and M. Luscher, "'Pheromones': A New Term for a Class of Biologically Active Substances," *Nature* 183 (1959): 55; *Dorland's Illustrated Medical Dictionary*, 27th ed., s.v. "Pheromones," 1279; J. Bancroft and J. M. Machover-Reinisch, *Adolescence and Puberty* (New York: Oxford University Press, 1990), 55–59; and W. B. Cutler, *Love Cycles: The Science of Intimacy* (New York: Villard, 1991). In the same year that the term *pheromone* was

introduced, Irving Bieber published "Olfaction in Sexual Development and Adult Sexual Organization" (*American Journal of Psychotherapy* 13 [1959]: 851–59). What makes Bieber's theory that the sense of smell is the primary sense involved in development of the human sexual response was his comment that ". . . there are instances where it can be demonstrated that most individuals react to an odor without awareness" (851).

8. This web linking pheromones with genes, hormones, and neurotransmitters with sexual development and behavior is complicated by the fact that pheromones are produced by the breakdown of cholesterol and pregnenolone produced by the adrenal glands, while at the same time the sex hormones derived from cholesterol and pregnenolone influence sexual development and behavior. Behind the dual influence of GnRH as a hormone and as a neurotransmitter on sexual development and sexual behavior is the trigger of pheromones.

9. G. K. Beauchamp, K. Yamazaki, and E. A. Boyse, "The Chemosensory Recognition of Genetic Individuality," *Scientific American* 253 (1985).

10. Musk or muscone, 3-methyl cyclopentadecanone, is obtained from the musk deer. Civet or civetone, cis-9-cyclopentadecanone, comes from the civet cat. Both compounds are similar in structure to the musk-smelling compounds found in both humans and boars. See B. H. Kingston, "The Chemistry and Olfactory Properties of Musk, Civet, and Castoreum," Proceedings of the Second International Congress on Endocrinology, 1964.

11. D. R. Melrose, H. C. B. Reed, and R. L. S. Patterson, "Androgen Steroids Associated with Boar Odour as an Aid to the Detection of Oestrus in Pig Artificial Insemination," *British Veterinary Journal* 127 (1971); M. Schleidt, "The Semiotic Relevance of Human Olfaction: A Biological Approach," in S. Van Toller and G. H. Dodd, eds., *Fragrance: The Psychology and Biology of Perfume* (Amsterdam: Elsevier Applied Science, 1992), 41.

12. R. C. Camphausen, *The Encyclopedia of Erotic Wisdom* (Rochester, Vermont: Inner Traditions International, 1991), 197; P. Langley-Danysz, "La Truffe, un Aphrodisiaque," *La Recherche* 136 (1982): 1059; P. Redgrove, *The Black Goddess and the Sixth Sense* (London: Bloomsbury, 1987).

13. R. T. Francouer, "Experimental Embryology as a Tool for Saving Endangered Animal Species," in R. D. Martin, ed., *Breeding Endangered Species in Captivity* (New York: Academic Press, 1975), 357–60.

14. A. LeGuerer, *Scent: The Mysterious and Essential Powers of Smell* (New York: Turtle Bay Books, 1992), 8.

15. F. H. Bronson, "Rodent Pheromones," *Biology of Reproduction* 4 (1971): 344–57.

16. While it is natural odor and not a pheromone, the noxious scent of rotten meat, mercaptan, attracts scavengers and warns off other animals not adapted to eating carrion. Gas companies add this alarm odor to odorless natural gas to warn us of the danger of leaking gas.

17. These structures include the hypothalamus and limbic system of the brain, where smells trigger emotions, initiate the sex hormone production system, and control various sexual behaviors.

18. The labels we use to classify different pheromones are arbitrary. In the literature, one finds various labels used by different researchers and writers. In addition to signaling or releaser pheromones and primer pheromones, some refer to
a kind of "imprinter" pheromone which exposes the developing individual to a
chemical messenger that may affect later adult sexual behavior. Some
researchers talk about "informer pheromones," which draw out information
stored in the memory and help influence a choice of behaviors; an example
would be the smell of gas from a leaking stove, which may alert one to escape
the danger. [D. Muller-Schwarze, "Complex Mammalian Behavior and Pheromone Bioassay in the Field," in D. Muller-Schwarze and M. M. Mozel, eds.,
Chemical Signals in Vertebrates (New York: Plenum Press, 1977)]. Other
researchers speak of "kinship pheromones." Some suggest that we distinguish
between "seducer," "enhancer," and "libido" pheromones as well. In reality, it
makes little difference what we call them. Whether they are consciously
smelled, or merely subliminally detected, all types of pheromones operate from
the same biological principles.

19. Most of the research and data on apocrine glands was done in the early part of
this century before the link between androgenic hormones and apocrine
glands was known. Early reports claimed that females have more apocrine
glands than males. This conflicts with more recent evidence that the presence
of apocrine glands depends on the level of androgenic hormones, which is
higher in males than in females. Some of the early research also speaks of
apocrine glands being associated with hair follicles outside the areola of the
breast and on the face and head.

20. In recent years, as the quest for human sex scents has flowered, pheromones
have provided recurring story lines for television series like "Lois and Clark
(The New Adventures of Superman)," "L. A. Law," "Northern Exposure," and
"Star Trek: The Next Generation," which push speculation to the border of
reality.

21. Schleidt, 40–42; H. Ellis, *Studies in the Psychology of Sex: Sexual Selection in
Man*, vol. 4 (Philadelphia: Davis, 1914), 62. "The predominance of the olfactory area in the nervous system of the vertebrates generally has inevitably
involved intimate psychic associations between smell stimuli and the sexual
impulse. For most mammals, not only are all sexual associations mainly olfactory, but the impressions received by this sense suffice to dominate all others"
(Ellis, 46).

22. Ibid., 59–60.

23. Ibid., 60–61.

24. Schleidt, 43–48; Fisher, 44.

25. Ellis, 48.

26. Schleidt, 41.

27. Ellis, 59.

28. D. Ackerman, *A Natural History of the Senses* (New York: Random House,
1990); Fisher, 41; J. L. Hopson, *Scent Signals* (New York: William Morrow and
Company, 1979).

CHAPTER 3: A BALL OF STRING

1. *Benet's Reader's Encyclopedia*, 3d ed. (New York: Harper and Row, 1987), 45, 653, 971.

2. "The first more highly organized sense to arise on the diffused tactile sensitivity of the skin is, in most cases, without doubt that of smell. . . . The sense of smell is gradually specialized, and when taste also begins to develop a kind of chemical sense is constituted. . . . The organ of smell, however, speedily begins to rise in importance as we ascend the zoological scale." [H. Ellis, *Studies in the Psychology of Sex: Sexual Selection in Man*, vol. 4 (Philadelphia: Davis, 1914), 44]

3. E. Dobb, "The Scents Around Us," *Sciences* (November–December 1989): 46–53.

4. G. Brum, L. McKane, and G. Karp, *Biology: Exploring Life*, 2d ed. (New York: John Wiley and Sons, 1994), 229–46.

5. In a dozen pages on "Perfume, Starlight and Melody," N. J. Berrill has a classic sketch of mating scents in various animals that remains a good introduction to the topic. See N. J. Berrill, *Sex and the Nature of Things* (New York: Dodd, Mead and Company, 1953), 70–82. German naturalist Herbert Wendt has also explored the natural history of sex in "Varieties of Come-Thither" and "Flirtation, Courtship, and Wedding Gifts." See Herbert Wendt, *The Sex Life of the Animals* (New York: Simon and Schuster, 1965)123–92. In a similar vein, see Wolfgang Wickler's *The Sexual Code: The Social Behavior of Animals and Men*, including the brief chapter on psychic castration in which pheromones play a major role (New York: Anchor/Doubleday, 1973). See also our discussion of "Aggressive Odors and Infanticide" in chapter 6.

6. Brum, McKane, and Karp, 486–92.

7. Ibid., 510–12.

8. David Freedman has provided an excellent, easy-reading summary of the sense of smell and how it works in *Discover*, June 1993. The reader interested in a summary of the evolution of the central nervous system and smell should consult any general biology or zoology text book currently used at a college. (A good example is the text cited in note 4 above.) In describing the natural history and functioning of the olfactory system, brain, genes, hormones, and neurosecretions, this text provides many illustrations of what we have termed "Ariadne's thread" of consistency and evolutionary efficiency.

9. Brum, McKane, and Karp, 786–800.

10. Ibid., 804.

11. S. S. Mader, *Biology: Evolution, Diversity, and the Environment*, 2d ed. (Dubuque, Iowa: W. C. Brown, 1987), 737; Brum, McKane, and Karp, 804.

12. One of the definitions of "behavior" in *Webster's Unabridged Dictionary* is: "The action or reaction of any material under given circumstances." It is in this context that we can speak of one-celled organisms with no brain or central nervous system as engaging in behavior, meaning they act, react, and function.

13. K. Stephens, "Pheromones among the Procaryotes," *Critical Reviews of Microbiology* 13 (1986): 309–34; D. B. Clewell and K. E. Weaver, "Sex Pheromones and Plasmid Transfer in *Enterococcus faecalis*," *Plasmid* 21 (1989): 175–84.

14. *Saccharomyces cerevisiae*, commonly known as brewer's or baker's yeast, makes bread rise and juice ferment into beer and wine.

15. G. F. Sprague, L. C. Blair, and J. Thorner, "Cell Interactions and Regulation of Cell Type in the Yeast *Saccharomyces cerevisiae*," *Annual Review of Microbiology* 37 (1983): 623–60; K. Yoshida, T. Hisatomi, and N. Yanagishima, "Sexual Behavior and its Pheromonal Regulation in Ascoporogenous Yeasts," *Journal of Basic Microbiology* 29 (1989): 99–128.

16. Mating types A and B yeast cells are haploid, with a single set of chromosomes. When A and B cells "mate," the resulting cell is diploid, with two complete sets of chromosomes. This diploid cell goes through a meiotic cell division, producing four haploid cells, each with a single set of chromosomes. In the higher animals, males and females have two sets of chromosomes: one from the mother, the other from the father. Males and females produce haploid eggs and sperm, and restore the diploid chromosome complement when egg and sperm unite at fertilization.

17. Brum, McKane, and Karp, 822–26.

18. While the common usage of "the sense of smell" involves odors dissolved in the air, aquatic and marine biologists commonly apply the term in an analogous way to fish and other animals that live in a water environment. Even in common usage, sharks are said to be attracted to the smell of blood diffused in water.

19. Brum, McKane, and Karp, 867–69.

20. C. I. Bargmann and H. R. Horvitz, "Control of Larval Development of Chemosensory Neurons in *Caenorhabditis elegans*," *Science* 251 (1991): 1243–46; Brum, McKane, and Karp, 869–71.

21. Brum, McKane, and Karp, 874–75; B. Gibbons, "The Intimate Sense of Smell," *National Geographic* 170 (1986): 334.

22. Dobb.

23. R. H. Wright, *The Sense of Smell* (Boca Raton: C. R. C. Press, 1982), 178.

24. "The name 'imprinting' has been given to a well-known phenomenon in which animals, birds, and fish become endowed with a lifelong trait or behavioral pattern as a result of being exposed to (or 'imprinted' with) a certain environmental factor at a certain critical period which is usually rather early in their development" (Wright, 174).

25. The specific scent used to imprint fingerling salmon is morpholine, a colorless liquid used chiefly as a solvent for dyes, resins, and waxes. See Gibbons, 349.

26. Wright, 178.

27. Female goldfish that have ovulated release steroid hormone-based prostaglandins into the water. This stimulates male spawning behavior. The relationship of the prostaglandins to a steroid maturational hormone that functions as a preovulatory "priming" pheromone suggests that hormones and their metabolites may commonly serve as reproductive pheromones in fish. See P. W. Sorensen et al., "F Prostaglandins Function as Potent Olfactory Stimulants that Comprise the Postovulatory Female Sex Pheromone in Goldfish," *Biology of Reproduction* 39 (1988): 1039–50.

28. "Male rainbow trout orientate to a 'releaser' pheromone emitted by an ovulated female." This priming pheromone acts through the hypothalamus-pituitary-

gonadal axis to cause changes in the hormone levels of the male. See K. H. Olsen and N. R. Liley, "The Significance of Olfaction and Social Cues in Milt Availability, Sexual Hormone Status, and Spawning Behavior of Male Rainbow Trout (*Oncorhynchus mykiss*)," *General and Comparative Endocrinology* 89 (1993): 107–18.

29. Brum, McKane, and Karp, 876–82.

30. Berrill, 70–82; Brum, McKane, and Karp, 878–81.

31. Gibbons, 324–61.

32. Biologists place spiders in the same phylum of arthropods as insects like the ant and bee, but in a different group, the arachnids. Because of their close relationship with insects, we include the pheromone abilities of the bolas spider here. Schulz and Toft provide a recent review of spider pheromone action. See S. Schulz and S. Toft, "Identification of a Sex Pheromone from a Spider," *Science* 260 (1993): 1635–37.

33. A sex pheromone has been recently identified in spiders of another species that causes web reduction behavior by males on the webs of unmated adult females. (See also Schulz and Toft).

34. N. Angier, "Finding Elusive Factors That Help Wire Up the Brain," *New York Times*, 16 August 1994.

35. Brum, McKane, and Karp, 486–89.

36. A dog's olfactory membrane can be as large as 150 centimeters square, while the same area in a man may be only 10 centimeters square. See Dobb.

37. W. J. Freeman and C. A. Skarda, "Spatial EEG Patterns, Non-Linear Dynamics and Perception: The Neo-Sherringtonian View," *Brain Research Reviews* 10 (1985): 147–75.

38. "The fact that olfactory information is coded as a pattern which requires a higher order of recognition means that animals with a greater neural backup have the potential for a more sophisticated pattern recognition. Since the olfactory bulb seems to be acting mainly as a filter, and decoding of the olfactory message is a more central event, animals with a greater neocortical support system have the greatest ability to make use of this system. Primates do not therefore have a poorly developed sense of olfactory perception, and the ways in which this is employed may well be the most evolved of all species." [E. B. Keverne, "Chemical Communication in Primate Reproduction," in J. G. Vandenbergh, ed., *Pheromones and Reproduction in Mammals* (New York: Academic Press, 1983]

39. Gibbons, 339.

40. Ibid., 344.

41. Dobb, 51.

42. Ibid.

CHAPTER 4: THE ANATOMY OF SMELLING

1. P. P. C. Graziadei, "Functional Anatomy of the Mammalion Chemoreceptor System," in D. Muller-Schwarze and M. M. Mozel, eds., *Chemical Signals in*

Vertebrates (New York: Plenum Press, 1977). Terminal nerves are also involved in our sense of smell, carrying impulses from the nasal passages to the medial septal and preoptic areas of the brain that regulate relaxation, appetite, anger, fear, and sexual desire. See B. Goldman, "The Essence of Attraction," *Health* 40 (March–April 1994): 3.

2. F. Stephenson, "The Smell of Sex," *Florida State University: Research in Review* 7 (Fall/Winter 1991): 9.

3. M. Meredith, "Patterned Response to Odor in Mammalian Olfactory Bulb: The Influence of Intensity," *Journal of Neurophysiology* 56 (1986): 572–97; M. Meredith and G. Howard, "Intracerebroventricular LHRH Relieves Behavioral Deficits Due to Vomeronasal Organ Removal,"*Brain Research Bulletin* 29 (1992): 75–79.

4. N. A. Bobrow, J. Money, and V. J. Lewis, "Delayed Puberty, Eroticism and Sense of Smell: A Psychological Study of Hypogonadotropinism, Osmatic and Anosmatic (Kallmann's Syndrome)," *Archives of Sexual Behavior* 1 (1971): 329–44; J. Money and A. A. Ehrhardt, *Man and Woman, Boy and Girl* (Baltimore: Johns Hopkins University Press, 1972), 205.

5. L. Magrassi and P. P. Graziadei, "Single Olfactory Organs Associated with Prosencephalic Malformation and Cyclopia in a *Xenopus Laevis* Tadpole," *Brain Research* 412 (1987): 386–90; A. G. Monti-Graziadei and P. P. Graziadei, "Experimental Studies on the Olfactory Marker Protein. V. Olfactory Marker Protein in the Olfactory Neurons Transplanted with the Olfactory Bulb," *Brain Research* 484 (1989): 157–67; T. Zigova, P. P. Graziadei, and A. G. Monti-Graziadei, "Olfactory Bulb Transplantation into the Olfactory Bulb of Neonatal Rats: An Autoradiographic Study," *Brain Research* 539 (1991): 51–58; A. G. Monti-Graziadei and P. P. Graziadei, "Sensory Reinnervation after Partial Removal of the Olfactory Bulb," *Journal of Comparative Neurology* 316 (1992): 32–44; Zigoya et al., "Olfactory Bulb Transplantation into the Olfactory Bulb of Neonatal Rats," *Brain Research* 513 (1990): 315–19.

6. For at least fifty years, embryologists have transplanted the primordia or anlage of embryonic legs, wings, eyes, ears and the brain in experiments to discover the various factors and influences on organ development. Graziadei has applied this standard and well-tested technique to some elegant neural experiments.

7. Quoted by Stephenson.

8. Each of these odor-sensitive cells is ten thousand times more sensitive than the sensory cells in our tongue that distinguish between sweet, sour, salty, and bitter. Moreover, there are only three hundred thousand taste cells, which says something about the relative importance of taste and smell.

9. The receptor may match either the aromatic molecule's structure or its vibration frequency. See G. H. Dodd and M. Skinner, "From Moods to Molecules: The Psychopharmacology of Perfumery and Aromatherapy," in S. Van Toller and G. H. Dodd, eds., *Fragrance: The Psychology and Biology of Perfume* (Amsterdam: Elsevier Applied Science, 1992), 127–29; 136–39.

10. Ibid., 129–36. Changeux provides an excellent description of "Chemical signaling in the brain" that provides important insights for readers interested in

the role of receptors and neurotransmitters in the brain." [Changeux, J. P., "Chemical Signaling in the Brain," *Scientific American* 269 (1993): 58–62.]

11. D. H. Freedman, "In the Realm of the Chemical," *Discover* 14, no. 9 (June 1993): 69–76; S. Firestein and G. M. Shepherd, "A Kinetic Model of the Odor Response in Single Olfactory Receptor Neurons," *Journal of Steroid Biochemistry and Molecular Biology* 39 (1991): 615–20.

12. L. Buck and R. Axel, "A Novel Multigene Family May Encode Odorant Receptors: A Molecular Basis for Odor Recognition," *Cell* 65 (1991): 175–87; J. Ngai et al., "The Family of Genes Encoding Odorant Receptors in the Channel Catfish," *Cell* 72 (1993): 657–66; K. J. Ressler, S. L. Sullivan, and L. B. Buch, "A Zonal Organization of Odorant Receptor Gene Expression in the Olfactory Epithelium," *Cell* 73 (1993): 597–609.

13. Freedman, 73.

14. Odors processed by the main olfactory system also affect production of other neurotransmitters such as dopamine, serotonin, and noradrenaline that also affect the functions of GnRH as a neurotransmitter changing our behavior.

15. Production of hormonal GnRH occurs in the medial basal circuits of the hypothalamus.

16. GnRH from the hypothalamus circulates in the blood to the nearby pituitary gland where it regulates the production of two major hormones, FSH and LH. Follicle stimulating hormone (FSH) is structurally the same in males as it is in females. Its main action is also similar in that it controls the early stages of egg growth in the ovarian follicle and sperm production in the seminiferous tubules. The other hormone, luteinizing hormone (LH), triggers maturation of the egg and its release from the ovarian follicle and movement of the mature sperm into the lumen of the seminiferous tubules and their maturation in the epididymis. In women this cascade of hormones in the hypothalamic-pituitary-gonad (HPG) axis also involves the uterus and its hormone production. In both men and women, feedback loops involving the hormones produced by the ovaries, testes, and adrenal glands control the hypothalamus' production of GnRH.

17. K. Schwenk, "Why Snakes Have Forked Tongues," *Science* 263 (1994): 1573–77.

18. The Danish anatomist Ludwig Levin Jacobson discovered the VNO in mammals in 1811, while Potiquet identified them in human infants in 1891. Karen Wright provides a detailed account of the research on the VNO and the recent documentation of its structure and olfactory functions in an article on "The Sniff of Legend," in *Discover* 15, no. 4 (1994):60–77.

19. G. Licht and M. Meredith, "Convergence of Main and Accessory Olfactory Pathways onto Single Neurons in the Hamster Amygdala," *Experimental Brain Research* 69 (1987): 7–18.

20. B. Goldman, "The Essence of Attraction," *Health* 3 (March/April 1994): 40; M. Meredith, "Sensory Processing in the Main and Accessory Olfactory Systems: Comparisons and Contrasts," *Journal of Steroid Biochemistry and Molecular Biology* 39 (1991): 601–14; R. Taylor, "Brave New Nose: Sniffing Out Human Sexual Chemistry," *Journal of NIH Research* 6 (1994): 47–51.

21. Blocking input to the VNO in male garter snakes completely eliminates any sexual behavior, an effect not seen when input to the main olfactory system is blocked. See J. L. Kubie, A. Vagvolgyi, and M. Halpern, "The Roles of the Vomeronasal and Olfactory Systems in the Courtship Behavior of Male Garter Snakes," *Journal of Comparative and Physiological Psychology* 92 (1978): 627–41.

22. M. Halpern, "The Organization and Function of the Vomeronasal System," *Annual Review of Neuroscience* 10 (1987): 325–62; R. T. Mason et al., "Sex Pheromones in Snakes," *Science* 245 (1989): 290–93.

23. Kubie, Vagvolgyi, and Halpern.

24. Halpern; Mason et al. Mason and colleagues noted that "Although pheromonal communication is evident in all orders of *Reptilia*, this is to our knowledge the first identification of sex pheromones in that class." Garter snake pheromones are not produced by a discrete gland but are components of skin lipids found in all land-dwelling vertebrates. They are similar to the lipids in the cuticles of insects that often serve a pheromonal function.

25. Mason et al.; B. Alstetter, "Snakes in Drag," *Discover* 11 (June 1990): 20.

26. Taylor; L. Monti-Bloch and B. I. Grosser, "Effect of Putative Pheromones on the Electrical Activity of the Human Vomeronasal Organ and Olfactory Epithelium," *Journal of Steroid Biochemistry and Molecular Biology* 39 (1991): 573–82; S. Takami et al., "Vomeronasal Epithelial Cells of the Adult Human Express Neuron-Specific Molecules," *Neuroreport* 4 (1993): 375–78.

27. E. C. Crosby and T. Humphrey, "Studies of the Vertebrate Telencephalon," *Journal of Comparative Neurology* 71 (1938): 121.

28. D. T. Moran, B. W. Jafek, and J. C. Rowley, "The Ultrastructure of the Human Olfactory Mucosa," in D. G. Laing, R. L. Doty, and W. Breipohl, eds., *The Human Sense of Smell* (New York: Springer-Verlag, 1991); Goldman.

29. J. Garcia-Velasco and M. Mondragon, "The Incidence of the Vomeronasal Organ in 1000 Human Subjects and Its Possible Clinical Significance," *Journal of Steroid Biochemistry and Molecular Biology* 39 (1991): 561–63; Moran, Jafek, and Rowley.

30. Garcia-Velasco and Mandragon.

31. L. J. Stensaas et al., "Ultrastructure of the Human Vomeronasal Organ," *Journal of Steroid Biochemistry and Molecular Biology* 39 (1991): 553–60.

32. Monti-Block and Grosser.

CHAPTER 5: LOVE APPLES AND
THE NOBLE PERFUME OF VENERY

1. One of the old varieties of apples common three or four hundred years ago in England, and still raised by some arbiculturalists, is a small apple known as the "Lady's Apple." Its size makes it perfect for carrying in the armpit.

2. R. C. Camphausen, *The Encyclopdia of Erotic Wisdom* (Rochester, Vermont: Inner Traditions International, 1991), 138.

3. H. E. Fisher, *Anatomy of Love* (New York: W. W. Norton, 1991) 40–43; E. Gregersen, *Sexual Practices: The Story of Human Sexuality* (London: Mitchell

Beazley, 1982); A. LeGuerer, *Scent: The Mysterious and Essential Powers of Smell* (New York: Turtle Bay Books, 1992), 9–11.

4. Alpha-androstenone and alpha-androstenol are respectively the ketone and alcohol forms of delta-16 steroids that have been identified as pig pheromones. For cross-species comparison, these steroids are of interest in humans because they are present in human male underarm sweat secreted by apocrine glands, which in lower animals are specialized for pheromone secretion. Also, the ratio of androstenone to testosterone in the blood of men is similar to that of the boar. Hence the term "boar's taint," and the expression "He stinks like a pig." Both androstenone and androstenol are found in the urine of men and women, but only after puberty. The ketone derivative, androstenone, has a urinous scent and is found in the urine, plasma, sweat, and saliva of both women and men, but in higher concentrations in males. The alcohol androstenol has a musky scent and is similarly found in the urine, plasma, sweat, and saliva in both men and women. Males have much higher levels of both these steroid metabolites than women. Although it is possibly less effective than androstenol in evoking a response, the ketone androstenone is more stable than the alcohol androstenol. For this reason, androstenone has been used more often than androstenol in clinical tests even though in real life, androstenol may be a more effective pheromone. See E. E. Filsinger, "Human Responses to the Pig Sex Pheromone Androstenol," *Journal of Comparative Psychology* 98 (1984): 219–22. See also: J. N. Labows and G. Preti, "Human Semiochemicals," in S. Van Toller and G. H. Dodd, eds., *Fragrance: The Psychology and Biology of Perfume* (Amsterdam: Elsevier Applied Science 1992), 70–73; M. Schleidt, "The Semiotic Relevance of Human Olfaction: A Biological Approach," in Toller and Dodd, eds., *Fragrance*, 44–45.

5. J. J. Cowley, A. L. Johnson, and W. L. Brooksbank, "The Effect of Two Odorous Compounds on Performance in an Assessment-of-People Test," *Psychoneuroendocrinology* 2 (1977): 159–72.

6. LeGruerer, 10; P. Langley-Danysz, "La Truffe, un Aphrodisiaque," *La Recherche* 136 (1982); J. D. Vincent, *Biologie des Passions* (Paris: Odile Jacob, 1986), 267.

7. Camphausen, 81.

8. Vincent, 267.

9. In 1986 John Money claimed that while pheromones could end or prevent a pregnancy in rodents, this effect did not occur in humans. See J. Money, *Lovemaps* (New York: Irvington Publishers, 1986). John, Savitz, and Shy have subsequently reported a similar effect in humans. In a five year study of licensed female cosmetologists ages twenty-two to thirty-six in North Carolina found a two-fold increase in the incidence of spontaneous abortions among pregnant women exposed to high levels of aromatic cosmetic chemicals. See E. M. John, D. A. Savitz, and C. M. Shy, "Spontaneous Abortions Among Cosmetologists," *Epidemiology* 5 (1994): 147–55.

10. M. McClintock, "Menstrual Synchrony and Suppression," *Nature* 229 (1971): 244–45; A. Comfort, "Communications May Be Odorous," *New Scientist and*

Science Journal (25 February, 1971) 412–14; "Likelihood of Human Phero-mones," *Nature* 230 (1971): 432–33.

11. J. L. Hopson, *Scent Signals* (New York: William Morrow and Company, 1979); J. Durden-Smith and D. DeSimone, *Sex and the Brain* (New York: Arbor House, 1983), 215.

12. M. J. Russell, G. M. Switz, and K. Thompson, "Olfactory Influences on the Human Menstrual Cycle," *Pharmacology Biochemistry and Behavior* 13 (1980): 737–38.

13. C. A. Graham and W. C. McGrew, "Menstrual Synchrony in Female Undergraduates Living on a Coeducational Campus," *Psychoneuroendocrinology* 5 (1980): 245–52; D. M. Quadagno et al., "Influence of Male Social Contacts, Exercise and All-Female Living Conditions on the Menstual Cycle," *Psychoneuroendocrinology* 6 (1981): 239–44.

14. G. Preti et al., "Human Axillary Secretions Influence Women's Menstrual Cycles: The Role of Donor Extract of Females," *Hormones and Behavior* 20 (1986): 474–82.

15. Normally, after an egg escapes the ruptured follicle in the ovary, it implants in the lining of the uterus if it is fertilized. The embryonic mass then sends hor-mone messages back to the follicle, stimulating it to become a corpus luteum and produce estrogen and progesterone to help maintain the early pregnancy. This also suppresses production of GnRH, the releasing hormone of the hypo-thalamus, which inhibits further egg production. If the egg is not fertilized and there is no pregnancy, the corpus luteum quickly degenerates. In this kind of scent-induced false pregnancy, the corpus luteum continues to develop and the egg-production cycle stops. This effect is known as the Lee-Boot Effect. S. Van der Lee and L. M. Boot, "Spontaneous Pseudopregnancy in Mice," *Acta Physiologica et Pharmacologica Neederlandica* 4 (1955): 442–44.

16. This scent-related effect is known in the literature as the Whitten Effect (Bronson & Whitten, 1968). See F. H. Bronson and W. Whitten, "Estrous Accelerating Pheromone of Mice: Assay, Androgen-Dependency, and Presence in Bladder Urine," *Journal of Reproduction and Fertility* 15 (1968): 131–34.

17. Veith et al., "Exposure to Men Influences the Occurrence of Ovulation in Women," *Physiology and Behavior* 31 (1983): 313–15.

18. W. B. Cutler, C. R. Garcia, and A. M. Krieger, "Luteal Phase Defects: Sporadic Sexual Behavior in Women," *Hormones and Behavior* 13 (1979): 214–18; "Sexual Behavior Frequency and Menstural Cycle Length in Mature Premenopausal Women," *Psychoneuroendocrinology* 4 (1979): 297–309; "Sporadic Sexual Behavior and Menstural Cycle Length in Women," *Hormones and Behavior* 14 (1980): 163–72.

19. Cutler et al.; Fisher, 1992, 42–43. In our research for this book we encountered two very tantalizing bits of unconfirmed research that could provide prococa-tive new answers and more questions. Twenty-five years ago, Persky, Lief, and colleagues reported finding a strong trend for a husband's blood level of tes-tosterone to peak soon after his wife's testosterone level reached its cyclic ovulatory peak. What positive effect this synchronization might have for the

woman's fertility, and on her husband's behavior, one can hardly speculate without confirmation and further research. However, Persky suggested either that: "(1) the husband's testosterone level had become entrained to the wife's menstrual cycle reflecting the pair-bonding of the two partners, or (2) a form of communication exists between the two partners whereby the female informs the male that she has ovulated and he responds, like the dominant rhesus monkey, with an increase in his testosterone level facilitating his entire response cycle." See: *Psychoendocrinology of Human Sexual Behavior* (New York: Praeger, 1987), 108. Is this form of communication based in human pheromones? Equally intriguing, Henderson found that young Australian husbands experienced a drop in basal body temperature followed by a rise that synchronized nicely with the wife's dip in basal body temperature at midcycle and its subsequent rise after ovulation. Henderson also reported a similar synchronization of basal body temperature in one male homosexual couple. See: "Evidence for a Male Menstrual Temperature Cycle and Synchrony With the Female Menstrual Cycle" (abstract). *New Zealand Medical Journal* 84 (1976): 164

20. John Money's use of "or" in this quote, i.e., "by way of pheromones or odors," is not disjunctive, meaning "either pheromones or odors" as if the two are opposed. The intent, rather, is to clarify that pheromones are odors. J. Money, *Love and Love Sickness: The Science of Sex, Gender Difference, and Pair-bonding* (Baltimore: Johns Hopkins, 1980), 122–23.

21. G. Epple, M. C. Alveario, and A. M. Belcher, "Copulatory Behavior of Adult Tamarins (*Sanguinus fuscicollis*) Castrated as Neonates of Juveniles: Effect of Testosterone Treatment," *Hormones and Behavior* 24 (1990): 470–83; Durden-Smith and D. DeSimone, 222–23.

22. Durden-Smith and DeSimone, 222–23.

23. H. Ellis, *Studies in the Psychology of Sex: Sexual Selection in Man*, vol. 4 (Philadelphia: Davis, 1914), 97–98.

24. Ibid., 96–97.

25. A. Forsythe, "Good Scents and Bad," *Natural History* (November 1985): 25–32.

26. For a definition of smegma, see: R. T. Francoeur, T. Perper, and N. Scherzer, *The Complete Dictionary of Sexology* (New York: Continuum, 1994), 620. When a female mouse smells the smegma produced by the apocrine glands around the edge of the penile glans of a male, she is strongly attracted to him even though she is not in heat. When the male then urinates on her, another pheromone in his urine apparently brings her into heat. The pheromone under the male's foreskin attracts the female, and his urinous pheromone makes her sexually receptive. Interestingly, virgin female mice who are not under the influence of postpubertal levels of estrogen are unaffected by the male's penile pheromone. [R. Winter, *The Smell Book. Scent, Sex and Society* (New York: Lippincott, 1976), 43].

27. P. Redgrove, *The Black Goddess and the Sixth Sense* (London: Bloomsbury, 1987), 65.

28. L. Watson, *Neophilia: The Tradition of the New* (London: Hodder and Soughton, 1989), 87.

29. Durden-Smith and DeSimone, 221.

30. T. Engen, *The Perception of Odors* (New York: Academic Press, 1982), 65–71.

31. Auguste Galopin, quoted in Winter, 35.

CHAPTER 6: FRIENDS, STRANGERS, AND LOVERS

1. R. L. Doty, "Psychophysical Measurement of Odor Perception in Humans," and "Olfactory Function in Neonates," in *The Human Sense of Smell* ed. D. G. Laing, R. L. Doty, and W. Breipohl (New York: Springer-Verlag, 1991).

2. R. D. Balogh and R. H. Porter, "Olfactory Preferences Resulting from Mere Exposure in Human Neonates," *Infant Behavioral Development* 9 (1986): 395–401.

3. M. Schleidt and C. Genzel, "The Significance of Mother's Perfume for Infants in the First Weeks of Their Life," *Ethology and Sociobiology* 11 (1990): 145–54.

4. M. J. Russell, G. M. Switz, and K. Thompson, "Olfactory Influences on the Human Menstrual Cycle," *Pharmacology Biochemistry and Behavior* 13 (1980). See also: A. Walsh, *The Science of Love: Understanding Love and Its Effects on Mind and Body* (New York: Prometheus Books, 1991), 57–75. Walsh's chapter on "The Chemistry of Mother Love" is particularly good, and quite relevant to our discussion here, although our focus is much more directly on the effects of pheromones.

5. Walsh, 57–75.

6. J. Money, *Lovemaps* (New York: Irvington Publishers, 1986), 94–95; Russell, Switz, and Thompson, "Olfactory Influences on the Human Menstural Cycle," *Pharmacology Biochemistry and Behavior* 13 (1980): 737–38.

7. J. N. Labows and G. Preti, "Human Semiochemicals," in S. Van Toller and G. H. Dodd, eds., *Fragrance: The Psychology and Biology of Perfume* (Amsterdam: Elsevier Applied Science 1992), 84–85; A. MacFarlane, "Olfaction in the Development of Social Preferences in the Human Neonate," *Ciba Foundation Symposium* 33 (1975): 103–13; M. J. Russell, "Human Olfactory Communication," *Nature* 260 (1976): 520–22.

8. J. M. Cernoch and R. H. Porter, "Recognition of Maternal Axillary Odors by Infants," *Child Development* 56 (1985): 1593–98.

9. R. T. Francoeur, T. Perper, and N. Scherzer, *The Complete Dictionary of Sexology* (New York: Continuum, 1994).

10. Money, 94.

11. Walsh.

12. F. A. Beach, "Sexual Attractivity, Proceptivity, and Receptivity in Female Mammals," *Hormones and Behavior* 7 (1976): 105–38; A. LeGuerer, Scent: *The Mysterious and Essential Powers of Smell* (New York: Turtle Bay Books, 1992), 24.

13. R. H. Porter, J. M. Cernoch, and R. D. Balogh, "Odor Signatures and Kin Recognition," *Physiology and Behavior* 34 (1985): 445–48.

14. R. J. H. Russell, P. A. Wells, and J. P. Ruston, "Evidence for Genetic Similarity Detection in Human Marriage," *Ethology and Sociobiology* 6 (1985): 183–87; P. Wallace, "Inidividual Discrimination of Humans by Odor," *Physiology and Behavior* 19 (1977): 577–79.

15. R. Winter, *The Smell Book. Scent, Sex and Society* (New York: Lippincott, 1976), 52.

16. G. K. Beauchamp, K. Yamazaki, and E. A. Boyse, "The Chemosensory Recognition of Genetic Individuality," *Scientific American* 253 (1985); R. L. Doty et al., "Endocrine, Cardiovascular, and Psychological Correlates of Olfactory Sensitivity Changes During the Human Menstrual Cycle," *Journal of Comparative and Physiological Psychology* 95 (1981); R. L. Doty, "Reproductive Endocrine Influences Upon Olfactory Perception: A Current Perspective," *Journal of Chemical Ecology* 12 (1986): 497–511.

17. M. Schleidt, "The Semiotic Relevance of Human Olfaction: A Biological Approach," in Van Toller and Dodd, eds., *Fragrance*, 40–47.

18. J. A. Mennella and G. K. Beauchamp, "Olfactory Preferences in Children and Adults," in D. G. Laing, R. L. Doty, and W. Breipohl, eds., *The Human Sense of Smell* (New York: Springer-Verlag, 1991).

19. R. W. Moncrieff, *Odour Preferences* (New York: John Wiley and Sons, 1966).

20. R. L. Doty, "An Examination of Relationships Between the Pleasantness, Intensity, and Concentration of 10 Odorous Stimuli," *Perceptual Psychophysiology* 17 (1975): 492–96.

21. K. M. Dorries et al., "Changes in Sensitivity to the Odor of Androstenone During Adolescence," *Developmental Psychobiology* 22 (1989): 423–35; C. J. Wysocki and A. N. Gilbert, "National Geographic Smell Survey: Effects of Age Are Heterogenous," in C. Murphy, W. S. Cain, and D. M. Hegsted, eds., *Nutrition and the Chemical Senses in Aging: Recent Advances and Current Research Needs* (New York: Academy of Sciences, 1989).

22. C. J. Wysocki and G. K. Beauchamp, "Ability to Smell Androstenone Is Genetically Determined," *Proceedings of the National Academy of Science USA* 81 (1984): 4899–902.

23. C. J. Wysocki et al., "Changes in Olfactory Sensitivity to Androstenone with Age and Experience," abstract in *Chemical Senses* 12 (1987): 710; Dorries et al.

24. C. J. Wysocki, K. M. Dorries, and G. K. Beauchamp, "Ability to Perceive Androsteone Can Be Acquired by Ostensibly Anosmic People," *Proceedings of the National Academy of Science USA* 86 (1989): 7976–78.

25. C. Van Toller et al., "Skin Conductance and Subjective Assessments Associated with the Odour of 5-Androstan-3-One," *Biological Psychology* 16 (1983): 85–107.

26. H. S. Koelega and E. P. Koster, "Some Experiments on Sex Differences in Odor Perception," *Annals of the New York Academy of Sciences* 237 (1974): 234–46.

27. J. D. Vincent, *Biologie des Passions* (Paris: Odile Jacob, 1986), 267.

28. J. A. Mennella and H. Moltz, "Pheromonal Emission by Pregnant Rats Protects Against Infanticide by Nulliparous Conspecifics," *Physiology and Behavior* 46 (1989): 591–95.

29. Winter, 52–53.

30. Ibid., 52.

31. Cited in J. Durden-Smith and D. DeSimone, *Sex and the Brain* (New York: Arbor House, 1983), 218–19.

32. Ibid.

33. W. K. Whitten, "Genetic Variation of Olfactory Function in Reproduction," *Journal of Reproductive Fertility* 19 (1973): 405–10; Winter, 44.

34. This scent-dependent effect is known in the literature as the Bruce Effect (H. M. Bruce, "Further Observations of Pregnancy Block in Mice Caused by Proximity of Strange Males," *Journal of Reproduction and Fertility* 2 (1960): 311–12. See also: Money, 95 and A. S. Parker and H. M. Bruce, "Olfactory Stimuli in Mammalian Reproduction: Odor Excites Neurohormonal Responses Affecting Oestrus, Pseudopregnancy, and Pregnancy in the Mouse," *Science* 134 (1961): 1049–54.

35. Whitten; Winter, 44.

36. M. Young, "Attitudes and Behavior of College Students Relative to Oral-Genital Sexuality," *Archives of Sexual Behavior* 9 (1980): 61–67.

37. R. P. Michael, "Neuroendocrine Factors Regulating Primate Behaviour," in L. Martini and W. F. Ganong, eds., *Frontiers in Neuroendocrinology* (New York: Oxford University Press, 1971); R. P. Michael and R. W. Bonsall, "Chemical Signals and Primate Behavior," in D. Muller-Schwarze and M. M. Mozel, eds., *Chemical Signals in Vertebrates* (New York: Plenum Press); R. P. Michael, R. W. Bonsall, and P. Warner, "Human Vaginal Secretions: Volatile Fatty Acid Content," *Science* 186 (1974): 1217–19.

38. J. E. Amoore, "Evidence for the Chemical Olfactory Code in Man," *Annals of the New York Academy of Sciences* 237 (1974): 137–43; J. E. Amoore and J. R. Popplewell, "Sensitivity of Women to Musk Odor: No Menstrual Variation," *Journal of Chemical Ecology* 1 (1975): 291–97; J. E. Amoore, P. Pelosi, and L. J. Forrester, "Specific Anosmias to 5A-androst-16-en-3-one and w-pentadecalactone: The Urinous and Musky Primary Odors," *Chemical Senses and Flavor* 2 (1977): 401–25.

39. A few weeks after Francoeur's discussions with Charles Sekuruumah and Dr. Noble, he uncovered another example of the folk use of vaginal secretions while talking with a Brazilian lawyer. She shared her own recollections of a white magic spiritualist potion popular in the rural areas of Brazil where some women serve a special coffee to a male friend. After brewing, she reported, the coffee is filtered through a woman's soiled underwear.

    Since Francoeur's initial conversation with Dr. Noble, she has spoken with several black women friends and colleagues from southern states. All of them recalled as children hearing about the love-smitten boy who had been "fixed" by having "fixin's" secretly dabbed on him or mixed in his food. Susan Goodman also reports that "In the Middle Ages, a maiden who wanted to attract a man sat naked in a tub of wheat, moving around so the grains touched her genitals. The wheat was then ground and baked into an intoxicating bread for her desired mate. (In another version, the loaf was kneaded upon her buttocks.)" See Susan Goodman, "Loving Spoonfuls," *New Woman* (1994): 109, 146.

40. J. Money, *Love and Love Sickness: The Science of Sex, Gender Difference, and Pair-bonding* (Baltimore: Johns Hopkins, 1980), 74.

41. H. Ellis, *Studies in the Psychology of Sex: Sexual Selection in Man*, vol. 4 (Philadelphia: Davis, 1914), 75.

42. Money, *Love and Love Sickness*, 56, 89.

43. J. R. Baker, *Race* (New York: Oxford University Press, 1974); M. B. L. Craigmyle, *The Apocrine Glands and the Breast* (Chichester: Wiley and Sons, 1984); K. J. Reamy and S. E. White, "Sexuality in the Puerperium: A Review," *Archives of Sexual Behavior* 16 (1987): 165–86.

44. Ellis, 74–75.

45. J. Money, *The Destroying Angel* (New York: Prometheus Books, 1985), 64–65; *Lovemaps*, 94–96.

46. Ellis, 101–2.

47. Ibid., 75.

48. A. Forsythe, "Good Scents and Bad," *Natural History* (November 1985).

49. Doty et al.; R. L. Doty, "Reproductive Endocrine Influences Upon Olfactory Perception: A Current Perspective," *Journal of Chemical Ecology* 12 (1986): 497–511.

50. Durden-Smith and DeSimone, 226.

51. H. S. Koelega and E. P. Koster, "Some Experiments on Sex Differences in Odor Perception," *Annals of the New York Academy of Sciences* 237 (1974): 234–46.

52. T. Perper, *Sex Signals: The Biology of Love* (Philadelphia: ISI Press, 1985); M. F. Small, *Female Choices: Sexual Behavior of Female Primates* (Ithaca: Cornell University Press, 1993); Winter, 53–54.

53. P. Rovesti and E. Colombo, "Aromatherapy and Aerosols," *Soap, Perfumery and Cosmetics* 46 (1973): 475–78.

CHAPTER 7: DEEP IN THE WOMB

1. L. Nilsson, *A Child is Born* (New York: Delacorte Press, 1990).

2. A comparison of the texts in the 1965 and 1990 editions of Lennart Nilsson's *A Child if Born* reflects the radical shift of perspective suggested by Martin. The description of egg and sperm in the 1965 edition is typically male-biased. The 1990 text reflects the newer interpretation, describing the aimless movement of the sperm until they receive a chemical messenger signaling the entrance of an egg into the fallopian tube. The third photograph in the 1990 book, for example, shows pheromone molecules magnified four hundred thousand times and an insert of a couple kissing. The caption reads: "POWERFUL SIGNALS: Although our sense of smell is inferior to that of most animals, human beings, like other species, have been found to secrete chemical 'lures,' substances called pheromones. The concentration of these varies, rising during a kiss for example." E. Martin, "The Egg and Sperm: How Science Has Constructed a Romance Based on Stereotypical Male-Female Roles," *Signs: Journal of Women in Culture and Society* 13, no. 3 (Spring 1991); D. H. Freedman, "The Aggressive Egg," *Discover* 13 (June 1992): 61–65.

3. Freedman (69–76) indicates some researchers believe that the stopover of the sperm in the cervical crypts allows time for the female to prepare for the release

of an egg. He does not, however, name the researchers nor give any further details for this curious link. It is true that reflex ovulation, in which coitus triggers ovulation, has been reported in several animal species. But it is not common. In humans, egg maturation and ovulation is essentially controlled by the female's hormone cycle, not the stimulus of coitus. Nonetheless, some research supports that coitus induced ovulation does occur in human females. W. Jochle, "Current Research in Coitus Induced Ovulation," Journal of Reproduction and Fertility suppl. 22 (1975): 165–207. See also: Nilsson, 42–46.

4. For a summary of various forms of parthenogenesis or "virgin conception" see R. T. Francoeur, "Parthenogenesis," in V. I. Bullough and B. Bullough, eds., *Human Sexuality: An Encylopedia* (New York: Garland Publishing, 1994), 437–38.

5. The balance of calcium and potassium ions, and the acidic or alkaline environment in various regions of the female reproductive tract, play a major role in triggering different responses from the sperm. These include "capacitation," the effect the vaginal environment has in making the sperm capable of propelling themselves through the female tract and eventually penetrating the egg.

6. D. Ansley, "Sperm Tales," *Discover* 13 (June 1992): 68.

7. G. Kolata, "From Fly to Man, Cells Obey Same Signal," *New York Times*, 5 January 1993, C1, C10.

8. N. Angier, "Finding Elusive Factors that Help Wire up the Brain," *New York Times*, 16 August 1994.

9. N. Angier, "Making an Embryo: Biologists Find Keys to Body Plan: From Worms to Cows, One Class of Genes Spells Out the Blue Print," *New York Times*, 23 February 1993, C1, C9; Kolata, "From Fly to Man." By early 1994, the animals used in research on the HOX and hedgehog genes included fruit flies, roundworms, zebra fish, chickens, mice, and humans.

10. D. C. Page et al., "The Sex-Determining Region of the Human Y Chromosome Encodes a Finger Protein," *Cell* 51 (1987): 1091–104; M. S. Palmer et al., "Genetic Evidence that ZFY is not the Testis-Determining Factor," *Nature* 342, no. 6252 (1989): 937–39; A. H. Sinclair, "A Gene From the Human Sex-Determining Region Encodes a Protein with Homology to a Conserved DNA-Binding Motif," *Nature* 346 (1990): 240–44.

11. R. T. Francouer, *Becoming a Sexual Person*, (New York: Macmillan Publishing, 1991), 79.

12. Ibid, 82–86.

13. Scientists use the term "default programming" to describe nature's basic plan for female development without any negative or derogatory connotation. The analogy is based on the defaults or basic language and instructions programmed into a computer's central processing unit. Instructions for the development of a female embryo/fetus are contained in the genetic code, and will operate unless androgenic hormones are present at a level high enough to override the genetic program for female development and bring into play a supplemental genetic program that interacts with testosterone and MIH to produce a male. See Francoeur, 75–78, 80–81

14. For brain estrogens derived from testosterone to have a masculizing effect seems illogical, but that is the way it works.

15. Perper [T. Perper, *Sex Signals: The Biology of Love* (Philadelphia: ISI Press, 1985), 15–17] defines a brain or neural template as a "prenatal hormonally determined substrate *which is then overlaid by and elaborated on by postnatal determinants, social scripting, and one's personal experiences.*" See also: Francoeur, 86–92. For summaries of the biological roots of sex differences in the brain that are not too technical, see Pool or Kimura. [R. E. Pool, *Eve's Rib: Searching for the Biological Roots of Sex Differences* (New York: Crown, 1994)]. [D. Kimura, "Sex Differences in the Brain," *Scientific American* (1992): 119–25].

16. What causes this migration is not known, but some HOX and/or hedgehog genes may well play a major role in it. See:T. W. Sadler, *Langman's Medical Embryology*, 6th ed. (Baltimore: Williams and Wilkins, 1990), 313; K. L. Moore and T. V. N. Persaud, *The Developing Human: Clinically Oriented Embryology*, 5th ed. (Philadelphia: W. B. Saunders, 1993), 206–10.

17. What we know about sexual differentiation in the womb during the first few months of fetal life is completely compatible with the idea that hormones activate genes (E. H. Davidson, "Hormones and Genes," *Scientific American* 212 (1965): 36–45.), which direct migration of GnRH-secreting nerve cells from the olfactory placode into the nose, olfactory bulbs, limbic structures, hypothalamus, and·other areas of the brain [L. Buck and R. Axel, "A Novel Multigene Family May Encode Odorant Receptors: A Molecular Basis for Odor Recognition," *Cell* 65 (1991): 175–87; K. M. Dorries et al., "Changes in Sensitivity to the Odor of Androstenone During Adolescence," *Developmental Psychobiology* 22 (1989): 423–35]. Geneticists and reproductive biologists have not begun to look for hedgehog genes in the human embryo because of the great difficulty of conducting such research, but their presence and role in fish, birds, and small mammals suggests that they also occur in humans, controlling early embryonic development in a similar way. While there is no direct evidence of HOX genes in humans, the consistency of DNA and genetic processes suggests this is certainly quite likely. See Angier (1993); Kolata; J. C. Smith, "Hedgehog, the Floor Plate, and the Zone of Polarizing Activity," *Cell* 76 (1994): 193–96.

18. It appears that reciprocal relationships between the GnRH pulse, hormone levels, and neuronal development allow either: (1) the cyclic pattern of hormone secretion which facilitates connections between neurons that allow positive feedback characteristic of the adult female; or (2) the tonic (continuous) pattern characteristic of the adult male. However, subtle variations in the degree of prepubertal tonic, or cyclic hormone control may determine development of the negative and positive feedback loops on LH secretion that are characteristic of adult men and women.

19. J. D. Weinrich, *Sexual Landscapes: Why We Are What We Are, Why We Love Whom We Love* (New York: Scribners, 1987).

20. Two studies, in our opinion, provide the most nuanced and careful evaluation of research findings of sex differences in the brain. The briefer of the two is Doreen Kimura's 1992 article on "Sex Differences in the Brain" in *Scientific*

American. Much more detailed and current is Robert Pool's 1994 book *Eve's Rib: Searching for the Biological Roots of Sex Differences*, which concentrates on the extensive research of female scientists who maintain strong feminist values with an openness to whatever their research turns up. See Christine Gorman's readable, quite balanced, but somewhat dated, summary "Sizing Up the Sexes," *Time*, (20 January 1992): 42–51.

21. Remember our chapter 4 discussion of Gradziadei's research with the nose and brain development in tadpoles, chicks, and mice, and his discovery that the olfactory system helps to regulate and direct the development of the brain. Increasing evidence suggests that the speed and strength of the early prenatal hypothalamic GnRH pulse may depend on the numbers and/or types of nerve cells that complete their migration during the first trimester (E. Knobil, "The GnRH Pulse Generator," *American Journal of Obstetrics and Gynecology* 163 (1990): 1721–26; W. F. Crowley and R. W. Whitcomb, "Gonadotropin-releasing Hormone Deficiency in Man: Diagnosis and Treatment with Exogenous Gonadotropin-releasing Hormone," *American Journal of Obstetrics and Gynecology* 163 (1990): 1752–58. It is clear, however, that once the fetal hypothalamus is functional, the GnRH pulse begins to control the HPG axis. And it has become increasingly apparent that a faster GnRH pulse causes the pituitary to release more LH than FSH. M. M. Grumbach and D. M. Styne, "Puberty: Ontogeny, Neuroendocrinology, Physiology and Disorders," in J. D. Wilson and D. W. Foster, eds., *Textbook of Endocrinology*, 8th ed. (Philadelphia: W. B. Saunders, 1992). Also, through complex interactions with developing receptor sites and other hormones that act as, or influence neuromodulators and neurotransmitters, GnRH controls the LH/FSH ratio that conditions the release of testosterone and estrogen from the testes or ovaries.

22. S. S. C. Yen and A. Lein, "The Apparent Paradox of the Negative and Positive Feedback Control System on Gonadotropic Secretion," *American Journal of Obstetrics and Gynecology* 126 (1976): 942–54.

23. A higher level of testosterone than estrogen may alter or destroy nerve cells, particularly those connected with sexual differentiation, which might otherwise allow the cyclic hormone fluctuations characteristic of the female. The result seems to be the characteristic male, tonic pattern of hormone control, which becomes operative in late fetal life. F. Neumann and H. Steinbeck, "Influence of Sexual Hormones on the Differentiation of Neural Centers," *Archives of Sexual Behavior* 2 (1972): 147–162.

24. G. Dorner, "Hormone-Dependent Brain Development and Neuroendocrine Prophylaxis," *Experimental Clinical Endocrinology* 94 (1989): 4–22; R. W. Dittmann et al., "Congenital Adrenal Hyperplasia II: Gender-Related Behavior and Attitudes in Female Salt-Wasting and Simple-Virilizing Patients," *Psychoneuroendocrinology* 15 (1990): 421–34; A. A. Ehrhardt et al., "Sexual Orientation After Prenatal Exposure to Exogenous Estrogen," *Archives of Sexual Behavior* 14 (1985): 57–77.

25. P. Corbier et al., "Sex Differences in Serum Luteinizing Hormone and Testosterone in the Human Neonate During the First Few Hours After Birth," *Journal of Clinical Endocrinology and Metabolism* 71 (1990): 1347–48.

26. Y. Arai, A. Matusumoto, and M. Nishizuka, "Synaptogenesis and Neuronal Plasticity to Gonadal Steroids," in D. Ganten and D. W. Pfaff, eds., *Morphology of Hypothalamus and Its Connections* (Berlin: Springer-Verlag, 1986).

27. Earlier we remarked that human infants are born about eighteen months premature and that developmental biologists commonly speak of a nine-month uterogestation (in the womb) followed by continued development outside the womb, a roughly eighteen-month exterogestation. Because a woman's birth canal cannot handle a fully developed infant's brain, we are born premature. See: A. Walsh *The Science of Love: Understanding Love and Its Effects on Mind and Body* (New York: Prometheus Books, 1991), 42–43.

28. D. W. Lincoln, "Translation of Hypothalamic Electrical Activity into Episodic Hormone Secretion," in W. F. Crowley and J. G. Hofler, eds., *The Episodic Secretion of Hormones* (New York: John Wiley and Sons, 1987); F. H. Bronson and E. F. Rissman, "The Biology of Puberty," *Biological Reviews of the Cambridge Philosophical Society* 61 (1986): 157–95. This ability to redirect the behavioral templates of our limbic and reptilian brains may, in part, be due to their common embryonic origins. The neurons of the brain, the olfactory system, and touch receptors in the skin all come from the same layer of embryonic tissue. The nerve fibers connecting the olfactory placodes and skin to the three brain systems are also better developed than are other nerve fibers, so that even minimal stimulation or a slight reduction in smell and touch stimulation during critical periods increases or reduces neural activity, growth of nerve cell branches, and neuron-nourishing glial cells. Changes in the structure, arrangement, and pathways of the neural system naturally affect behavior, often throughout life. See M. Rutter, *Maternal Deprivation Reassessed* (Middlesex, England: Penguin, 1972), 57; Walsh, 49–51.

29. The sexual dimorphism between a tonic pattern involving a negative feedback system with two hormones in males and a cyclic pattern involving positive feedback with three hormones in females is not as simple as it seems. The cyclic hormone control characteristic of the female incorporates both positive and negative feedback although it is not readily apparent until later in life. Accordingly, current hypotheses on the development of hormone control systems recognize only the presence of tonic hormone control in prepubertal males and females. However, there is evidence from Hansen, Hoffman & Ross [J. W. Hansen, H. J. Hoffman, and G. T. Ross, "Monthly Gonadotropin Cycles in Premenarcheal Girls," *Science* 190 (1975): 161–63] that an undetected cyclic pattern in the female fetus and in prepubertal girls conditions the release of higher levels of FSH, and E, that will eventually help promote transient increases in LH secretion in women. This is commonly referred to as the "positive feedback" of estrogen on LH. Additionally, it is unlikely that the tonic pattern characteristic of the adult male matures in the complete absence of its adult female (cyclic) counterpart. Since there is also evidence that the positive feedback mechanism matures during adolescence in human males and females [H. Kulin and E. O. Reiter, "Gonadotropin and Testosterone measurements After Estrogen Administration to Adult Men, Prepubertal and Pubertal Boys, and Men with Hypogonadism," *Pediatric Research* 10 (1976): 46–51], it seems more likely that the cyclic pattern of hormone control is masked by the

predominance of prepubertal tonic hormone control. While immature follicles in the ovaries of women secrete low levels of estrogen that suppress LH release (negative feedback), mature follicles normally secrete enough estrogen to induce a surge of LH release (positive feedback) that is indicative of ovulation. Thus, the positive feedback of estrogen on LH becomes characteristic of an ovulatory menstrual cycle. In men, the testes produce testosterone that suppresses LH secretion (negative feedback). Higher testosterone levels in the male fetus and tonic hormone control via the negative feedback of testosterone on LH in prepubertal boys appears to partially destroy the capacity for positive feedback in men. Ultimately, however, the development of characteristic male and female hormone control systems seems to proceed from, and depend most upon, the speed of the prenatal hypothalamic GnRH pulse generator.

30. Grumback and Styne.

31. T. B. Van Wimersma Greidanus and D. DeWied, "Neuropeptides, Brain Function and Reproductive Behavior," in A. R. Genazzani et al., eds., *The Brain and Female Reproductive Function* (Park Ridge, N. J.: Parthenon, 1987).

32. Luteinizing hormone takes its name from the hormone-producing corpus luteum or "yellow body" that develops in a ruptured ovarian follicle after the egg is released. Hence, the name "yellow hormone."

33. D. M. Stoddart, *The Scented Ape: The Biology and Culture of Human Odor* (Cambridge: Cambridge University Press, 1990), 84.

34. Ibid., 110.

CHAPTER 8: FROM GENES TO BEHAVIOR AND BACK

1. Keep in mind that no one saw a mammalian egg or sperm until the 1670s, and the role of the union of egg and sperm was not discovered until 1776. The near-universal explanation of reproduction from ancient Greek philosophers and scientists to medieval and Renaissance biologists and theologians, depended on where a particular animal fit into "the Great Chain of Being." At the bottom of the Great Chain of Life, the creatures of dank swamps and dark night reproduced by spontaneous generation, asexually. For birds and reptiles in the middle of the Chain, mating was needed only to trigger development of the egg which contained everything needed for producing a new offspring. These animals were quite capable of producing fertile eggs without the male. As for the higher animals, warm-blooded mammals, primates, and humans, well, the male's seed or semen was all-important. When injected into a handy female "incubator," the hot male semen molded the menstrual blood to produce a newborn in the image of the parents. At the top of the Great Chain were sexless angels and God, none of whom had bodies or ever reproduced. (R. T. Francoeur, *Utopian Motherhood: New Trends in Human Reproduction* [New York: A. S. Barnes, 1970, 1977], 1–20.) As for explaining how the mother or father produced an offspring in her or his image and likeness, that was a simple matter of "preformation." In the Garden, the Creator packaged miniature models for all subsequent generations until the end of time into the ovaries and testes of the original male and female pairs. In each generation, a preformed

offspring was unpacked like the latest in a series of wooden Russian dolls, nestled one inside the other. In the early 1700s, philosophers like Leibnitz and Emmanuel Kant, and biologists like Marcello Malpighi, a papal physician, and Anton Leeuwenhoek, who discovered the human sperm, argued whether the Creator had packed all models for all generations into Eve's eggs or Adam's seed. Improvements in the microscope soon revealed neither Adam nor Eve had priority, and the preformed homunculus or "tiny human" scientists thought they saw in the sperm or egg was really the product of powerfully biased imaginations. In 1776 Lazzaro Spalanzanni experimented with artificial insemination and proved that both semen and egg were needed for any animal to reproduce. In the late 1800s, Charles Darwin offered an ingenious theory of heredity he called "pangenesis." According to Darwin, offspring always looked very much like their parents because every organ and structure in the parent's body continually dispatched microscopic "invisible germs," each with its own blueprint of that body part, to the ovaries or testes. Each sperm and egg was then packed with a complete set of "blue prints." Gregor Mendel's experiments with sweet peas in 1866 produced the first scientific laws of heredity, even though his research was not widely known or understood until early in this century. The genetic code of DNA/RNA was unraveled by James Watson and Francis Crick only forty years ago, in 1953.

2. B. S. McEwen, "Steroid Hormones and the Brain: Linking 'Nature and Nurture'," *Neurochemical Research* 13 (1988): 663.

3. Ibid.

4. D. Kimura, "Sex Differences in the Brain," *Scientific American* (1992): 119–125; C. Tavris, *The Mismeasure of Woman* (New York: Simon and Shuster, 1992); A. Fausto-Sterling. *Myths of Gender: Biological Theories about Women and Men* (New York: Basic Books, 1992).

5. Kimura, 118.

6. A Rossi, "Gender and Parenthood: American Sociological Association, 1983 Presidential Address," *American Sociological Review* 49 (1984): 1–19.

7. McEwen, 663.

8. J. Cohen and I. Stewart, *The Collapse of Chaos* (New York: Viking Penguin, 1994). Despite our inability to recover all the DNA of a preserved prehistoric animal and reproduce it, the fragments of ancient DNA scientists continue to recover can provide important insights into the rates of evolutionary change and the relationships between different organisms.

9. McEwen, 664.

10. Adrenaline is also known as noradrenaline, epinephrine, and norepinephrine.

11. John Money's comments on the role of opponent-process theory in explaining certain paraphilic behavior may shed some light on this condition. Opponent-process theory was proposed by Richard Solomon to augment traditional stimulus-response learning theory, according to which a powerful aversion or attraction to a particular activity or experience undergoes a reversal in the brain. For example, pain becomes pleasure, tragedy becomes triumph, terror turns into euphoria, or the forbidden turns into the prescribed. See J. Money, *Lovemaps* (New York: Irvington Publishers, 1986), 194, 196, 292.

12. The effects of low MAO on specific areas of the brain have been shown with PET scans, and linked with manic depression and psychopathologies. See Anthony Walsh's discussion of "Casanova; Casanovism" in V. L. Bullough and B. Bullough, eds. *Human Sexuality: An Encyclopedia* (New York & London: Garland Publishing, Inc., 1994), 85–86.

13. The full technical name of the enzyme is delta-4-steroid-5-alpha steroid reductase.

14. J. Diamond, "Turning a Man," *Discover* 13 (June 1992): 70–77; R. T. Francouer, *Becoming a Sexual Person* (New York: Macmillan Publishing, 1991), 99–100; J. Imperato-McGinley et al., "The Impact of Androgens on the Evolution of Male Gender Identity," in Z. DeFries et al., eds., *Sexuality: New Perspectives* (Westport, Conn.: Greenwood Press, 1985), 125–40; R. E. Pool, *Eve's Rib: Searching for the Biological Roots of Sex Differences* (New York: Crown, 1994), 72–73.

15. The opening of the urethra will be in or behind the scrotum, so that even though vaginal penetration is possible, ejaculation will occur outside the vagina of the female partner.

16. In Sambia, in the high lands of New Guinea, where this mutation has also been reported and studied, parents are much more concerned about the sex of their infants. Despite the lack of medical sophistication, infants with 5AR-DHT deficiency are raised as boys with a birth defect or as a third gender known as "turnim," meaning "expected to become a man." These boys are rejected by both parents, teased, and humiliated. Even after their penis and male secondary sex traits develop at puberty, they are not accepted as real males. Whether they are raised as boys or girls, these Sambian children seldom adapt to a normal adult sexual life. Diamond, 75–77.

17. The gene behind familial precocious male puberty is an autosomal, dominant, male-limited mutant gene.

18. I. Boekhoff et al., "Olfaction Desensitization Requires Membrane Targeting of Receptor Kinase Mediated by Beta Gamma-Subunits of Heterotrimeric G Proteins," *Journal of Biological Chemistry* 269 (1994): 37.

19. A. Shenker et al., "A Constitutively Activating Mutation of the Luteinizing Hormone Receptor in Familial Male Precocious Puberty," *Nature* 365 (1993): 652–54.

20. J. Money. *Gay, Straight and In-Between.* New York: Oxford University Press, 1988, 38–40.

21. Pool, 1994, and Kimura, 1992, provide clear and balanced summaries and commentaries on the evidence of the biological roots of some key human gender differences in the brain. Pool is particularly useful because the author cites the findings of a wide range of female feminist researchers that clearly support the contention of biological roots for gender differences in the brain. Some of the more valuable commentaries on the latest evidence for a biological basis for sexual orientations include: M. Barinaga, "Is Homosexuality Biological?," *Science* 253 (1991): 956–57; C. Burr, "Homosexuality and Biology," *The Atlantic Monthly* 271 (1993): 47–65; W. Byne and B. Parsons, "Human Sexual Orientation: The Biologic Theories Reappraised," *Archives of General Psychiatry*

50 (1993): 228–39; D. Gelman et al., "Mind: Born or Bred?," *Newsweek* (24 February): 46–53.

22. "Analyses of 24-hr urines from young healthy adult males for androsterone and etiocholanolone produced values which when subjected to linear discriminant analysis gave a clear discrimination between heterosexual and homosexual groups." M. S. Margolese, "Homosexuality: A New Endocrine Correlate," *Hormones and Behavior* 1 (1970): 151.

23. Margolese, 1970; M. S. Margolese and O. Janiger, "Androsterone-Etiocholanolone Ratios in Male Homosexuals," *British Medical Journal* 207 (1973): 207–210; Letter to the editor, *Nature* (1973): 244, 329; *Newsweek* (26 April 1971): 54–55.

24. Margolese and Janiger, 210.

25. Ibid., 208.

26. Heino Meyer-Bahlburg, a prominent researcher in this area, wrote in 1977 (314) that: "Margolese and Janiger (1973) speculate that this result may indicate a shift in metabolic pathway, toward the female side, which would then raise interesting questions of possible enzyme induction by prenatal hormone conditions. However, there are no standards available for male or female A/E ratios; the patterns of the levels of androsterone and of etiocholanolone across the Kinsey scale categories vary among the four studies, and the A/E ratios are very sensitive to other influences, especially diseases." ["Sex Hormones and Male Homosexuality in Comparative Perspective," *Archives of Sexual Behavior* 6 (1977): 297–325.]

27. A. P. Bell, M. S. Weinberg, and S. K. Hammersmith, *Sexual Preference: Its Development in Men and Women* (Bloomington: Indiana University Press, 1981).

28. Francouer, *Becoming a Sexual Person*, 71–101, 431–48.

29. R. C. Pillard and J. D. Weinrich, "Evidence of Familial Nature of Male Homosexuality," *Archives of General Psychiatry* 43 (1986): 808–12.

30. J. M. Bailey and R. C. Pillard, "A Genetic Study of Male Sexual Orientation," *Archives of General Psychiatry* 48 (1991): 1089–95.

31. J. M. Bailey et al., "Heritable Factors Influence Sexual Orientation in Women," *Archives of General Psychiatry* 50 (1993): 217–23.

32. F. L. Whitam, M. Diamond, and J. Martin, "Homosexual Orientation in Twins: A Report on 61 Pairs and Three Triplet Sets," *Archives of Sexual Behavior* 22 (1993): 187–206.

33. These recent studies confirm several genetics studies from the 1950s and 1960s that were, like Margolese's early findings, widely ignored or rejected in favor of the belief that sexual orientation was a social construction and a matter of free choice or preference. In 1952 and 1963, J. Kallmann reported on ten identical and forty-five fraternal twin pairs in which at least one twin admitted homosexual behavior. In every pair, Kallmann found the twin was also homosexual. Moreover, if the first identified twin was predominantly or exclusively homosexually oriented—Kinsey 5 or 6, there was a 90 percent chance the other twin would also be Kinsey 5–6. Usually, the twins were within one or two

points on the Kinsey six-point scale. Although Schlegel (1962) and others confirmed Kallmann's findings of a strong heritability and dominance of some biological factor, this explanation was not popular in the 1960s and 1970s. In the 1980s, the genetic and familial heritability began to emerge as the most likely and best documented explanation.

34. J. E. Bishop, "Research Points Toward a 'Gay' Gene," *Wall Street Journal* (16 July 1993): B1, B8; D. Hamer et al., "A Linkage Between DNA Markers on the X Chromosome and Male Sexual Orientation," *Science* 261 (1993): 321–27; Pool.

35. S. LeVay, *The Sexual Brain* (Cambridge, Mass.: MIT Press, 1993); S. LeVay and D. H. Hamer, "Evidence For a Biological Influence in Male Homosexuality," *Scientific American* (May 1994): 44–49.

36. Barinaga; Burr; Gelman; S. LeVay, "A Difference in Hypothalamic Structure Between Heterosexual and Homosexual Men," *Science* 253 (1991): 1034–37; *The Sexual Brain*; LeVay and Hamer; D. Y. Rist, "Are Homosexuals Born that Way?: Sex on the Brain," *The Nation* 255 (1992): 424–29.

37. C. L. Moore, "Interaction of Species-Typical Environmenal and Hormonal Factors in Sexual Differentiation of Behavior," *Annals of the New York Academy of Science* 474 (1986): 111.

38. "In older animals, there is the possibility that 16-androstenes might be involved in dominance relationships in both heterosexual and homosexual (boars) groups of pigs." D. B. Gower and W. D. Booth, "Salivary Pheromones in the Pig and Human in Relation to Sexual Status and Age," in W. Breipohl, ed., *Ontogeny of Olfaction* (Berlin: Springer-Verlag, 1986), 261.

39. N. Angier, "Making an Embryo: Biologists Find Keys to Body Plan. From Worms to Cows, One Class of Genes Spells Out the Blue Print," *New York Times*, 23 February 1993, C1, C9.

40. A. Booth et al., "Testosterone, and Winning and Losing in Human Competition," *Hormones and Behavior* 4 (1989): 556–71; Mazur, from Booth et al., 125–46.

41. N. Angier, "Finding Elusive Factors That Help Wire up the Brain," *New York Times*, 16 August 1994, C1, C7.

42. A similar marked consistency has been found in the locations and organization of GnRH neurosecretory neurons in the olfactory pathways and limbic system of many species. In the rat, GnRH neurons form a Y-shaped field oriented with the base along the midline of the rostral forebrain in a rostral-caudal plane. "[The arms of the 'Y'] first extend upwards through the diagonal band of Broca to the medial septum, and then turn ventrally into the preoptic area as they fan out laterally. They pass through the junction of the medial and lateral preoptic areas, the region just lateral to the suprachiasmatic nuclei, and then extend into the ventro lateral anterior hypothalamus where they lie just medial to the supraoptic nuclei" [See G. E. Hoffman et al., "Neuroendocrine Projections to the Median Eminence." In *Morphology of the Hypothalamus and its Connections*, ed., D. Ganten and D. W. Pfaff (Berlin: Springer-Verlag, 1986), 169]. This general pattern is found throughout vertebrate classes, and in most mammals, but the number of cells in specific regions varies. Although GnRH neurons are

found primarily in the hypothalamus, their distribution in the preoptic area, and outside the hypothalamus, in the hippocampus, cingulate cortex, and olfactory bulb, coupled with the ability of GnRH to enhance or depress the electrical activity of certain nerve cells and the wide distribution of receptors for GnRH, suggests a link between olfaction, GnRH, emotions, and behavior. See S. Reichlin, "Neuroendocrinology," in J. D. Wilson and D. W. Foster, eds., *Textbook for Endocrinology*, 8th ed. (Philadelphia: W. B. Saunders, 1992).

CHAPTER 9: THE EMOTIONAL MIND

1. E. H. Galluscio, *Biological Psychology* (New York: Macmillan Publishing, 1990), 105.

2. Paul MacLean ["Brain Evolution: The Origins of Social and Cognitive Behaviors," in M. Frank, ed., *A Child's Brain: The Impact of Advanced Research on Cognitive and Social Behaviors* (New York: Haworth Press, 1984), 9–22; *Journal of Children in Contemporary Society* 16, no. 1–2 (Fall/Winter 1983): 9–22] lists more than twenty behaviors that are key to self-preservation and survival which are moderated by the reptilian brain in all animals from snakes and lizards to humans. These include: (1) homesite selection and preparation; (2) establishment of domain or territory; (3) "marking" of domain or territory; (4) showing place-preferences; (5) ritualistic display in defense of territory (commonly involving color and adornment); (6) formalized intraspecific fighting in defense of territory; (7) triumphal display after successful defense; (8) assumption of distinctive postures and coloration signalling surrender; (9) routinization of daily activities; (10) foraging; (11) hunting; (12) homing; (13) hoarding; (14) use of defecation posts; (15) formation of social groups; (16) establishment of social hierarchy by ritualistic display and other means; (17) greeting; (18) grooming; (19) courtships with coloration and adornment displays; (20) mating; (21) breeding and in isolated instances, attending offspring; (22) flocking.

3. Developmental biologists describe human pregnancy as having two stages, a nine-month uterogestation in the womb and a year or more of exterogestation before the human infant reaches the level of neural development the offspring of four-legged mammals enjoy when they are born. The human infant is born premature at nine months because if he or she stayed in the womb another year his or her head would be too large to pass through the birth canal. A. Walsh *The Sciece of Love: Understanding Love and Its Effects on Mind and Body* (New York: Prometheus Books, 1991), 42–43.

4. The smile is also genetically programmed to trigger certain brain cells to releases natural opiates, or endorphins. These produce a natural psychological "high," much as some drugs do. That reward reinforces the smile reflex by making the infant feel good. Once the connection is made between feeling good and smiling, the infant keeps smiling when it learns that smiling will bring a cuddle, hug, or a thirst-quenching spell at the breast. Abused or neglected children seldom develop this reflex smile, and gradually learn to withdraw emotionally into their own shell.

5. L. Lipsit, "Critical Conditions in Infancy: A Psychological Perspective," *American Psychologist* 34 (1979): 973–80; Walsh, 80–81.

6. MacLean, 13.

7. Ibid., 14–15.

8. The GnRH neurons which migrate to the hypothalamus somehow generate a GnRH pulse, though how this is done remains a significant mystery. It seems that a loosely connected network of GnRH found in various parts of the limbic system affects the pulse generation. As mentioned elsewhere, the speed of the hypothalamic GnRH pulse generator sets the ratio of LH to FSH secretion, which in turn determines the amount of androgens and estrogens secreted by the ovaries and testes.

9. C. W. Malsbury, "Facilitation of Male Rat Copulatory Behavior by Electrical Stimulation of the Medial Preoptic Area," *Physiology and Behavior* 7 (1971): 797–805.

10. M. Numan, "Neuronal Basis of Maternal Behavior in the Rat," *Psychoneuro-endocrinology* 13 (1988): 47–62.

11. R. A. Gorski et al., "Evidence for a Morphological Sex Difference Within the Medial Preoptic Area of the Rat Brain," *Brain Research* 143 (1978): 333–46; G. W. Arendash and R. A. Gorski, "Effects of Discrete Lesions of the Sexually Dimorphic Regions on the Sexual Behavior of Male Rats," *Brain Research* 10 (1983): 147–54. See also Robert Pool's *Eve's Rib* (New York: Crown, 1994) especially 110–24 and 166–67. This book, as its subtitle *Searching for the Biological Roots of Sex Differences* indicates, is invaluable because it provides a very readable review of what we know and don't know based on the latest research on sex differences in the human brain. The fact that most of the research reviewed by Pool has been done by female feminist psychologists and biologists certainly makes a difference in the way we evaluate the research data.

12. D. W. Pfaff and Y. Sakuma, "Deficit in the Lordosis Reflex of Female Rats Caused by Lesions in the Ventromedial Nucleus of the Hypothalamus," *Journal of Physiology* 288 (1979): 203–10; E. T. Pleim and R. J. Barfield, "Progesterone Versus Estrogen Facilitation of Female Sexual Behavior by Intracranial Administration to Female Rats," *Hormones and Behavior* 22 (1988): 150–59.

13. LeVay's preliminary sample included only sixteen males and six females, so confirmation in larger samples will be a crucial test of his theory. S. LeVay, "A Difference in Hypothalamic Structure Between Heterosexual and Homosexual Men," *Science* 253 (1991): 1034–37; *The Sexual Brain* (Cambridge, Mass.: MIT Press, 1993); S. LeVay and D. H. Hamer, "Evidence For a Biological Influence in Male Homosexuality," *Scientific American* (May 1994): 44–49; W. Byne and B. Parsons, "Human Sexual Orientation: The Biologic Theories Reappraised," *Archives of General Psychiatry* 50 (1993): 228–39.

14. D. Hamer and P. Copeland, *The Science of Desire* (New York: Simon and Schuster, 1994), 163.

15. These structures include the thalamus in the inner walls of the cerebral hemispheres and the nearby paraolfactory area. Psychologist Anthony Walsh [*The Science of Love: Understanding Love and Its Effects on Mind and Body* (Buffalo,

New York: Prometheus Books, 1991), 37–95] provides an excellent summary of the many connections between altruism and love and the chemistry of the reptilian and limbic minds in his chapters on "The Neurophysiology of Touch and Love," "The Chemistry of Mother Love," and "Love and the Triune Brain."

16. The research on Somatosensory Affectional Deprivation (SAD) syndrome compiled in convincing detail by James W. Prescott provides an excellent example of our ability to reprogram the limbic system's pleasure and violence circuits. See "Affectional Bonding for the Prevention of Violent Behaviors: Neurological, Psychological and Religious/Spiritual Determinants," in L. J. Hertzberg, G. F. Ostrum, and J. R. Field, eds., *Violent Behavior*, vol. 1 of *Assessment and Intervention*, (New York: PMA Publishing, 1990).

17. MacLean, 11.

18. Walsh, 87.

19. M. Long, "Visions of a New Faith," *Science Digest* 89 (1981): 36–42; G. Ogden, *Women Who Love Sex* (New York: Pocket Books, 1994); J. W. Prescott, "Affectional Bonding for the Prevention of Violent Behaviors: Neurological, Psychological and Religious/Spiritual Determinants," in L. J. Hertzberg, G. F. Ostrum, and J. R. Field, eds., *Violent Behavior*, vol. 1 of *Assessment and Intervention* (New York: PMA Publishing, 1990), 115–17.

20. We should point out a common but misleading simplification of the link between genes and their specific effects. While it is true that genes directly affect hormones which directly influence behavior, that odors affect the expression of certain genes, and that many specific genes carry the same identical information, we must also remember that the same identical gene can have slightly different expressions when it is in a chimpanzee cellular environment and when it is translated in a human cell loaded with a distinctly human combination of proteins and enzymes. This very important qualification has been well detailed by Jack Cohen and Ian Steward in their 1994 book *The Collapse of Chaos* (New York: Viking Penguin, 1994). See also Cohen and Stewart's article "Our Genes Aren't Us" in *Discover* 15 (April 1994): 78–84.

21. D. H. Freedman, "In the Realm of the Chemical," *Discover* 14, no. 9 (June 1993): 73.

22. S. Van der Lee and L. M. Boot, "Spontaneous Pseudopregnancy in Mice," *Acta Physiologica et Pharmacologica Neederlandica* 4 (1955): 442–44.

23. F. H. Bronson and W. Whitten, "Estrous Accelerating Pheromone of Mice: Assay, Androgen-Dependency, and Presence in Bladder Urine," *Journal of Reproduction and Fertility* 15 (1968): 131–34.

24. H. M. Bruce, "Further Observations of Pregnancy Block in Mice Caused by Proximity of Strange Males," *Journal of Reproduction and Fertility* 2 (1960): 311–12.

25. This increase in the risk of spontaneous abortion was found only in women who worked full-time and were directly exposed to the many chemicals in hair-permanent solutions, dyes, and disinfectants. To reduce this risk, researchers recommended use of gloves, proper ventilation, not eating and drinking at work, and avoiding products containing formaldehyde. See: Associated Press Release, 28 February 1994. 22:05 EST VO714; and E. M.

John, D. A. Savitz, and C. M. Shy, "Spontaneous Abortions Among Cosmetologists," *Epidemiology* 5 (1994): 147–55.

26. MacLean, 11.

27. Ibid., 11.

28. Ibid., 19–20.

29. Ibid., 12.

30. Walsh, 69–70. The long-term effects of the oxytocin on human and animal behavior prompted psychophysiologist Niles Nelson ["Terribly Sensuous Woman," *Psychology Today* (July 1971): 68] to honor this hormone as "the hormone of love." Angier ["A Potent Peptide Prompts an Urge to Cuddle," *New York Times*, 22 January 1991, C1, C10] provides a fine non-technical overview of recent research on "the cuddling hormone." See also, P. Klopfer, "Mother Love: What Turns It On? Studies of Maternal Arousal and Attachment in Ungulates May Have Implications for Man," *American Scientist* 59 (1971): 404–7.

31. Prescott.

32. R. Ader, D. Felten, and N. Cohen, "Interactions Between the Brain and the Immune System," *Annual Review of Pharmacology and Toxocology* 30 (190): 561–602. The effects of pleasuring touches on basic human physiology have been studied by many researchers interested in enhancing the survival and development of infants born prematurely. In one typical study, an eight-month experiment with premature infants kept in isolettes, some were massaged for fifteen minutes three times a day while the controls were not massaged. Massaged babies gain weight forty-seven percent faster than unmassaged babies. Massaged babies are more alert, more active, and more responsive than unmassaged babies. Massaged babies are better able to tolerate noise than unmassaged babies. Massaged babies are "better able to calm and console themselves." The nervous systems of massaged babies mature more rapidly. Massaged preemies are discharged from hospitals an average of six days earlier than unmassaged preemies. When tested eight months later, massaged infants did better in tests of mental and motor ability. See D. Ackerman, *A Natural History of the Senses* (New York: Random House, 1990).

33. Ader, Felten, and Cohen.

34. K. Olness and R. Ader, "Conditioning as an Adjunct in the Pharmacotheraphy of Lupus Erythematosus," *Journal of Developmental and Behavioral Pediatrics* 13 (1992): 124–25.

35. Precisely how the influence of pheromones on GnRH may be involved in learning and memory is beyond the scope of this book. Moreover, current biological knowledge of primates makes it difficult to model or test hypotheses about the sense of smell in human learning and memory. On the other hand, if we examine animal models, particularly the rat, concentrations of GnRH receptors are found in the hippocampus. Predictably then, pheromones may have an influence on the amount of GnRH that reaches these receptors. The olfactory system then appears to be the sensory system with the most direct access to the hippocampus, a structure very important to learning and memory. See B. Marchetti et al., "Age-Dependent Changes of LHRH Receptor

Systems: Role of Central and Peripheral LHRH in the Decline of Reproductive Function," in A. R. Genazzani et al., eds., *The Brain and Female Reproductive Function* (New Jersey: Parthenon, 1988; M. Shipey and P. Reyes, "Anatomy of the Human Olfactory Bulb and Central Olfactory Pathways," in D. Laing, R. L. Doty, and W. Breipohl, eds., *The Human Sense of Smell* (New York: Springer-Verlag,1991).

36. See also: A. K. Francoeur and R. T. Francoeur, *Hot and Cool Sex: Cultures in Conflict* (New York: Harcourt, 1974), 104.

37. MacLean, "The Brain's Generation Gap."

38. M. Proust, *Remembrance of Things Past* (New York: Random House, 1934).

CHAPTER 10: NATURAL OPIATES, INFATUATIONS, AND BONDING

1. B. Gibbons, "The Intimate Sense of Smell," *National Geographic* 170 (1986): 324–61; J. Money, *Lovemaps* (New York: Irvington Publishers, 1986), 94–95; M. J. Russell, G. M. Switz, and K. Thompson, "Olfactory Influences on the Human Menstrual Cycle," *Pharmacology, Biochemistry and Behavior* 13 (1980): 737–38.

2. Some female reptiles, notably crocodiles, will defend the eggs in their nests from predators.

3. Money, 94–95.

4. M. F. Small, "What's Love Got to Do With It?," *Discover* 13 (June 1992): 46–51; *Female Choices: Sexual Behavior of Female Primates* (Ithaca: Cornell University Press, 1993).

5. H. E. Fisher, *Anatomy of Love* (New York: W. W. Norton, 1992), 129–30.

6. F. DeWaal, *Chimpanzee Politics: Power and Sex Among Apes* (New York: Harper and Row, 1982); "Tension Regulation and Non-Reproductive Function of Sex in Captive Bonobos (*Pan paniscus*)," *National Geographic Research* 3 (1987): 318–35; C. S. Ford and F. A. Beach, *Patterns of Sexual Behavior* (New York: Harper and Row, 1951); M. Goodall, *The Chimpanzees of Gombe: Patterns of Behavior* (Cambridge, Mass.: Belknap, 1986); S. B. Hrdy, *The Woman That Never Evolved* (Cambridge, Mass.: Harvard University Press, 1987); T. Kano and M. Mulavwa, "Feeding Ecology of the Pygmy Chimpanzees (*Pan paniscus*) of Wamba," in R. L. Susman, ed., *The Pygmy Chimpanzee* (New York: Plenum Press, 1984); S. Kuroda, "Interaction Over Food Among Pygmy Chimpanzees," in R. L. Susman ed., *The Pygmy Chimpanzee* (New York: Plenum Press, 1984); N. Thompson-Handler et al., "Sexual Behavior of *Pan paniscus* under Natural Conditions in the Lomako Forest, Equateur, Zaire," in R. L. Susman ed., *The Pygmy Chimpanzee* (New York: Plenum Press, 1984).

7. Money, 94.

8. For details on how neurons use receptors and neurotransmitters to signal each others, see Changeux.

9. M. R. Leibowitz, *The Chemistry of Love* (Boston: Little Brown, 1983), 49.

10. "Lacking in experiences that prepare them for loving relationships with people, addicts find their warmth and pleasure pharmacologically. Lacking attachments, heroin substitutes for the brain's own endorphins; lacking romantic attraction, cocaine and other stimulants stand in for the brain's own phenylethylamine." A. Walsh *The Science of Love: Understanding Love and Its Effects on Mind and Body* (New York: Prometheus Books, 1991), 134.

11. Ibid., 188.

12. Ibid., 189.

13. "Biologists [have] long believed . . . that up to 94 percent of bird species were monogamous, with one mother and one father sharing the burden of raising their chicks. Now, using advanced techniques [involving DNA probes] to determine the paternity of offspring, biologists are finding that, on average, 30 percent or more of the baby birds in any nest were sired by someone other than the resident male. Indeed, researchers are having trouble finding bird species that are not prone to such evident philandering." N. Angier, "Mating for Life? It's Not for the Birds," *New York Times*, 22 January 1991, C1, C10.

14. Walsh, 189–90.

15. This endorphin effect is produced mainly in the locus ceruleus.

16. Quite independently, another psychiatrist, Hector Sabelli, came to a similar conclusion about the link between PEA and being in love. Sabelli found high levels of PEA metabolites in the urine of thirty three men and women who reported positive feelings about their relationship with a significant other. One man and one woman who were going through a divorce, showed low levels of PEA metabolites, Sabelli suggests, probably because they were experiencing a low grade depression in a painful breakup. See H. C. Sabelli, A. Carlson-Sabelli, and J. I. Javaid, "The Thermodynamics of Bipolarity: A Bifurcation Model of Bipolar Illness and Bipolar Character and Its Therapeutic Applications," *Psychiatry* 53 (1990): 356–68; H. C. Sabelli, "Rapid Treatment of Depression with Selegiline-Phenylalanine Combination [Letter to the Editor]," *Journal of Clinical Psychiatry* 52 (1991): 3.

17. Walsh, 121–27 and 144–45; E. Coleman and J. Cesnik, "Skoptic Syndrome: The Treatment of an Obsessional Gender Dysphoria with Lithium Carbonate and Psychotherapy," *American Journal of Psychotherapy* 44 (1990): 204–17; E. Coleman, "Compulsive Sexual Behavior: New Concepts and Treatments," *Journal of Psychology and Human Sexuality* 4 (1991): 37–52.

18. Liebowitz, 179–89.

19. J. Money, *Love and Love Sickness: The Science of Sex, Gender Difference, and Pair-Bonding* (Baltimore: Johns Hopkins, 1980), 79, 152, 193.

20. Endorphins, like other neuroactive substances referred to as enkephalins and dynorphins, are derived from much larger peptides. Some neuroscientists believe that the anesthetic effects of acupuncture may involve the release of endorphins triggered by fine needles being inserted at certain points on the meridians of the body detailed thousands of years ago by early Chinese healers. See H. Akil et al., "Endogenous Opioids: Biology and Function," *Annual Review of Neuroscience* 7 (1984): 223–55; J. Olds and P. Milner, "Positive Reinforcement Produced by

Electrical Stimulation of Septal Area and Other Regions of the Rat Brain," *Journal of Comparative and Physiological Psychology* 47 (1954): 419–27.

21. Angier, "Mating for Life? It's Not for the Birds," C1, C10.

22. Ovulating female mice injected with oxytocin are 60 to 80 percent more attentive in finding a male to mount and impregnate them than noninjected females. Gregarious field mice are known to have more natural oxytocin than mice of another species who prefer living alone and getting together only to mate. When gregarious field mice are given extra oxytocin they become even more cuddly. Oxytocin has no effect on the closely related, but standoffish and withdrawn mice. Their brain structure is much less sensitive to oxytocin. Perhaps their brain cells do not have as many oxytocin receptors, but other factors may also contribute to the different responses.

23. L. Tiger and R. Fox, *The Imperial Animal* (New York: Holt, Rinehart and Winston, 1971).

24. R. I. Shtarkshall, "Israel: Section of Kibbutz Movement," in R. T. Francouer, ed., *International Encyclopedia of Sexuality* (New York: Continuum Press, in press).

25. See also: A. K. Francoeur and R. T. Francoeur, *Hot and Cool Sex: Cultures in Conflict* (New York: Harcourt, 1974), 99–100.

26. "Choosing the Perfect Mate a Matter of Who Smells Best." An Associated Press News Release from the 1993 annual meeting of the American Society of Human Genetics, New Orleans. Published in the *Las Vegas Review-Journal/Sun*, 10 October 1993.

27. W. Beamer, G. Bermant, and M. Clegg, "Copulatory Behavior of the Ram," *Animal Behavior* 17 (1969): 795–800; E. H. Galluscio, *Biological Psychology* (New York: Macmillan Publishing, 1990), 161. In 1952, Jerome Grunt and William Young, at University of Kansas School of Medicine, first confirmed the Coolidge Effect as operating on the sexual responsiveness of both male and female guinea pigs. It has since been confirmed to exist in both male and female mice, rats, dairy cattle, water buffaloes, sheep, pigs, and cats.

28. Francoeur and Francoeur, 98. William Masters and Virginia Johnson pioneered the first use of sexual surrogates for erectile problems in their Sexual and Marital Therapy Clinic in St. Louis in the early 1960s. After a few years, they discontinued the practice although other therapists continued its use. There was even an International Professional Surrogates Association. The emergence of the AIDS epidemic in the 1980s spelled the end of this form of therapy. See R. T. Francoeur, T. Perper, and N. A. Scherzer, *A Descriptive Dictionary and Atlas of Sexology* (New York: Greenwood Press, 1991; Francoeur, Perper, and Scherzer, *The Complete Dictionary of Sexology*, New Expanded Edition (New York: Continuum, 1994), 610, 641.

29. Quoted in Francoeur and Francoeur, 105.

CHAPTER 11: MAKING HUMAN PHEROMONES

1. Each type of gland is actually part of a glandular system that may be activated or inactivated by a number of different factors.

2. Eccrine glands in the palms and soles respond primarily to psychogenic stimuli, while those on the rest of the body respond to thermal stimulation. The larger eccrine glands in the soles of our feet are, in part, responsible for the distinctive odor of our feet. "Given sufficient thermal stimulation, an individual through his two to three million sweat glands can produce two to three liters of sweat per hour for a short interval. An increase in body heat arouses temperature-sensitive centers in the hypothalamus and serves as a potent stimulus for generalized sweating." See M. L. Johnson, "Skin Diseases," in *Cecil Textbook of Medicine*, vol. 2, ed. J. B. Wyngaarden and J. B. Smith Jr. (Philadelphia: W. B. Saunders, 1982).

3. Sebaceous glands are a major source of pheromones in other mammals [J. N. Labows and G. Preti, "Human Semiochemicals," in S. Van Toller and G. H. Dodd, eds., *Fragrance: The Psychology and Biology of Perfume* (Amsterdam: Elsevier Applied Science 1992)]. The secretion from eccrine glands reflects the chemical composition of plasma in a diluted form. It contains proteins, enzymes, glycoproteins, lactic acid, glucose, amino acids, and inorganic salts. Secretions from the sebaceous glands are rich in cholesterol, cholesterol esters, squalene, fatty acids, and triglycerides. See W. Monagna, "The Evolution of Human Skin," *Journal of Human Evolution* 14 (1985): 19.

4. Eccrine glands develop first and appear in the sixth week of embryogenesis. Sebaceous glands differentiate at thirteen to fifteen weeks gestation and immediately begin to produce sebum in all hairy areas. "Apocrine glands originate from and empty into the hair follicles, just above the sebaceous glands. At seven to eight months' gestation, they start to produce a milky white fluid containing water, lipids, protein, reducing sugars, ferric iron, and ammonia. Decomposition of this fluid by skin bacteria produces a characteristic odor." S. Blackburn and D. L. Loper, *Maternal, Fetal, and Neonatal Physiology* (Philadelphia: W. B. Saunders, 1992), 506.

5. Unlike sebaceous glands that open directly to the exterior by spirally wound ducts, apocrine glands have straight ducts and, as a rule, open into a hair follicle. Once apocrine secretions are in solution, they appear to pass through the intact cell membrane to the hair follicle. See: J. R. Baker, *Race* (New York: Oxford University Press, 1974).

6. The presence of apocrine glands has (at one time or another) been reported in skin from the following areas: axilla (underarm), umbilical region (around the navel or bellybutton), suprapubic region (above the genitals), perianal region (around the anus), hairy part of the chest, areola (the area surrounding the nipple of the breast), hypogastric region (lower abdomen), inguinal region (the groin), prepuce (the skin that surrounds the tip of the penis, or covers the clitoris), scrotum (the pouch that contains the testes), labium majus (the larger lips of the vagina), labia minora (the smaller lips of the vagina), scalp, eyebrow, malar region (the cheeks of our face), forehead, bearded portion of face, nasal vestibule (at the base of the nose), and in the scalp. [M. B. L. Craigmyle, *The Apocrine Glands and the Breast* (Chichester: Wiley and Sons, 1984), 11]. "The breast is actually a modified apocrine gland, as are the ceruminous (wax) glands of the ear and Moll's glands of the eyelid" (at the base of the eyelashes).

M. L. Johnson, "Skin Diseases," in *Cecil Textbook of Medicine*, vol. 2, ed. J. B. Wyngaarden and J. B. Smith Jr. (Philadelphia: W. B. Saunders, 1982).

7. Baker.

8. Man has more sebaceous glands than any other mammal. Men have more sebaceous glands than women paralleling the same dimorphism in mammals generally. B. Nicholson, "Does Kissing Aid Human Bonding by Semiochemical Addiction?," *British Journal of Dermatology* 111 (1984): 623–27.

9. Reports that women have more apocrine glands than men, indicate that estrogens may even increase the number of apocrine glands that are formed in the fetus. "We do, however, know that there are 75 percent more apocrine glands in the female of our species than in the male, and it is interesting to recall that in lower mammals during sexual encounters the male sniffs the female more than she sniffs him" D. Morris. *The Naked Ape*. (London: Jonathan Cape, 1967), 77. "Women have 75 percent more apocrine glands than men" B. Brody, "The Sexual Significance of the Axillae," *Psychiatry* 38 (1975): 279. And finally, Craigmyle (1984, p. 34) agrees with "Schiefferdecker (1922) and Homma (1926) [who] claimed that apocrine glands were better developed and occurred with twice the frequency in women compared with men."

10. The high levels of the adrenal hormones DHEA and DHEAS in newborns is important to their aromatic secretions because these hormones are precursors of testosterone and increase apocrine and sebaceous gland secretions. G. B. Culter et al., "The Adrenarche (Human and Animal)," in M. M. Grumback, P. C. Sizonenko, and M. L. Aubert, eds., *Control of the Onset of Puberty* (Baltimore: Williamson and Wilkens, 1990), 513.

11. "Normal pubertal development in humans involves two distinct processes: 'adrenarche' (i.e., maturation of adrenal androgen secretion), involving the hypothalamic-pituitary-adrenal (HPA) axis; and 'gonadarche,' reactivation of the hypothalamic-pituitary-gonadal (HPG) axis and maturation of gonadal sex steroid secretion. Adrenarche usually occurs at ages six to eight. Adrenal androgen secretion increases gradually, continues to rise through puberty, and reaches asymptote in late adolescence. No physiological role has been ascribed as yet to adrenal androgens, other than stimulation of growth of small amounts of pubic hair. Gonadarche usually occurs at ages nine to thirteen. Gonadotropin levels rise first, followed by gonadal sex steroids, the levels of which rise more steeply than adrenal androgens and reach asymptote around midadolescence. The gonadal sex steroids are responsible for the development of secondary sex characteristics. Testosterone and its active metabolite 5-dihydrotestosterone masculinize boys, and estradiol is the hormone primarily responsible for feminizing girls." E. D. Nottelmann et al., "Hormones and Behavior at Puberty," in J. Bancroft and J. Machover-Reinisch, eds., *Adolescence and Puberty* (New York: Oxford University Press, 1990), 89.

12. A branched, loose meshwork in the base of the apocrine gland produces oily secretions that are then transported to the skin surface by a duct. These secretions, though colorless to the naked eye, contain large, brownish-yellow globules made from fatty material, which consists of phospholipids and cholesterol esters (Baker). Because DHEA and DHEAS come almost entirely from

adrenal secretion, plasma levels of these two hormones are the most useful biochemical markers of adrenarche. In addition to DHEA and DHEA sulfate, adrenarche causes an increase in the adrenal secretion of several other hormones involved in pheromone production. There is, however, no scientific evidence suggesting that DHEA acts as a pheromone. The fact that the levels of DHEA vary only slightly between males and females, makes it a very unlikely candidate for a sex pheromone, or any other kind of pheromone. DHEA levels are important in our context only because they are metabolized differently in men and women to other potential human pheromones.

13. E. E. Filsinger and W. C. Monte, "Sex History, Menstrual Cycle, and Psychophysical Ratings of Alpha Androstenone, a Possible Human Sex Pheromone," *Journal of Sex Research* 22 (1986): 243–48.

14. "The odor which develops in the axillae has been shown to be a function of the resident microorganism present there. Correlations of odor quality and bacterial populations have been found in recent studies; these results show that when a faint or acid odor was present micrococcaceae were present in 100% of subjects. A more pungent odor similar to that of C19-delta-16 steroids [such as androstenone] is produced by lipophilic diphtheroids, a different species of bacteria. These more pungent substances were found in 85% of males and 66 % of females examined" [G. Preti et al., "Human Axillary Secretions Influence Women's Menstrual Cycles: The Role of Donor Extract of Females," *Hormones and Behavior* 20 (1986): 475]. Halpin adds that "Among the environmental factors that may affect individual odors, both bacterial flora and diet have been shown to be important." Z. T. Halpin, "Individual Odors Among Mammals," in *Advances in the Study of Behavior*, vol. 16, J. S. Rosenblatt, C. Beer, M. Busner, and P. J. B. Slater, eds. (Orlando: Academic Press, 1986), 51.

15. Early investigators claimed that the apocrine glands enlarge and secrete more actively just before menstruation. Later, some investigators agreed and others disagreed. Although the majority opinion seems to be that apocrine glands enlarge and exhibit increased activity with pregnancy, there is also disagreement on whether apocrine glands alter during pregnancy.

16. "The sebaceous gland depends upon and is extremely receptive to androgenic hormones. Maternal androgens ensure full development and function at birth. The vernix caseosa covering the neonate is mostly sebum. Normally the gland then atrophies until the child's pubertal hormones stimulate it once more. Sebaceous gland activity in children can result from congenital adrenal hyperplasia or anabolic hormone therapy as given in aplastic anemia. Disorders of androgen excess in adult women are associated with increased sebaceous gland activity. Androgen insufficiency in either sex such as hypogonadism or adrenal insufficiency is associated with decreased activity. Androgens increase the sebaceous gland size, increase the secretion of sebum, and increase sebaceous gland mitotic rate. Estrogens decrease gland size and secretion but do not decrease the mitotic rate. Their effect may be from the suppression of androgens primarily at sites of androgen synthesis rather than at the glandular level. In women, adrenal androgens in addition to gonadal androgens are a source of sebaceous stimulation.

Progesterone in physiologic amounts has no effect, and the role of the pituitary is most likely indirect through tropic hormones. With severe caloric deprivation sebum secretion levels decrease.

"The function of sebaceous gland lipid is in question. Although variously touted as a barrier to microbes or other hostile environment, as a regulator of percutaneous absorption, and as a vitamin D precursor, all these roles have been challenged. Further, skin conditions characterized by dry skin, such as ichthyosis or asteatosis, are allegedly associated with decreased sebum production, but without supporting data."

"What is known is that sebaceous gland maturation, which begins at age eight to ten and continues through adolescence, remains fairly unchanged through adult life until it decreases some time past the fifth decade in women and the seventh decade in men. Patients with Parkinson's disease and postmenopausal women with breast cancer have statistically higher rates of sebum secretion that the average. Because the distribution of sebum levels overlaps with normal values, an individual reading has limited diagnostic importance." M. L. Johnson, "Skin Diseases" in J. B. Wyngaarden and J. B. Smith, eds., *Cecil Textbook of Medicine*, vol. 2 (Philadelphia: W. B. Saunders, 1982), 2252.

17. "Hurley & Shelley (1960) state that apocrine secretion occurs only in response to emotional stimuli and not in response to heat, whereas eccrine glands respond to both. A very good case has been made by Way & Memmesheimer (1938) and by Higginson & McDonald (1949) for classifying apocrine glands as accessory sexual glands, and Montagna & Parakkal (1974) suggest that the glands in fact produce odorous pheromones. I am in complete agreement with these stances and feel the time has now come when we should cease to refer to the apocrine glands as sweat glands" (Craigmyle, 35).

18. Brody, 279.

19. Filsinger and Monte.

20. S. Takami et al., "Vomeronasal Epithelial Cells of the Adult Human Express Neuron-Specific Molecules," *Neuroreport* 4 (1993): 378.

21. L. A. Goldsmith, "My Organ is Bigger than Your Organ," *Archives of Dermatology* 126 (1990): 301–2. The skin is the largest organ of the body. For example, it encompasses over 1.7 square meters on a 70 kilogram man.

22. D. L. Berliner, "Biotransformation of Steroids by the Skin," *Advances in the Biology of the Skin*, annual series, vol. 12 (New York: Pergamon, Symposium Publications, 1972), 357; Berliner, J. R. Pasqualini, and A. J. Gallegos, "The Formation of Water Soluble Steroids by Human Skin," *Journal of Investigative Dermatology* 50 (1968): 220–24; A. I. Mallet et al., "Applications of Gas Chromatography-Mass Spectometry in the Study of Androgen and Odorous 16-androstene Metabolism by Human Axillary Bacteria," *Journal of Chromatography* 562 (1991): 657.

23. Other organs (the liver, adrenals, intestines, kidneys, ovaries, testes, various fetal tissues, and the placenta) also help metabolize the steroid hormones (including corticosteroids). And when it comes to cause and effect, our skin cells mimic the gonads, adrenals, and other hormone-secreting organs that function under varying degrees of control by the hypothalamus and the pituitary.

24. "... it is extremely unlikely that any two individuals will make exactly the same substances in exactly the same proportions. Slight normal variations in enzyme concentrations, pH, body temperature, or cofactor concentrations, for example, could easily and markedly affect the final concentration of each fatty chain and thus provide an individual with a 'chemical signature.' This would be the distinctive odor by which a dog that had once sniffed a person would recognize and remember the person thereafter." N. Nicolaides and J. M. B. Apron, "The Saturated Methyl Branched Fatty Acids of Adult Human Skin Surface Lipid," *Biomedicine and Mass Spectrometry* 4 (1977): 186.

25. "Perhaps these acids serve a pheromonal function and contribute to our distinctive 'chemical signature' just as the skin gives each of us a distinctive fingerprint." Ibid, 347.

26. Alpha-androstenone and alpha-androstenol are found in the urine of both human sexes after puberty, with much greater concentrations in male urine. The ratio of alpha-androstenone to testosterone in the blood of men is similar to the ratio in boars. Filsinger.

27. A number of different enzymes and bacteria found in the mouth contribute to the odor of our breath, which may provide others with knowledge about the levels of our sex hormones. Saliva is similar in composition to plasma and clinical studies show that for many steroid hormones, serum, and saliva values correlate well. Saliva samples are used to measure testosterone, progesterone, estriol, and estradiol. S. M. Miller, "Saliva Testing—A Nontraditional Diagnostic Tool," *Clinical Laboratory Science* 7 (1994): 39–44.

28. S. Bird and D. B. Gower, "Validation and Use of RIA for Androstenone in Axillary Collection," *Journal of Steroid Biochemistry and Molecular Biology* 14 (1981): 213–19.

29. "The body in reality gives off a number of different odors. The most important of these are: (1) the general skin odor, a faint, but agreeable, fragrance often to be detected on the skin even immediately after washing; (2) the smell of the hair and scalp; (3) the odor of the breath; (4) the odor of the armpit; (5) the odor of the feet; (6) the perineal odor; (7) in men the odor of the preputial smegma; (8) in women the odor of the mons veneris, that of vulvar smegma, that of vaginal mucus, and the menstrual odor. All these are odors which may usually be detected, though sometimes only in a very faint degree, in healthy and well-washed persons under normal conditions" [H. Ellis, *Studies in the Psychology of Sex: Sexual Selection in Man*, vol. 4 (Philadelphia: Davis, 1914), 62].

30. Montagna.

31. P. R. Abramson and E. H. Pearsall, "Pectoral Changes During the Sexual Response Cycle: A Thermographic Analysis," *Archives of Sexual Behavior* 12 (1983): 357–68.

32. Berliner, "Biotransformation of Steroids by the Skin."

33. Exposed regions of the body are more susceptible to skin-cell loss due to friction, even if this friction is merely the result of air passing over the skin surface.

34. Why do we call these dogs, with their acute sense of smell, "bloodhounds"? Is this because they can detect the hormone levels in our blood with their sense of smell?

35. D. L. Berliner, C. Jennings-White, and R. M. Lavker, "The Human Skin: Fragrances and Pheromones," *Journal of Steroid Biochemistry and Molecular Biology* 39 (1991): 671–79.

36. M. S. Margolese and O. Janiger, "Androsterone-Etiocholanolone Ratios in Male Homosexuals," *British Medical Journal* 207 (1973): 207–10.

37. "The possibility that pentane in exhaled air could serve as a sensitive and specific test for acute myocardial infarction requires further study". Ze'Ev W. Weitz et al., "High Breath Pentane Concentrations During Acute Myocardial Infarction," *Lancet* 337 (1991): 933–35. See also: D. Bilton, J. Madison, and A. K. Webb, "Cystic Fibrosis, Breath Pentane, and Lipid Peroxidation," *Lancet* 337 (1991): 1420.

38. L. Keith, A. Dravicks, and B. Krotoszinski, "Olfactory Study: Human Pheromones," *Archiv fur Gynaekologie* 218 (1975) 203–4.

39. "It is concluded from these and other observations that male sex-attractant pheromones, with powerful behavioral effects, are present in ether extracts of oestrogen-stimulated vaginal secretions . . ." E. B. Keverne and R. P. Michael, "Sex Attractant Properties of Ether Extracts of Vaginal Secretions from Rhesus Monkeys," *Journal of Endocrinology* 51 (1971) 313.

40. "Human vaginal secretions are thought to consist of several components: (1) vulval secretions from sebaceous, sweat, Bartholin's and Skeen's glands, (2) mucus secretions from the cervix, (3) endometrial and oviductal fluids, (4) transudate through the vaginal walls, and (5) exfoliated cells of the vaginal mucosa. The type and amounts are dependent on sex steroid levels; consequently, metabolic by-products of these processes should also vary with sex steroid levels" G. Preti and G. R. Huggins, "Cyclical Changes in Volatile Acidic Metabolites of Human Vaginal Secretions and their Relation to Ovulation," *Journal of Chemical Ecology* 1 (1975): 362. See also: R. P. Michael and E. B. Keverne, "Primate Sex Pheromones of Vaginal Origin," *Nature* 225 (1970): 84–85.

41. "That sexual releaser pheromones have been identified in rhesus monkeys is significant because rhesus monkeys, having menstrual rather than estrus cycles, are reproductively more closely related to humans" [J. J. Sokolov, R. T. Harris, and M. R. Hecker, "Isolation of Substances from Human Vaginal Secretions Previously Shown to be Sex Attractant Pheromones in Higher Primates," *Archives of Sexual Behavior* 5 (1976): 270].

42. R. P. Michael, R. W. Bonsall, and P. Warner, "Human Vaginal Secretions: Volatile Fatty Acid Content," *Science* 186 (1974): 1217–19.

43. Michael and Keverne.

44. Preti and Huggins, 373.

45. In similar experiments, ". . . data demonstrate that vaginal odors are normally neither sufficient nor necessary to induce copulation. In addition, anosmia in the male rhesus achieved by chemical means was found to have no detrimental influence on sexual performance. Further clarification of the importance of aliphatic acids for sexual behavior remains to be elaborated. Alternatively, these results could indicate that the particular odor of a partner is not the determining characteristic which initiates sexual activity. Rather, either by innate mechanism, or, much more likely, by associative learning, particular

odor may be one additional cue, not always reliable, which tells the male something about his chances of success with a potential sexual partner." D. A. Goldfoot et al., "Lack of Effect of Vaginal Lavages and Aliphatic Acids on Ejaculatory Responses in Rhesus Monkeys: Behavior and Chemical Analyses," *Hormones and Behavior* 7 (1976): 24–25.

46. R. L. Doty, M. Ford, and G. Preti, "Changes in the Intensity and Pleasantness of Human Vaginal Odor During the Menstrual Cycle," *Science* 190 (1975): 1316–18.

47. "Of greater importance for diagnosis [of *Gardnerella vaginalis*] is the addition of 10% KOH to vaginal discharge. This produces a fishy, aminelike odor" [S. M. Finegold and W. J. Martin, *Diagnostic Micorbiology*, 6th ed., (St. Louis: C. V. Mosby, 1982), 110].

"Medical textbooks refer to the malodorous aspects of many infectious, nutritional, and mental diseases, such as yellow fever, smallpox, typhoid fever, diphtheria, plague, measles, impetigo, scurvy, and schizophrenia. Historically, specific odor qualities have been ascribed to a series of medical conditions: diphtheria (sweetish), yellow fever (butcher shop), scurvy (putrid), scrofula (stale beer), typhoid fever (fresh-baked brown bread), and diabetic coma (fruity). The urine and sweat in some more recently identified disorders of amino acid and fatty acid metabolism have also been described as having distinctive odors: phenylketonuria (musty, barny, wolf-like, 'Like stale, sweaty locker-room towels'), maple-syrup-urine disease, oatshouse syndrome (like dried malt or hops), hypermethioninemia (fishy, sweet fruity, like rancid butter or boiled cabbage), isovaleric acidemia syndrome (cheesy, like sweaty feet), and odor-of-sweaty-feet syndrome" [S. S. Schiffman, "Taste and Smell in Disease, Part 2," *New England Journal of Medicine* 308 (1983): 1341].

CHAPTER 12: A KISS ISN'T JUST A KISS

1. B. Brody, "The Sexual Significance of the Axillae," *Psychiatry* 38 (1975): 279.

2. Recall our discussion in chapter 5 about love apples and the male's use of sweat-soaked handkerchiefs as part of the courtship ritual of dancing in Balkan and Mediterranean cultures.

3. Preliminary work indicates that 5alpha-androst-16-en-3-one is present in the pooled saliva of men at a level of approximately 160pmol/l [See D. B. Gower and W. D. Booth, "Salivary Pheromones in the Pig and Human in Relation to Sexual Status and Age," in W. Breipohl, ed., *Ontogeny of Olfaction* (Berlin: Springer Verlag, 1986), 261]. "Androstenone is a steroid found most abundantly in boars; it influences the female pigs' sexual response in a manner approximating a strict definition of a mammalian pheromone. It is also found in urine, sweat, saliva, fatty tissue, and blood plasma of human males. In females, it occurs at much lower concentrations, if at all" [K. M. Dorries et al., "Changes in Sensitivity to the Odor of Androstenone During Adolescence," *Developmental Psychobiology* 22 (1989): 424].

4. "Kissing is almost ubiquitous throughout the cultures of man, but what is it for? This paper proposes that kissing may be a mechanism by which semiochemicals

[pheromones] are exchanged between human beings to induce bonding or love" [B. Nicholson, "Does Kissing Aid Human Bonding by Semiochemical Addiction?," *British Journal of Dermatology* 111 (1984): 623]. Few would deny that kissing provides an arousing tactile (touch) sensation. However, that primary effect does not eliminate all other effects. We know it is nearly impossible to hide alcohol on the breath; the odor is fairly obvious. Since we also know that androstenone, the ketone form of a sex hormone, is found in our saliva, it seems very likely that androstenol, the alcohol form of the same sex hormone, is also found in our saliva. Do ketones and alcohols like androstenone and androstenol send kissing messages about your body's reproductive condition?

5. B. Ehrenreich, E. Hess, and G. Jacobs, *Re-Making Love: The Feminization of Sex* (New York: Doubleday/Anchor, 1987), 153; G. Ogden, *Women Who Love Sex* (New York: Pocket Books, 1994).

6. "Oral-genital contact, while relatively taboo in Victorian-oriented cultures, is relatively widespread in many other cultures" [J. J. Sokolov, R. T. Harris, and M. R. Hecker, "Isolation of Substances from Human Vaginal Secretions Previously Shown to be Sex Attractant Pheromones in Higher Primates," *Archives of Sexual Behavior* 5 (1976): 270]. Also, according to Young [M. Young, "Attitudes and Behavior of College Students Relative to Oral-Genital Sexuality," *Archives of Sexual Behavior* 9 (1980): 61–7]. "Gadpaille (1975) suggests that for some people old taboos against oral-genital sex are not taboos anymore" while ". . . according to Hunt (1974) it is in these 'formerly all-but-unmentionable oral-genital acts' that the most dramatic changes in sexual behavior have taken place." Today's high standards of personal hygiene reduce the amount of pheromones distributed from other parts of the body. Having reduced or eliminated pheromone distribution from more accessible areas of the body, it would seem likely that we might wish to seek them out in other—even formerly forbidden—areas. See also: S. S. Janus and C. L. Janus, *The Janus Report on Sexual Behavior* (Sommerset, N. J.: Wiley and Sons, 1992), 311.

7. S. Brown, *French Silk* (New York: Warner Books, 1992), 194.

8. "Thus, cunnilingus and fellatio derive part of their attraction, more especially in some individuals, from a predilection for the odors of the sexual parts" H. Ellis, *Studies in the Psychology of Sex: Sexual Selection in Man*, vol. 4 (Philadelphia: Davis, 1914), 75.

9. Oddly, having sex when fully clothed, a condition that also severely limits pheromone distribution, is linked to the Victorian era. In the Middle Ages and Elizabethan era, when bathing was widely viewed as unhealthy, Europeans commonly limited bathing to washing the hands, feet, and face only. This obviously leaves pheromonal and other body odors to build up and decay, with unavoidable consequences. Hence the immense popularity of perfumes.

10. In Iran the Farsi term for the head veil is *chador*, although this term is also used for the full-body garment. *Burka* is a general term for the full-body garment worn by both men and women in the Middle East. In Egypt, the simple covering for the hair is known as the *hajib*, while the full-body covering for women is known as *niqaab*. Parrinder provides an interesting history of Moslem veiling

and interpretation of the several reasons offered to explain its origins. See: G. Parrinder, *Sex in the World's Religions* (Ontario: Don Mills, 1980), 174–77.

11.   1 Cor 11:1–7.

12.   Quoted in K. Wright, "The Sniff of Legend. Human Pheromones: Chemical Sex Attractants? And a Sixth Sense Organ in the Nose? What Are We Animals?," *Discover* 15 (April 1994): 60–77.

13.   J. DeMeo, "Desertification and the Origins of Amouring: The Saharasian Connection," *Journal of Orogonymy* 21 (1989): 185–213; B. Z. Goldberg, *The Sacred Fire: The Story of Sex in Religion* (New York: University Books, 1958); G. A. Larue, "Religious Traditions and Circumcision," *The Truth Seeker* 1 (1989): 4–8.

14.   For a brief discussion of the history of male and female circumcision, see R. T. Francoeur, T. Perper, and N. A. Scherzer, *The Complete Dictionary of Sexology* (New York: Continuum, 1994), 101–3. The July/August 1989 issue of *The Truth Seeker* (a humanist freethinker publication) contains several excellent articles on "crimes of genital mutilation." The best study of female castration is Alice Walker and Pratibha Parmar's *Warrior Mark: Female Genital Mutilation and the Sexual Blinding of Women* (New York: Harcourt Brace Jovanovich, 1994).

15.   The popularity of male circumcision in the United States was motivated more by a Victorian need to reduce the opportunities for young boys to masturbate while washing under the foreskin. Male circumcision is about as popular in the United States as it is unpopular in Canada and European countries. J. Money, *The Destroying Angel* (New York: Prometheus Books, 1985), 99–102; R. T. Francouer, *Becoming a Sexual Person*, (New York: Macmillan Publishing, 1991), 163–65.

16.   D. Steel, *Heartbeat* (New York: Delacorte Press, 1991), 109.

17.   "Think of the men or women that you find sexually attractive. If you're a man, for instance, do you prefer women who are blond or brunette, flat-chested or buxom, and with big or small eyes? If you're a woman, do you like men who are bearded or smooth-shaven, tall or short, and smiling or scowling. Probably you don't go for anyone, but only certain types attract you. Everyone can name friends who got divorced, then chose a second spouse who was the exact image of the first one." J. Diamond, "Turning a Man," *Discover* 13 (June 1992): 100.

18.   C. S. Coon, *Racial Adaptations* (Chicago: Nelson Hall, 1982), 95.

19.   Ibid., 85–86. "Adult women of all races are, on the average, shorter than their men by about 6 percent and, excepting the obese, they are about 8 percent lighter in weight. American men stand about 5 feet, 8 inches (172.7 cm) and women about 5 feet, 4 1/2 inches (164 cm)."

20.   I. Bloch, *Odoratus Sexualis: A Scientific and Literary Study of Sexual Scents and Erotic Perfumes* (New York: American Anthropological Society, 1933), 52–53; Ellis, 80.

21.   Ellis, 81.

22.   Jared Diamond reminds us that the subject of human races is so explosive that Darwin excised all discussion of it from his famous 1859 book *On the Origin of*

Species. This sensitivity has hardly changed since the time of Ellis. Diamond also cites Darwin's observation that we pay inordinate attention to breasts, hair, eyes, and skin color in selecting our mates and sex partners. He also noted that people in different parts of the world define beautiful breasts, hair, eyes, and skin by what is familiar to them. J. Diamond, *The Third Chimpanzee* (New York: Harper Collins, 1992), 111, 119.

23. B. Gibbons, "The Intimate Sense of Smell," *National Geographic* 170 (1986): 348–49.

24. Ellis, 59.

25. Ibid., 60.

26. What may be even more surprising, given this age of political correctness, is that anyone would mention a racial difference at all.

27. "Homma (1926) found Negroes to possess three times as many apocrine glands as Caucasians. . . . Hurley & Shelly (1960) claim that the apocrine glands are larger in Negroes and produce more and thicker secretion." M. B. L. Craigmyle, *The Apocrine Glands and the Breast* (Chichester: Wiley and Sons, 1984), 34.

28. "Men have more and larger apocrine glands than women, blacks more than Caucasians, Caucasians more than Orientals." (Gibbons, 348). We question whether men have more apocrine glands than women. Though men do have larger apocrine glands than women, at least two other sources state that women have more apocrine glands than men.

29. "The axillary organ produces and propagates specific human odors; this 'organ' is found only in man and in chimpanzees and gorillas. In other primates the skin of the axilla is not particularly different from the skin elsewhere on their bodies. Many other primates have scent-producing organ systems, but these are not in the axillae. All mammalian scent glands, whether those of carnivores, ungulates or primates, consist of apocrine glands and sebaceous glands usually together." W. Montagna, "The Evolution of Human Skin," *Journal of Human Evolution* (1985): 17–18.

30. Ibid.

31. Odor production in the Japanese is considered to be an inherited trait from ancestors of other subraces who produced more odor.

32. "Mean testosterone levels in blacks were 19% higher than in whites, and free testosterone levels were 21% higher. We are uncertain whether the difference in circulating testosterone levels persists with aging. However, the 2:1 ratio in prostate cancer incidence between blacks and whites remains throughout life, suggesting that these differences may be long standing." [R. Ross et al., "Serum Testosterone Levels in Healthy Young Black and White Men," *Journal of the National Cancer Institute* 76 (1986): 45–48] "We have now compared serum testosterone concentrations in young adult Japanese men with those of young adult whites and blacks, but found no significant differences. However, these white and black men had significantly higher values of 3alpha, 17 beta androstanediol glucuronide (31% and 25% higher, respectively) and androsterone glucuronide (50% and 41% higher, respectively) than Japanese subjects.

These two androgens are indices of 5alpha-reductase activity. Black women have testosterone values that are almost 50% higher than those of white women during early gestation. This excess of testosterone in early gestational black women might predispose their male offspring to altered steroid hormone secretion . . ." [R. K. Ross et al., "5-A-Reductase Activity and Risk of Prostate Cancer Among Japanese and U. S. White and Black Males," *Lancet* 339 (1992): 887–89.] "In fact, the mean FSH value at the peak in Japanese women (17.6 +/– 7.9 mIU/ml) was not only considerably lower than in the groups of Nigerian mothers with singletons (peak value, 27.1 mIU/ml), but also the mean LH value at the peak in Japanese women (75.2 +/–26.0 mIU/ml) was lower than in Nigerian women with singletons (peak value, 126.3 mIU/ml) and in Americans (peak value, 91.2 +/– 9.7 mIU/ml)." [H. Soma et al., "Serum Gonadotropin Levels in Japanese Women," *Obstetrics and Gynecology* 46 (1975): 311.]

33. J. R. Baker, *Race* (New York: Oxford University Press), 1974.

34. Sniffing to perceive an odor better operates in the same manner as a shorter, wider nose, as it provides a rapid burst of air through a shortened passageway more directly to the smell center.

35. S. Bird and D. B. Gower, "Validation and Use of RIA for Androstenone in Axillary Collection," *Journal of Steroid Biochemistry and Molecular Biology* 14 (1981): 213–19; R. Claus and W. Alsing, "Occurrrence of 5A-androst-16-en3-one, a Boar Pheromone in Man and Its Relationship to Testosterone," *Journal of Endocrinology* 68 (1976): 483–84; E. E. Filsinger, "Human Responses to the Pig Sex Pheromone Androstenol," *Journal of Comparative Psychology* 98 (1984): 219–22; S. S. Schiffman, "Taste and Smell in Disease," *New England Journal of Medicine* 308 (1983): 1337–43.

CHAPTER 13: THE JOY OF ODOR

1. R. A. Schneider, "Anosmia: Verification and Etiologies," *Annals of Otology, Rhinology and Laryngology* 81 (1972): 272.

2. T. Engen, *The Perception of Odors* (New York: Academic Press, 1982), 80.

3. Sarnat, cited by Engen.

4. H. F. Blakeslee, "Unlike Reactions of Different Individuals to Fragrance in Verbena Flowers," *Science* 48 (1918): 298–99.

5. K. McWhirter, "Ethnography of Specific Anosmia," *Canadian Journal of Genetics and Cytology* 11 (1969) 479.

6. J. E. Amoore, "Specific Anosmias and the Concept of Primary Odors," *Chemical Senses and Flavor* 2 (1977): 267–81.

7. A. N. Gilbert and C. J. Wysocki, "The Smell Survey Results," *National Geographic* 171 (1987): 514–25.

8. Engen, 92–93.

9. J. C. Henkin and G. F. Powell, "Increased Sensitivy of Taste and Smell in Cystic Fibrosis," *Science* 138 (1962): 1107–8; S. Wotman et al., "Salt

Thresholds and Cystic Fibrosis," *American Journal of Disease in Children* 108 (1964): 372–74; J. Hertz et al., "Olfactory and Taste Sensitivity in Children with Cystic Fibrosis," *Physiology and Behavior* 14 (1975): 89–94.

10. Schneider.

11. R. S. Sparkes, R. W. Simpson, and C. A. Paulsen, "Familiar Hypogonadotropic Hypogonadism with Anosmia," *Archives of Internal Medicine* 121 (1968): 534–38; R. A. Schneider, "Newer Insights into the Role and Modifications of Olfaction in Man Through Clinical Studies," *Annals of the New York Academy of Sciences* 237 (1974): 217–23; N. A. Bobrow, J. Money, and V. J. Lewis, "Delayed Puberty, Eroticism and Sense of Smell: A Psychological Study of Hypogonadotropinism, Osmatic and Anosmatic (Kallmann's Syndrome)," *Archives of Sexual Behavior* 1 (1971): 329–44; E. I. Rugarli and A. B. Ballabio, "Kallman Syndrome: from Genetics to Neurobiology," *Journal of the American Medical Association* 270 (1993): 2713–16.

12. J. Durden-Smith and D. DeSimone, *Sex and the Brain* (New York: Arbor House, 1983), 217.

13. C. J. Wysocki and G. K. Beauchamp, "Ability to Smell Androstenone is Genetically Determined," *Proceedings of the National Academy of Science USA* 81 (1984): 4899–902; C. J. Wysocki et al., "Changes in Olfactory Sensitivity to Androstenone with Age and Experience," abstract in *Chemical Senses* 12 (1987): 710; C. J. Wysocki, K. M. Dorries, and G. K. Beauchamp, "Ability to Perceive Androsteone Can Be Acquired by Ostensibly Anosmic People," *Proceedings of the National Academy of Science USA* 86 (1989): 7976–78.

14. Engen, 87.

15. Douek, cited by Engen, 88.

16. D. T. Moran, B. W. Jafek, and J. C. Rowley, "The Ultrastructure of the Human Olfactory Mucosa," in D. G. Laing, R. L. Doty, and W. Breipohl, eds., *The Human Sense of Smell* (New York: Springer-Verlag, 1991); L. Monti-Bloch and B. I. Grosser, "Effect of Putative Pheromones on the Electrical Activity of the Human Vomeronasal Organ and Olfactory Epithelium," *Journal of Steroid Biochemistry and Molecular Biology* 39 (1991): 573–82; J. Garcia-Velasco and M. Mondragon, "The Incidence of the Vomeronasal Organ in 1000 Human Subjects and its Possible Clinical Significance," *Journal of Steroid Biochemistry and Molecular Biology* 39 (1991): 561–63.

17. Quoted in T. Monmaney, "Are We Led by the Nose?," *Discover* 8 (September 1987): 48.

18. A. N. Gilbert and C. J. Wysocki, "The Smell Survey Results," *National Geographic* 171 (1987): 519.

CHAPTER 14: THE HEALING POWER OF AROMATIC OILS

1. R. Winter, *The Smell Book. Scent, Sex and Society* (New York: Lippincott, 1976), 93.

2. The comfort with which the early Moslems integrated the sensual and erotic in their places of worship reminded us of David Schnarch's experience in visiting

the thousand-year-old "erotic love temples" of northern India. After noting how Hindu Tantric Yoga stresses the merging of sexual energies with another individual as a cosmic experience and the most intense awakening of human consciousness, Schnarch commented that "While the [exquisite sculptures on the] exterior of the walls [of the temples] depicted every conceivable manifestation of erotic behavior, the interior chamber was unadorned. At the center of this circular chamber, some 15 feet in diameter, was a simple ceremonial bed platform, around which one could barely walk without brushing the plain stone walls. Inside the chamber, there was nothing to suggest it represented the culmination of a society that had developed sexuality as its religious core and as a means of spiritual worship and transcendence.

"And yet, the *aroma* of the eight or ten sexually aroused visitors within the temple was striking. It was as if there were a sexual radiance, such as people experience during embarrassing adolescent arousal, coming from each of us; each of us vibrated in harmony with a sexual energy that seemed to come out of nowhere and everywhere. There were simple, knowing, friendly smiles between the men and women tourists who resonated with the moment. . . . It was a very unusual experience, *being highly aroused for nothing or anyone in particular*. There was no impulse to start an orgy or even pair up. There was this peculiar sense of eroticism and sexual desire emanating from each of us, in the context of an intense spirituality. It was not that any of us became more attractive at that moment; we simply became *desirous without an apparent object of that desire*." [D. M. Schnarch, *Constructing the Sexual Crucible: An Integration of Sexual and Marital Therapy* (New York: W. W. Norton, 1991), 548–49] Such is the power of the sexual aroma when it is free to link with limbic memories in an accepting religious atmosphere.

3. Business and stock prospectus provided by EROX Corporation to James Kohl.

4. T. K. Lacy, "Aromatherapy," *Las Vegas Review-Journal*, 13 June 1994, 1C, 3C.

5. "Secrets That Have Been Sniffed Out," *Las Vegas Review-Journal/Sun*, 2 July 1994, 14B; reprinted from the *Los Angeles Times*.

6. "Researcher Nosing Around for Clues to How Smell Works," *Las Vegas Review-Journal/Sun*, 2 July, 1994, 14B. Reprinted from the *Los Angeles Times*.

7. Lacy, 1C.

8. L. Sawahata, "The Sweet Smell of Success: Fragrance and Athletic Performance," *Self* (July 1994): 32.

9. J. Steingarten, "The Sweet Smell of Sex?," *Vogue* (June 1993): 204–7.

10. Peter Born, "A Feel-Good Fragrance Set to Bow," *Women's Wear Daily Accessories Beauty Report* (9 April, 1993). Copy supplied by EROX Corporation.

11. Business and stock prospectus provided by EROX Corporation to James Kohl.

12. "Montel Williams Show." Transcript #47. Air Date: 16 November, 1993. Copyright 1993 by Viacom International, Inc.

13. Information taken from an October 10, 1993 FAX of pheromone brochures from Marilyn Miglin to James Kohl. See also: M. Menter, "The Secret Messages of Scent," *Redbook* (January 1993): 30–32.

14. J. Jones, "Labs Conjure Up Fragrances and Flavors to Add Allure," *New York Times*, New Jersey Section, New Jersey Weekly Desk, 26 December 1993, 1.

15. "Secrets That Have Been Sniffed Out," *Las Vegas Review-Journal/Sun*, 2 July 1994, 14B.

16. Lacy, 1C.

17. C. A. Dudley, G. Rajendren, and R. L. Moss, "Induction to FOS Immuno-reactivity in Central Accessory Olfactory Structures of the Female Rat Following Exposure to Conspecific Males," *Molecular and Cellular Neurosciences* 3 (1992): 360–69.

18. G. Rajendren, C. A. Dudley, and R. L. Moss, "Role of the Vomeronasal Organ in the Male-induced Enhancement of Sexual Receptivity in Female Rats," *Neuroendocrinology* 52 (1990): 368–72. G. Rajendren, C. A. Dudley, and R. L. Moss, "Influence of Male Rats on the Luteinizing Hormone-releasing Hormone Neuronal System in Female Rats: Role of the Vomeronasal Organ," *Neuroendocrinology* 57 (1993): 898–906. G. Rajendren, and R. L. Moss, "The Role of the Medial Nucleus of Amygdala in the Mating-induced Enhancement of Lordosis in Female Rats: The Interaction With Luteinizing Hormone-releasing Hormone Neuronal System," *Brain Research* 617 (1993): 81–86.

19. A. Perkins, J. A. Fitzgerald, and G. Moss, "A Comparison of LH Secretion and Brain Estradiol Receptors in Heterosexual and Homosexual Rams and Female Sheep," *Hormones and Behavior* (1995): in press.

20. See: S. LeVay, *The Sexual Brain* (Mass.: MIT Press, 1993), and S. LeVay and D. H. Hamer, "Evidence for a Biological Influence in Male Homosexuality," *Scientific American* (May 1994): 44–9.

21. B. S. McEwen, and H. M. Schmeck Jr., *The Hostage Brain* (New York: Rockefeller University Press, 1994).

22. H. Ellis, *Studies in the Psychology of Sex: Sexual Selection in Man*, vol. 4 (Philadelphia: Davis, 1914), 55.

23. J. Money, *The Destroying Angel* (New York: Prometheus Books, 1985), 195.

GLOSSARY

16-ANDROSTENES: A family of steroid hormones related to sex hormones. They are found in human urine, saliva, and in axillary secretions. Most produce strong odors.

ACCESSORY OLFACTORY SYSTEM (AOS): A system for the unconscious processing of chemical messages, particularly pheromones. In most mammals, it consists of the vomeronasal organ (VNO), the accessory olfactory bulb (AOB), axons of the AOB that connect with the amygdala, and the bed nucleus of the stria terminalis. From these structures, output is directed to other parts of the brain that help to process olfactory information and that influence the hormone levels and the behavior of many species.

ADRENAL GLANDS: Two small glands—one atop each kidney—that secrete several steroid hormones, including important precursors of the sex hormones.

ADRENOCORTICOTROPIC HORMONE (ACTH): A hormone secreted by the pituitary that stimulates the growth of the adrenal cortex and its secretion of corticosteroid hormones, some of which are converted into sex hormones.

ALIPHATIC ACIDS: A group of carbon-based chemical compounds found in the vaginal secretions of primates, which are believed to function as pheromones.

AMBERGRIS: A waxy, grayish substance formed in the intestines of sperm whales and found floating at sea or washed ashore; or, a synthetic product used in perfumes.

AMINO ACID: A simple organic compound containing both an amino group and a caroxylic acid group linked together by a chemical bond called a peptide bond.

AMPHETAMINE: A central nervous system stimulant produced naturally by secretory cells in the brain, or a synthetic chemical with a similar effect.

AMYGDALA: An almond-shaped group of nerve cells found in the temporal lobe of the brain (basal forebrain). It processes sensory input and is linked to recognition and the generation of aggressive, sexual, and other emotion-laden behaviors.

ANDROGEN INSENSITIVITY SYNDROME (AIS): A genetic condition in which a male with testes and normal hormone balance cannot produce androgen receptors. As a consequence, the male has external female anatomy and, usually, a female gender identity.

ANDROGENS: Steroid hormones that control the development and the maintenance of masculine characteristics, driving development in a male direction. Testosterone and DHT are potent androgens.

ANDROSTENOL: The alcohol form of a chemically active substance, derived from a steroid hormone, which may function as a human pheromone.

ANDROSTENONE: The ketone form of a chemical substance, derived from a steroid hormone, which functions as a mammalian pheromone.

ANDROSTERONE: A steroid hormone derived from the breakdown of dehydroepiandrosterone (DHEA) and excreted in urine. It functions as a weak androgen to reinforce masculine characteristics and may also function as a human pheromone.

ANLAGE: The initial cluster of cells in an embryo which develops into particular parts or organs.

ANOSMIA: Complete loss of the sense of smell, or the inability to smell a particular odor. Many adults are anosmic to musk; they do not consciously smell it.

APHRODISIAC: A substance that arouses or intensifies sexual desire.

APOCRINE: A type of glandular secretion in which part of the secreting cell is released along with its products. See apocrine glands.

APOCRINE GLANDS: Specialized glands, part of the hair-gland complex, that secrete a milky substance with properties that allow bacterial action to convert the substance to pheromones. In human beings, apocrine glands are found (with hair glands) around the nipples, in the genital area, in the armpits, and in the area of the navel. They may also be found in the scalp, on the forehead, on the cheeks, under the nose, at the base of the eyelashes, in the bearded portion of the face (in males), and in several other areas.

AREOLA: A small ring of darkly-colored tissue around the nipple of the breast.

AUTOIMMUNE: An immune response by the body to one of its own tissues or types of cells.

AXILLA: The underarm area or armpit.

AXON: The part of a nerve cell that generally conducts impulses away from the body of the nerve cell.

BARTHOLIN'S GLANDS: Two small glands in the vagina that secrete a lubricating mucus.

BRUCE EFFECT: Pregnancy block due to pheromones. When a recently impregnated female mouse is placed in a cage with a unfamiliar male, the pheromones of the male may cause a spontaneous abortion.

CASTOREUM (CASTORUM) (CASTOR): An oily, brown, substance from the glands in the groin of the beaver or a synthetic product used in perfumes.

CASTRATION: Removal of a male's testes or a female's ovaries.

CELIBATE: Someone who abstains from sexual intercourse.

CHEMOTAXIS: The movement of an organism or cell either toward or away from a chemical stimulus.

CHROMOSOME: A threadlike strand of DNA and associated proteins in the nucleus of a cell. Chromosomes carry the genes that transfer the hereditary information necessary for cell life.

CILIUM (PL. CILIA): A hairlike process extending from the surface of a cell or from a one-celled organism. Cilia act in unison to move either the cell or the surrounding medium.

CIVETONE (CIVET): The thick, yellowish, musky-smelling fluid secreted by civet cats, or a synthetic product used in perfumes.

CLITORIS: The elongated protruding erectile organ that lies in front of the urethra where the labia minor fuse at the midline. It is comparable to the head of the penis as a major site of sexual excitability.

COITUS: Inserting the male penis into the female vagina; sexual intercourse.

CONTRACEPTION: Intentional prevention of conception and pregnancy.

COOLIDGE EFFECT: A shortening of the lag-time for sexual excitability caused by the presence of a novel female. Colloquialism: "Variety is the spice of life."

COPULATION: Sexual intercourse; usually in reference to sex in "animals" rather than humans.

CORTEX: The outer layer of an internal organ like the brain or the adrenal glands. The cortex of the brain is comprised of several layers of nerve cells.

CUNNILINGUS: Oral stimulation of the clitoris or vulva.

DENDRITES: The branched extensions of a nerve cell that conduct impulses toward the cell body.

DEOXYRIBONUCLEIC ACID (DNA): A nucleic acid that carries a cell's genetic information and determines individual hereditary characteristics. It consists of two long chains of nucleotides twisted into a double helix and joined by hydrogen bonds between the complementary bases adenine and thymine or cytosine and guanine. DNA is capable of self-replication and synthesis of RNA. See gene.

DHT: See dihydrotestosterone .

DIFFERENTIATE: To cause a distinction between through alteration of structure and concurrent modification of function, often in a progressive, developmental manner that results in a more specialized form or function or in different characteristics.

DIHYDROTESTOSTERONE (DHT): A modified form of testosterone that is responsible for masculinization of the male external genitals. It may also be involved in other masculinization processes.

DOPAMINE: A monoamine neurotransmitter formed in the brain that is essential to the normal functioning of the central nervous system.

ECCRINE GLANDS: Glands that secrete a watery sweat onto the skin. Eccrine glands are found over most of the body; their secretions help to keep the body cool.

ELECTROCHEMICAL: The interaction or the conversion of electrical and chemical processes.

EMBRYO: (1) An organism in its early stages of development, prior to the time when it acquires a recognizable form. (2) In human beings: the product of conception from the time of implantation in the uterus through the eighth week of development.

ENDOCRINE CELL/GLAND: A cell or a ductless gland that secretes its protein product internally and directly into the bloodstream as a hormone.

ENDORPHINS: Naturally produced peptide hormones that bind to opiate receptors. They have actions similar to opiates, which reduce sensations of pain and affect emotions. Also known as opioids.

ENZYME: A protein that promotes a specific chemical reaction in a living organism.

ESTROGENS: A class of steroid hormones produced mainly by follicles in the ovary. They are responsible for completion of female sexual development at puberty, the estrous cycle, or the human female's menstrual cycle; and the development and the maintenance of female secondary sex characteristics. Estradiol is a potent estrogen. In males, estrogens are made from androgens by some cells in the brain, and they play a role in the male sexual development of the brain.

ESTROUS CYCLE: A sexual cycle in female animals comparable to the menstrual cycle in women. It is marked by recurring changes in hormone levels and in behavior from one period of estrus or "heat" to the next.

ETIOCHOLANOLONE: A steroid hormone derived from the chemical breakdown of dehydroepiandrosterone and excreted in urine. It has no known function, but evidence suggests it may be a human pheromone.

EXOCRINE GLAND: A gland that secretes its protein product through a duct. For example, a salivary gland or a sweat gland.

EXTRAHYPOTHALAMIC: A substance that is produced outside the hypothalamus.

FATTY ACIDS: A group of acids that combine with glycerol to produce the fats, oils, and waxes found outside the body. Most have rank vinegar-like or goat-like odors.

FELLATIO: Oral stimulation of the penis.

FETISH: An obsessive preoccupation with or attachment to a material object or non-sexual part of the body that arouses sexual desire.

FETUS: The distinctly recognizable form an organism acquires during development. A human embryo becomes a distinctively recognizable fetus eight weeks after conception.

FIVE ALPHA REDUCTASE (5AR): The enzyme that is responsible for the modification of testosterone to dihydrotestosterone (DHT).

FIXATIVE: A substance added to a perfume to slow the rate of evaporation.

FLAGELLUM (PL. FLAGELLA): A threadlike extension of a one-celled organism that helps the organism move.

FOLLICLE STIMULATING HORMONE (FSH): A hormone, secreted by the pituitary gland, which stimulates the growth of egg-bearing follicles in women or of spermatogenesis in men.

FOREBRAIN: The part of the adult brain that includes the cerebrum, thalamus, and the hypothalamus.

FORESKIN: The loose fold of skin covering the glans of the penis.

FSH: See follicle stimulating hormone .

G-PROTEIN: A particular type of protein essential to intercellular communication. When found in olfactory receptor nerve cells, G-proteins are activated by chemical stimuli from the outer environment.

GAMONE: A chemical messenger, produced by ova and by spermatozoa that is believed to facilitate their union.

GENE: A functional unit of heredity occupying a specific location—a stretch or sequence of DNA—on a chromosome. Genes determine and transfer particular characteristics of organisms, exist in a number of different forms, and can mutate or recombine. They generally code for a protein, several adjoining regulatory sequences, and some sequences that appear to have no function.

GLAND: A cell, group of cells, or an organ that produces a secretion for use elsewhere in the body, or for elimination from the body.

GnRH: See gonadotropin releasing hormone .

GONADOTROPIN RELEASING HORMONE (GnRH): A hormone produced by nerve cells in the hypothalamus and in structures of the limbic and olfactory systems that signals the pituitary gland to secrete LH and FSH.

GONADS: The testes or the ovaries of mammals. The gonads produce sex cells and sex hormones.

HIPPOCAMPUS: A part of the brain's limbic system containing nerve cells that play a central role in memory processes.

HISTOCOMPATIBILITY: (1) The absence of the immunological interference that would cause tissue rejection. (2) A matching tissue type.

HLA: See Human Leucocyte Antigen system.

HORMONE: A protein produced by a tissue; it is comprised of specialized endocrine or neuroendocrine cells and conveyed by the bloodstream to another tissue where it alters physiological activity like growth or metabolism at the cellular level, and behavior through activation and organization.

HPG AXIS: See hypothalamic-pituitary-gonadal axis .

HUMAN LEUCOCYTE ANTIGEN SYSTEM: The system that determines genetic individuality or "tissue type." It consists of recognizable locations for specific "MHC-linked" genes that are known to affect growth and reproduction in humans. These genes also have been linked to unique pheromone signatures and to mate selection for genetic diversity in humans and other mammals. One human study also demonstrated that changing mates could eliminate recurrent spontaneous abortions in some women.

HYPOGONADISM: Below-normal size gonads and amounts of male or female hormones.

HYPOSMIA: The reduced ability to smell certain odors. It may be either a temporary or a permanent condition.

HYPOTHALAMIC-PITUITARY-GONADAL AXIS (HPG) AXIS: The interactive system of glands that regulates concurrent development of the neuroendocrine and reproductive systems of mammals and of other species. GnRH from the hypothalamus triggers the release of LH and FSH from the pituitary, which regulate production of sex hormones from the gonads.

HYPOTHALAMUS: A small region at the base of the brain that regulates body temperature, certain metabolic processes, instinctual drives, the levels of many different hormones, and other autonomic activities.

IMMUNE SYSTEM: The integrated body system of organs, tissues, cells, and cell products that differentiates self from nonself and neutralizes potentially pathogenic organisms or substrates.

INBORN: Present at birth, inherited, or hereditary.

INBRED: A trait that is either produced by inbreeding or that is fixed in the character or disposition of an organism.

INSEMINATION: The introduction or injection of semen into the reproductive tract of a female.

KALLMANN'S SYNDROME: A hereditary condition characterized by reduced GnRH secretion, delayed puberty, and anosmia.

KETONE: A class of organic compounds with a carbonyl group that is linked to a carbon atom in each of two hydrocarbon radicals.

LABIUM (PL. LABIA): Any of the four folds of tissue that make up the female external genitalia.

LEE-BOOT EFFECT: Suppression of estrus by the pheromones of other females. Female mice housed together in the absence of male tend not to ovulate.

LH: See luteinizing hormone .

LH SURGE: The GnRH-induced release of relatively large amounts of LH from the pituitary. Occurring with ovulation in female mammals, the LH surge prompts testosterone levels to peak and it is often associated with increases in sexual behavior.

LIBIDO: (1) Psychic and emotional energy associated with instinctual biological drives. (2) The manifestation of the sexual drive. (3) Sexual desire.

LIMBIC SYSTEM: A group of interconnected structures deep in the brain which are common to all mammals. They are involved in olfaction, emotion, motivation, behavior, and in various autonomic functions.

LUTEINIZING HORMONE (LH): A hormone produced by the pituitary gland that stimulates ovulation in the female and the production of testosterone in both the male and the female.

MAIN OLFACTORY SYSTEM (MOS): A system for the conscious processing of chemical messages that are generally detected as odors. This system may also detect and respond to pheromones when they are found in high concentration. It allows a variety of situations in which odors are present to trigger appropriate responses, which include changes in hormone levels and in behavior. As compared to those found in the accessory olfactory system, nerve cells of the main olfactory system have broad pathways to wide areas of the brain.

MAJOR HISTOCOMPATIBILITY COMPLEX (MHC): A group of genes that confer olfactory individuality and immune function in mice. A similar set of genes probably exists in all vertebrates. The HLA system in human beings shares similar functions with the MHC in mice. These may include pheromonal functions important in imprinting, mate preference, and hormone regulation, which affects implantation, lactation, and various behaviors.

MAMMAL: A warm-blooded animal with an internal skeleton and with other characteristics like a covering of hair on the skin and—in females—milk-producing mammary glands for nourishing the young.

MAO: See monoamine oxidase .

MENSES: The monthly flow of blood and cellular debris from the uterus which begins at puberty in women and ceases at menopause.

MENSTRUAL CYCLE: The monthly cycle of changing hormone levels in women and in rhesus monkeys.

MENSTRUAL SYNCHRONY: A pheromone-induced phenomena causing women who spend time in close proximity to have menstrual cycles that coincide. Both the onset of menses and peak fertility occur in synchrony. See sexual synchrony.

MENSTRUATION: Discharge of the menses. Colloquialism: "having her period."

MERCAPTAN: A sulfur-containing organic compound.

METABOLISM: The physical and chemical synthesis and breakdown of substances that must occur within a cell or in an organism to maintain life.

METABOLITE: A substance produced through metabolism that may either take part in a life-sustaining process or be discharged from the body.

MID-CYCLE: The middle of the menstrual cycle; when ovulation occurs.

MIH: See Mullerian inhibiting hormone.

MISCARRIAGE: Premature expulsion of a nonviable fetus from the womb.

MONOAMINE OXIDASE (MAO): An enzyme found in the cells of most tissues that catalyzes the oxidation of monoamines like norepinephrine and serotonin.

MUCOUS MEMBRANES: Membranes that line all body passages communicating with the air. Also called mucosa, as in the olfactory mucosa.

MULLERIAN INHIBITING HORMONE (MIH): A hormone produced in the testes of fetal and newborn males, which defeminizes internal sexual anatomy. It causes the regression of the Mullerian ducts which would otherwise help to form a female's vagina, uterus, and fallopian tubes.

MUSK (MUSCONE): (1) A greasy secretion with a powerful odor, produced by animals, or a synthetic product used in perfumes. (2) The odor of musk or an odor similar to musk.

NATURE: The internal processes and functions that determine an organism's essential characteristics as they are found in its primitive state of existence, untouched and uninfluenced artificially or by socialization. Genes determine an organism's nature.

NERVE: A cordlike bundle of axons that allows sensory stimuli and motor impulses to pass between the brain or other parts of the central nervous system and other parts of the body.

NERVE CELL (NEURON): Any impulse-conducting cell of the brain, spinal column, or in nerves, that consists of a cell body, one or more dendrites, and a single axon.

NETRINS: Proteins that diffuse through cells and attract axons to their targets during development of the vertebrate nervous system.

NEURAL PATHWAY: A network of nerves that conducts information throughout the body.

NEUROHORMONE: A hormone secreted by a nerve cell or that acts on part of the nervous system.

NEUROTRANSMITTERS: A class of hormone that conveys or allows the transmission of impulses as messages across a synapse, between a nerve cell and receptor sites on the target nerve cells to which these chemical messengers attach.

NORADRENALINE: A substance that acts both as a hormone and as a neurotransmitter, which is secreted by the adrenals and the nerve endings of the sympathetic nervous system. It causes vasoconstriction and increases heart rate, blood pressure, and the sugar level of the blood.

NOREPINEPHRINE: See noradrenaline .

NUCLEUS (NUCLEI): (1) A centrally located large, membrane-bound structure within a living cell that contains most of its genetic material and controls its metabolism, growth, and reproduction. (2) In neuroanatomy: a group of specialized nerve cells recognizable as a discrete structure. The nerve cells of a nucleus are generally similar to each other in structure, chemistry, connections, and function.

NURTURE: The total effect of the environmental influences, including those social influences or conditions that act on an organism. Socialization is a primary factor in the nurture of mammals.

ODOR: (1) The property or quality of a thing that affects, stimulates, or is perceived by the sense of smell. (2) A sensation, stimulation, or perception of the sense of smell.

OLFACTION: The sense of smell. The act or the process of smelling.

OLFACTORY: A part of, or that which contributes to, the sense of smell.

OLFACTORY BULBS: The bulblike ends of the olfactory lobes where the olfactory nerves begin. They are found just above the nose in the floor of the brain.

OLFACTORY LOBE: A projection from the lower portion of each cerebral hemisphere; the part of the olfactory system closest to the brain.

OLFACTORY MEMBRANE: The mucous membrane that lines body passages leading to the olfactory system.

OLFACTORY NERVES: The first pair of cranial nerves. They conduct impulses from the mucous membranes of the nose to the olfactory bulb.

OLFACTORY RECEPTOR: A specialized group of nerve endings that responds to chemical stimuli like the odors we smell or the pheromones we may or may not consciously detect.

OPIATES (OPIOIDS): Sedative narcotics containing opium or its natural or synthetic derivatives. Natural opiates, which dull the senses and induce relaxation or apathy, are found in the brain. Also known as endorphins.

ORGANIC: A substance containing carbon compounds from a living organism or related to a living organism.

OVARIES: Paired female reproductive organs that produce ova and, in vertebrates, estrogen and progesterone.

OVULATE: To produce ova (eggs) or to discharge them from the ovary.

OXYTOCIN: A hormone released from the pituitary gland that stimulates the contraction of the uterus during labor and facilitates milk ejection from the breast during nursing. Colloquial expressions in associated behaviors: the "bonding" or the "cuddling" hormone.

PEA: See phenylethylamine .

PEPTIDE: Any natural or synthetic compound that contains two or more amino acids linked by the carboxyl group of one amino acid and the amino group of another.

PHENYLETHYLAMINE (PEA): A neurotransmitter that acts as a natural amphetamine to stimulate the brain, transform the senses, and perhaps, alter reality. It is linked to the emotion of falling in love.

PHEROMONE: A chemical message produced by one member of a species that influences the physiology and the behavior of another member of the same species. Whether or not this chemical message is consciously detected (smelled), pheromones have the same effect. Mammalian pheromones, in the form of "social odors" that one member of a species is exposed to during interaction with another member of the species, cause changes in hormone levels and in behavior.

PITUITARY GLAND (HYPOPHYSIS): A small, oval endocrine gland attached to the base of the vertebrate brain. Its secretions control the secretions from other endocrine glands and influence growth, metabolism, and maturation.

PLASMA: The clear, yellow-colored fluid portion of blood, lymph, or intramuscular fluid in which cells are suspended.

PREGNENOLONE: The steroid hormone from which most biologically active steroid hormones are derived.

PRIMATE: A mammal in the order Primates, characterized by refined development of the hands and feet, a short snout, and a large brain.

PROGESTERONE: A steroid hormone secreted by the ovaries and by the placenta that prepares the uterus for implantation of the fertilized ovum, maintains pregnancy, and promotes development of the mammary glands. Natural or synthetic progesterone is used to prevent miscarriage and to treat menstrual dysfunction.

PROSTAGLANDINS: Substances derived from amino acids that are produced in various mammalian tissues and which act like hormones to mediate a wide range of physiological functions like metabolism, smooth muscle activity, and nerve cell transmission.

PROTEINS: Large, complex organic molecules containing carbon, hydrogen, oxygen, nitrogen, and usually sulfur in one or more chains of amino acids. They are the most basic components of all living cells and include many substances, like the enzymes, hormones, and receptors (as well as antibodies), required for the proper functioning of an organism.

PUBERTY: The stage of adolescence in which an individual becomes physiologically capable of sexual reproduction; the approach to maturity.

RECEPTOR: A protein structure or molecular site on either the surface or the interior of a cell. Receptors bind with substances like hormones, antigens, drugs, or neurotransmitters.

RECEPTOR CELLS: A specialized cell or a group of dendrites that responds to sensory stimuli.

RECESSIVE TRAIT: A trait that is expressed only when two copies of the determining gene are present, rather than when only one dominant gene is present with a recessive gene.

SALIVARY GLAND: A gland that produces saliva.

SEBACEOUS GLANDS: Various glands in the dermis of the skin that open into a hair follicle and produce and secrete sebum.

SEBUM: An oily secretion (from sebaceous glands) that helps the bacteria on our skin to grow and increase their numbers.

SEMEN: A white, viscous secretion of the male reproductive organs that contains sperm and serves as their transport medium.

SEMIOCHEMICAL: A signalling chemical; a pheromone.

SEROTONIN: An organic compound found in the brain and other tissues that is active in vasoconstriction, stimulation of the smooth muscles, nerve cell transmission, and regulation of cyclic body processes.

SEX HORMONES: Steroid hormones, like estrogens, androgens, or progesterone, which affect the growth or the function of the reproductive organs, behavior, and the development of secondary sex characteristics.

SEX PHEROMONES: Pheromones derived from the sex hormones of one member of a species that alter levels of sex hormones and behavior in another member of the same species.

SEXUAL SYNCHRONY: A pheromone-induced effect on the hormone levels of couples through which peak levels of testosterone coincide with peak fertility in the female. One report suggests that a similar phenomena occurs in homosexual male couples.

SMEGMA: A sebaceous secretion, especially the cheesy secretion that collects under the foreskin or around the clitoris.

SPAWN: To deposit eggs or to produce offspring in large numbers as do aquatic animals.

SPECIES-SPECIFIC: A characteristic or trait that is found in only one species.

SPONTANEOUS ABORTION: See miscarriage.

STEROID HORMONES: Naturally occurring or synthetic fat-soluble compounds that contain 17 carbon atoms arranged in four rings. Steroid hormones include the sterols, bile acids, adrenal hormones, sex hormones, certain natural drugs, and the precursors of some vitamins.

SUBLIMINAL: A stimulus with an effect that lies below the threshold of conscious perception, producing a response which is not perceived.

SYNAPSE: The junction across which a nerve passes from an axon to the dendrites of another nerve cell, a muscle cell, or a gland cell.

SYNCHRONY: Occurring at the same time, as in menstrual synchrony or in sexual synchrony.

TESTIS (PL. TESTES): The reproductive gland of a male vertebrate; it is the source of both spermatazoa and androgens.

TESTOSTERONE: A steroid hormone that is produced primarily in the testes and is responsible for the development and maintenance of male secondary sex characteristics.

THALAMUS: A large ovoid mass of nerve cells situated in the forebrain; it relays sensory impulses to the cerebral cortex.

TRIGEMINAL NERVES: The fifth pair of cranial nerves. They have sensory and motor functions in the face, teeth, mouth, and nasal cavity.

TRIMETHYLAMINE: A substance with a fishy odor that is found in menstrual blood.

TRIUNE: Three in one, as in the conscious brain (mind), limbic brain (mind), and reptilian brain or the brain stem.

URETHRA: The canal that allows urine to be discharged from the bladder and through which semen is discharged in males.

UTERUS: The hollow muscular organ that is located in the pelvic cavity of female mammals and in which the fertilized egg implants and develops.

VANDENBERGH EFFECT: Pheromone-induced acceleration of the onset of puberty.

VENERY: The acts of, or the pursuit of, sex.

VERTEBRATE: An animal with a backbone or spinal column.

VOMERONASAL ORGAN (VNO): A structure in the roof of the mouth or in the nose. It generally consists of two small sacs lined with chemically sensitive nerve cells. The VNO provides mammals and many other species with a means for pheromone detection. The human VNO consists of two small sacs about 2 millimeters deep that open into shallow pits on either side of the upper one third of the nasal septum. Increasing evidence shows that the human VNO functions as a pheromone detector, just as it does in many other species.

VULVA: The external genital organs of the female, which include the labia majora, labia minora, clitoris, and vestibule of the vagina.

WHITTEN EFFECT: The suppression of fertility due to a pheromone. Female mice housed together in relatively crowded conditions experience a longer estrous cycle, or cessation of estrus and ovulation.

WOMB: See uterus.

BIBLIOGRAPHY

Abramson P. R., and E. H. Pearsall. "Pectoral Changes During the Sexual Response Cycle: A Thermographic Analysis." *Archives Of Sexual Behavior* 12 (1983): 357–68.

Ackerman, D. *A Natural History of the Senses.* New York: Random House, 1990.

Ader, R., D. Felten, and N. Cohen. "Interactions Between the Brain and the Immune System." *Annual Review of Pharmacology and Toxocology* 30 (1990): 561–602.

Akil, H., S. J. Watson, E. Young, M. E. Lewis, H. Khachaturian, and J. M. Walker. "Endogenous Opioids: Biology and Function." *Annual Review of Neuroscience* 7 (1984): 223–55.

Allstetter, B. "Snakes in Drag." *Discover* 11 (June 1990): 20.

Amoore, J. E. "Evidence for the Chemical Olfactory Code in Man." *Annals of the New York Academy of Sciences* 237 (1974): 137–43.

———."Specific Anosmias and the Concept of Primary Odors." *Chemical Senses and Flavor* 2 (1977): 267–81.

———, P. Pelosi, and L. J. Forrester. "Specific Anosmias to 5a-androst-16-en-3-one and w-pentadecalactone: The Urinous and Musky Primary Odors." *Chemical Senses and Flavor* 2 (1977): 401–25.

——— and J. R. Popplewell. "Sensitivity of Women to Musk Odor: No Menstrual Variation." *Journal of Chemical Ecology* 1 (1975): 291–97.

Angier, N. "Mating for Life? It's Not For the Birds." *New York Times*, 21 August 1990, C1, C8.

———. "A Potent Peptide Prompts an Urge to Cuddle." *New York Times*, 22 January 1991, C1, C10.

———. "In Fish, Social Status Goes Right to the Brain." *New York Times*, 12 November 1991, C1, C12.

———. "Making an Embryo: Biologists Find Keys to Body Plan. From Worms to Cows, One Class of Genes Spells Out the Blue Print." *New York Times*, 23 February 1993, C1, C9.

———. "Finding Elusive Factors That Help Wire Up the Brain." *New York Times*, 16 August 1994, B7, B12.

Ansley, D. "Sperm Tales." *Discover* 13 (June 1992): 66–9.

Arai, Y., A. Matusumoto, and M. Nishizuka. "Synaptogenesis and Neuronal Plasticity to Gonadal Steroids." In *Morphology of Hypothalamus and Its Connections.* Edited by D. Ganten and D. W. Pfaff. Berlin: Springer-Verlag, 1986.

Arendash, G. W., and R. A. Gorski. "Effects of Discrete Lesions of the Sexually Dimorphic Nucleus of the Preoptic Area of the Medial Preoptic Regions on the Sexual Behavior of Male Rats." *Brain Research* 10 (1983): 147–54.

Bailey, J. M., and R. C. Pillard. "A Genetic Study of Male Sexual Orientation." *Archives of General Psychiatry* 48 (1991): 1089–95.

———, R. C. Pillard, M. C. Neale, and Y. Agyei. "Heritable Factors Influence Sexual Orientation in Women." *Archives of General Psychiatry* 50 (1993): 217–23.

Baker, J. R. *Race*. New York: Oxford University Press, 1974.

Balogh, R. D. and R. H. Porter. "Olfactory Preferences Resulting From Mere Exposure in Human Neonates." *Infant Behavioral Development* 9 (1986): 395–401.

Bancroft, J., and J. M. Reinisch. *Adolescence and Puberty*. New York: Oxford University Press, 1990.

Bargmann, C. I., and H. R. Horvitz. "Control of Larval Development by Chemosensory Neurons in *Caenorhabditis elegans*." *Science* 251 (1991): 1243–46.

Barinaga, M. "Is Homosexuality Biological?" *Science* 253 (1991): 956–57.

Beach, F. A. "Sexual Attractivity, Proceptivity, and Receptivity in Female Mammals." *Hormones and Behavior* 7 (1976): 105–38.

Beamer, W., G. Bermant, and M. Clegg. "Copulatory Behavior of the Ram." *Animal Behavior* 17 (1969): 795–800.

Beauchamp, G. K., K. Yamazaki, and E. A. Boyse. "The Chemosensory Recognition of Genetic Individuality." *Scientific American* 253 (1985): 86–92.

Bell, A. P., M. S. Weinberg, and S. K. Hammersmith. *Sexual Preference: Its Development in Men and Women*. Bloomington: Indiana University Press, 1981.

Benet's Reader's Encyclopedia, 3d ed. New York: Harper and Row, 1987.

Berliner, D. L. "Biotransformation of Steroids by the Skin." *Advances in the Biology of Skin*. Vol. 12 (1972). Annual Series. New York: Pergamon, Symposium Publications.

Berliner, D. L., C. Jennings-White, and R. M. Lavken. "The Human Skin: Fragrances and Pheromones." *Journal of Steroid Biochemistry and Molecular Biology* 39 (1991): 671–79.

———, J. R. Pasqualini, and A. J. Gallegos. "The Formation of Water Soluble Steroids by Human Skin." *Journal of Investigative Dermatology* 50 (1968): 220–24.

Berrill, N. J. *Sex and the Nature of Things*. New York: Dodd, Mead and Company, 1953.

Bieber, I. "Olfaction in Sexual Development and Adult Sexual Organization." *American Journal of Psychotherapy* 13 (1959): 851–59.

Bilton, D., J. Madison, and A. K. Webb. "Cystic Fibrosis, Breath Pentane, and Lipid Peroxidation." *Lancet* 337 (1991): 1420.

Bird, S. and D. B. Gower. "Validation and Use of RIA for Androstenone in Axillary Collection." *Journal of Steroid Biochemistry and Molecular Biology* 14 (1981): 213–19.

———. "Estimation of the Odorous Steroid, 5a-androst-16-en-3-one in Human Saliva." *Experientia* 39 (1983): 790–92.

Bishop, J. E. "Research Points Toward a 'Gay' Gene." *Wall Street Journal*, 16 July 1993, B1, B8.

Blackburn, S. and D. L. Loper. *Maternal, Fetal, and Neonatal Physiology*. Philadelphia: W. B. Saunders, 1992.

Blakeslee, H. F. "Unlike Reactions of Different Individuals to Fragrance in Verbena Flowers." *Science* 48 (1918): 298–99.

Bloch, I. *Odoratus Sexualis: A Scientific and Literary Study of Sexual Scents and Erotic Perfumes.* New York: American Anthropological Society, 1933.

Bobrow, N. A., J. Money, and V. J. Lewis. "Delayed Puberty, Eroticism and Sense of Smell: A Psychological Study of Hypogonadotropinism, Osmatic and Anosmatic (Kallmann's Syndrome)." *Archives of Sexual Behavior* 1 (1971): 329–44.

Boekhoff, I., J. Inglese, S. Schleicher, W. J. Koch, R. J. Lefkowitz, and H. Breer. "Olfaction Desensitization Requires Membrane Targeting of Receptor Kinase Mediated by Beta Gamma-Subunits of Heterotrimeric G Proteins." *Journal of Biological Chemistry* 269 (1994): 37–40.

Booth, A., G. Shelley, A. Mazur, G. Tharp, and R. Kittok. "Testosterone, and Winning and Losing in Human Competition." *Hormones and Behavior* 4 (1989): 556–71.

Brody, B. "The Sexual Significance of the Axillae." *Psychiatry* 38 (1975): 278–89.

Bronson, F. H. "Rodent Pheromones." *Biology of Reproduction* 4 (1971): 344–57.

Bronson, F. H. and E. F. Rissman. "The Biology of Puberty." *Biological Reviews of the Cambridge Philosophical Society* 61(1986): 157–95.

——— and W. Whitten. "Estrous Accelerating Pheromone of Mice: Assay, Androgen-Dependency, and Presence in Bladder Urine." *Journal of Reproduction and Fertility* 15 (1968): 131–34.

Brown, S. *French Silk.* New York: Warner Books, 1992.

Bruce, H. M. "Further Observations of Pregnancy Block in Mice Caused by Proximity of Strange Males." *Journal of Reproduction and Fertility* 2 (1960): 311–12.

Brum, G., L. McKane, and G. Karp. *Biology: Exploring Life.* 2d ed. New York: John Wiley and Sons, 1994.

Buck, L., and R. Axel. "A Novel Multigene Family May Encode Odorant Receptors: A Molecular Basis for Odor Recognition." *Cell* 65 (1991): 175–87.

Burr, C. "Homosexuality and Biology." *The Atlantic Monthly* 271 (1993): 47–65.

Byne, W. "The Biological Evidence Challenged." *Scientific American* 68 (May 1994): 50–55.

Byne, W. and B. Parsons. "Human Sexual Orientation: The Biologic Theories Reappraised." *Archives of General Psychiatry* 50 (1993): 228–39.

Camphausen, R.C. *The Encyclopedia of Erotic Wisdom.* Rochester, Vermont: Inner Traditiona Internationa, 1991.

Cernoch, J. M. and R. H. Porter. "Recognition of Maternal Axillary Odors by Infants." *Child Development* 56 (1985): 1593–98.

Changeaux, J. P. "Chemical Signalling in the Brain." *Scientific American* 269 (1993): 58–62.

Claus, R. and W. Alsing. "Occurrence of 5a-androst-16-en-3-one, a Boar Pheromone in Man and its Relationship to Testosterone." *Journal of Endocrinology* 68 (1976): 483–84.

Clewell, D. B., and K. E. Weaver. "Sex Pheromones and Plasmid Transfer in *Enterococcus faecalis.*" *Plasmid* 21 (1989): 175–84.

Cohen, J. and I. Stewart. *The Collapse of Chaos.* New York: Viking Penguin, 1994.

———. "Our Genes Aren't Us." *Discover* 15 (April 1994): 78–84.

Coleman, E. and J. Cesnik. "Skoptic Syndrome: The Treatment of an Obsessional Gender Dysphoria with Lithium Carbonate and Psychotherapy." *American Journal of Psychotherapy* 44 (1990): 204–17.

Coleman, E. "Compulsive Sexual Behavior: New Concepts and Treatments." *Journal of Psychology and Human Sexuality* 4 (1991): 37–52.

———. "The Role of Psychotropic Medications on Hormonal Pathways and in Human Sexual Behavior." Symposium Presentation: Annual Meeting of the Society for the Scientific Study of Sex, Chicago, Illinois, 1993.

Comfort, A. "Communications May be Odorous." *New Scientist and Science Journal* (25 February 1971): 412–14.

———. "Likelihood of Human Pheromones." *Nature* 230 (1971): 432–33.

Coon, C. S. *Racial Adaptations.* Chicago: Nelson Hall, 1982.

Corbier, P., L. Dehennin, M. Castanier, et al. "Sex Differences in Serum Luteinizing Hormone and Testosterone in the Human Neonate During the First Few Hours After Birth." *Journal of Clinical Endocrinology and Metabolism* 71 (1990): 1347–48.

Cowley, J. J., A. L. Johnson, and W. L. Brooksbank. "The Effect of Two Odorous Compounds on Performance in an Assessment-of-People Test." *Psychoneuroendocrinology* 2 (1977): 159–72.

Craigmyle, M. B. L. *The Apocrine Glands and the Breast.* Chichester: Wiley and Sons, 1984.

Crosby, E. C., and T. Humphrey. "Studies of the Vertebrate Telencephalon." *Journal of Comparative Neurology* 71 (1938): 121.

Crowley, W. F. and R. W. Whitcomb. "Gonadotropin-Releasing Hormone Deficiency in Man: Diagnosis and Treatment with Exogenous Gonadotropin-Releasing Hormone." *American Journal of Obstetrics and Gynecology* 163 (1990): 1752–58.

Cutler, G. B., R. J. Schiebinger, B. D. Albertson, F. G. Cassorla, and G. P. Chrousos. "The Adrenarche (Human and Animal)." In *Control of the Onset of Puberty.* Edited by M. M. Grumback, P. C. Sizonenko, and M. L. Aubert, Baltimore: Williams and Wilkens, 1990.

Cutler, W. B. *Love Cycles: The Science of Intimacy.* New York: Villard, 1991.

———, C. R. Garcia, and A. M. Krieger. "Luteal Phase Defects: Sporadic Sexual Behavior in Women." *Hormones and Behavior* 13 (1979): 214–18.

———. "Sexual Behavior Frequency and Menstrual Cycle Length in Mature Premenopausal Women." *Psychoneuroendocrinology* 4 (1979): 297–309.

———. "Sporadic Sexual Behavior and Menstrual Cycle Length in Women." *Hormones and Behavior* 14 (1980): 163–72.

Cutler, W. B., G. Preti, A. M. Krieger, G. R. Huggins, G. R. Garcia, and H. J. Lawley. "Human Axillary Secretions Influence Women's Menstrual Cycles: The Role of Donor Extract from Men." *Hormones and Behavior* 20 (1986): 463–73.

Davidson, E. H. "Hormones and Genes." *Scientific American* 212 (1965): 36–45.

Dawkins, R. *The Selfish Gene.* New York: Oxford University Press, 1989.

DeMeo, J. "Desertification and the Origins of Amouring: The Saharasian Connection." *Journal of Orogonymy* 21 (1989): 185–213.

DeWaal, F. *Chimpanzee Politics: Power and Sex Among Apes.* New York: Harper and Row, 1982.

———. "Tension Regulation and Nonreproductive Function of Sex in Captive Bonobos (*Pan paniscus*)." *National Geographic Research* 3 (1987): 318–35.

Diamond, J. "Turning a Man." *Discover.* 13 (June 1992): 70–7.

———. *The Third Chimpanzee.* New York: Harper Collins, 1992.

———. "Guest Opinion." *Playboy* 40 (September 1993): 38.

Diamond, M. "Bisexualities: A Biological Perspective. From a Presentation at the Third International Berlin Conference of Sexology, July 10–15." In *Bisexualities.* Vol. 4 of *Social-Scientific Sex Research.* Edited by E. Haeberle. Berlin: W. de Gruyter, 1990.

Dittmann, R. W., M. H, Kappes, M. E. Kappes, D. Borger, H. F. Meyer-Bahlburg, H. Stegner, R. H. Willig, and H. Wallis. "Congenital Adrenal Hyperplasia II: Gender-Related Behavior and Attitudes in Female Salt-Wasting and Simple-Virilizing Patients." *Psychoneuroendocrinology* 15 (1990): 421–34.

Dobb, E. "The Scents Around Us." *Sciences* (November-December 1989): 46–53.

Dodd, G. H., and M. Skinner. "From Moods to Molecules: The Psychopharmacology of Perfumery and Aromatherapy." In *Fragrance: The Psychology and Biology of Perfume.* Edited by S. Van Toller and G. H. Dodd. Amsterdam: Elsevier Applied Science, 1992.

Dorland's Illustrated Medical Dictionary. 27th ed. Philadelphia: W. B. Saunders, 1985.

Dorner, G. "Hormone-Dependent Brain Development and Neuroendocrine Prophylaxis." *Experimental Clinical Endocrinology* 94 (1989): 4–22.

Dorries, K. M., H. J. Schmidt, G. K. Beauchamp, and C. J. Wysocki. "Changes in Sensitivity to the Odor of Androstenone During Adolescence." *Developmental Psychobiology* 22 (1989): 423–35.

Doty, R.L. "An Examination of Relationships Between the Pleasantness, Intensity, and Concentration of 10 Odorous Stimuli." *Perceptual Psychophysiology* 17 (1975): 492–96.

———. "Psychophysical Measurement of Odor Perception in Humans." In *The Human Sense of Smell.* Edited by D. G. Laing, R. L. Doty, and W. Breipohl. New York: Springer-Verlag, 1991.

———. "Olfactory Function in Neonates." In *The Human Sense of Smell.* Edited by D. G. Laing, R. L. Doty, and W. Breipohl. New York: Springer-Verlag, 1991.

———. "Influences of Aging on Human Olfactory Function." In *The Human Sense of Smell.* Edited by D. G. Laing, R. L. Doty, and W. Breipohl. New York: Springer-Verlag, 1991.

———. "Olfactory Capacities in Aging and Alzheimer's Disease. Psychophysical and Anatomic Considerations." *Annals of the New York Academy of Sciences* 640 (1991): 20–7.

———. "Reproductive Endocrine Influences Upon Olfactory Perception: A Current Perspective." *Journal of Chemical Ecology* 12 (1986): 497–511.

———, M. Ford, and G. Preti. "Changes in the Intensity and Pleasantness of Human Vaginal Odor During the Menstrual Cycle." *Science* 190 (1975): 1316–18.

Doty, R.L., P. J. Snyder, G. R. Huggins, and L. D. Lowry. "Endocrine, Cardiovascular, and Psychological Correlates of Olfactory Sensitivity Changes During the Human Menstrual Cycle." *Journal of Comparative and Physiological Psychology* 95 (1981): 45–60.

Durden-Smith, J., and D. deSimone. *Sex and the Brain.* New York: Arbor House 1983.

Ehrenreich, B., E. Hess, and G. Jacobs. *Re-Making Love: The Feminization of Sex.* New York: Doubleday/Anchor, 1987.

Ehrhardt A. A., H. F. L. Meyer-Bahlburg, L. R. Rosen, J. F. Feldman, N. P. Veridiano, I. Zimmerman, and B. S. McEwen. "Sexual Orientation After Prenatal Exposure to Exogenous Estrogen." *Archives of Sexual Behavior* 14 (1985): 57–77.

Ellis, H. *Studies in the Psychology of Sex: Sexual Selection in Man.* Vol. 4. Philadelphia: Davis, 1914.

Engen, T. *The Perception of Odors.* New York: Academic Press, 1982.

Epple, G., M. C. Alveario, and A. M. Belcher. "Copulatory Behavior of Adult Tamarins (Sanguinus fuscicollis) Castrated as Neonates of Juveniles: Effect of Testosterone Treatment." *Hormones and Behavior* 24 (1990): 470–83.

Fausto-Sterling, A. *Myths of Gender: Biological Theories about Women and Men.* New York: Basic Books, 1992.

Filsinger, E. E. "Human Responses to the Pig Sex Pheromone Androstenol." *Journal of Comparative Psychology* 98 (1984): 219–22.

———— and W. C. Monte. "Sex History, Menstrual Cycle, and Psychophysical Ratings of Alpha Androstenone, a Possible Human Sex Pheromone." *Journal of Sex Research* 22 (1986): 243–48.

Finegold, S. M. and W. J. Martin. *Diagnostic Microbiology.* 6th ed. St. Louis: C. V. Mosby, 1982.

Firestein, S. and G. M. Shepherd. "A Kinetic Model of the Odor Response in Single Olfactory Receptor Neurons." *Journal of Steroid Biochemistry and Molecular Biology* 39 (1991): 615–20.

Fisher, H. E. *Anatomy of Love.* New York: W. W. Norton, 1992.

Ford, C. S. and F. A. Beach. *Patterns of Sexual Behavior.* New York: Harper and Row, 1951.

Forsythe, A. "Good Scents and Bad." *Natural History.* (November 1985): 25–32.

Francoeur, R. T. "Experimental Embryology as a Tool For Saving Endangered Animal Species." In *Breeding Endangered Species in Captivity.* Edited by R. D. Martin. New York: Academic Press, 1975.

————. *Utopian Motherhood: New Trends in Human Reproduction.* New York: A. S. Barnes, 1970, 1977.

————. *Becoming a Sexual Person.* New York: Macmillan Publishing, 1991.

————. "On the Scent of a Lover." *Forum.* (November 1993): 40–5.

————. "Parthenogesis." In *Human Sexuality: An Encyclopedia.* V. L. Bullough and B. Bullough. New York: Garland Publishing, 1994.

Francoeur, A. K. and R. T. Francoeur. *Hot and Cool Sex: Cultures in Conflict.* New York: 1974.

Francoeur, R. T., A. Perkins, J. V. Kohl, and E. Coleman. "Hormones and Human Sexual Behavior." Symposium: Annual Meeting of the Society for the Scientific Study of Sex, Chicago, Illinois, 1993.

————, T. Perper, and N. A. Scherzer. *A Descriptive Dictionary and Atlas of Sexology.* New York: Greenwood Press, 1991.

————, M. Cornog, T. Perper, and N.A. Scherzer. *The Complete Dictionary of Sexology.* New Expanded Edition. New York: Continuum, 1994.

Freedman, D. H. "The Aggressive Egg." *Discover* 13 (June 1992): 61–5.

————. "In the Realm of the Chemical." *Discover* 14, no. 9 (June 1993): 69–76.

Freeman, W. J. and C. A. Skarda. "Spatial EEG Patterns, Non-Linear Dynamics and Perception: The Neo-Sherringtonian View. *Brain Research Reviews* 10 (1985): 147–75.

Gadpaille, W. *The Cycles of Sex.* New York: Scribner, 1975.

Galluscio, E. H. *Biological Psychology.* New York: Macmillan Publishing, 1990.

Garcia-Velasco, J. and M. Mondragon. "The Incidence of the Vomeronasal Organ in 1000 Human Subjects and its Possible Clinical Significance." *Journal of Steroid Biochemistry and Molecular Biology* 39 (1991): 561–63.

Gedda, L., D. Casa, and M. Comparetti. "Twin Zygosity Diagnosis: Experiments with Bloodhounds." *Rivista di Biologica* 73 (1980): 95–7.

Gelman, D., D. Foote, T. Barrett, and M. Talbot. "Mind: Born or Bred?" *Newsweek* (24 February 1992): 46–53.

Gibbons, B. "The Intimate Sense of Smell." *National Geographic* 170 (1986): 324–61.

Gilbert, A. N. and C. J. Wysocki. "The Smell Survey Results." *National Geographic* 171 (1987): 514–25.

Gilbert, A. N., K. Yamazaki, G. K. Beauchamp, and L. Thomas. "Olfactory Discrimination of Mouse Strains (*Mus musculus*) and Major Histocompatibility Types by Humans (*Homo sapiens*)." *Journal of Comparative Psychology* 100 (1986): 262–65.

Goldberg, B. Z. *The Sacred Fire: The Story of Sex in Religion.* New York: University Books, 1958.

Goldfoot, D. A., M. A. Kravets, R. W. Goy, and S. K. Freeman. "Lack of Effect of Vaginal Lavages and Aliphatic Acids on Ejaculatory Responses in Rhesus Monkeys: Behavioral and Chemical Analyses." *Hormones and Behavior* 7 (1976): 1–27.

Goldman, B. "The Essence of Attraction." *Health* 3 (March/April 1994): 40.

Goldsmith, L. A. "My Organ is Bigger Than Your Organ." *Archives of Dermatology* 126 (1990): 301–2.

Goodall, J. *The Chimpanzees of Gombe: Patterns of Behavior.* Cambridge, Mass.: Belknap, 1986.

Gorman, C. "Sizing Up the Sexes." *Time* (20 January 1992): 42–51.

Gorski, R. A., H. H. Gordon, J. E. Shryne, and A. M. Southam. "Evidence For a Morphological Sex Difference Within the Medial Preoptic Area of the Rat Brain." *Brain Research* 143 (1978): 333–46.

Gower, D. B. and W. D. Booth. "Salivary Pheromones in the Pig and Human in Relation to Sexual Status and Age." In *Ontogeny of Olfaction.* Edited by W. Breipohl. Berlin: Springer-Verlag, 1986.

Graham, C. A. and W. C. McGrew. "Menstrual Synchrony in Female Under-graduates Living on a Coeducational Campus." *Psychoneuroendocrinology* 5 (1980): 245–52.

Graziadei, P. P. C. "Functional Anatomy of the Mammalian Chemoreceptor System." In *Chemical Signals In Vertebrates*. Edited by D. Muller-Schwarze and M. M. Mozel. New York: Plenum Press, 1977.

Gregersen, E. *Sexual Practices: The Story of Human Sexuality*. London: Mitchell Beazley, 1982.

Grumbach, M. M. and D. M. Styne. "Puberty: Ontogeny, Neuroendocrinology, Physiology and Disorders." In *Textbook of Endocrinology*. 8th ed. Edited by J. D. Wilson and D. W. Foster. Philadelphia: W. B. Saunders, 1992.

Halpern, M. "The Organization and Function of the Vomeronasal System." *Annual Review of Neuroscience* 10 (1987): 325–62.

Halpin, Z. T. "Individual Odors Among Mammals." In *Advances in the Study of Behavior*, vol. 16. Edited by J. S. Rosenblatt, C. Beer, M. Busner, and P. J. B. Slater. Orlando: Academic Press, 1986.

Hamer, D., and P. Copeland. *The Science of Desire*. New York: Simon and Schuster, 1994.

———, S. Hu, V. L. Magnuson, N. Hu, and A. M. L. Pattatucci, A.M.L. "A Linkage Between DNA Markers on the X Chromosome and Male Sexual Orientation." *Science* 261 (1993): 321–27.

Hansen, J. W., H. J. Hoffman, and G. T. Ross. "Monthly Gonadotropin Cycles in Premenarcheal Girls." *Science* 190 (1975): 161–63.

Henderson, M. E. "Evidence for a Male Menstrual Temperature Cycle and Synchrony With the Female Menstrual Cycle" (abstract). *New Zealand Medical Journal* 84 (1976): 164.

Henkin, J. C. and G. F. Powell. "Increased Sensitivity of Taste and Smell in Cystic Fibrosis." *Science* 138 (1962): 1107–8.

Hertz, J., W. S. Cain, L. Bartoshuk, and T. F. Dolan, Jr. "Olfactory and Taste Sensitivity in Children with Cystic Fibrosis." *Physiology and Behavior* 14 (1975): 89–94.

Hoffman, G. E., C. J. Phelps, H. Khachaturian, and J. R. Sladek. "Neuroendocrine Projections to the Median Eminence." In *Morphology of the Hypothalamus and its Connections*. Edited by D. Ganten and D. W. Pfaff. Berlin: Springer-Verlag, 1986.

Holldobler, B. and E. O. Wilson. *The Ants*. Cambridge, Mass.: Harvard University Press, 1990.

Hopson, J. L. *Scent Signals*. New York: William Morrow and Company, 1974.

Hrdy, S. B. *The Woman That Never Evolved*. Cambridge, Mass.: Harvard University Press, 1987.

Hunt, M. M. *Sexual Behavior in the 1970's*. Chicago: Playboy Press, 1974.

Imperato-McGinley, J., R. E. Peterson, T. Gautier, and E. Sturla. "The Impact of Androgens on the Evolution of Male Gender Identity." In *Sexuality: New Perspectives*. Edited by Z. DeFries, R. C. Friedman, and E. Corn. Westport, Conn.: Greenwood Press, 1985.

Jacobson, M. *Insect Sex Attractants*. New York: Interscience Publishers, 1965.

Janus, S. S. and C. L. Janus. *The Janus Report on Sexual Behavior*. Sommerset, N. J.: Wiley and Sons, 1992.

Jochle, W. "Current Research in Coitus Induced Ovulation," *Journal of Reproduction and Fertility* 22 (1975): 165–207.

John, E. M., D. A. Savitz, and C. M. Shy. "Spontaneous Abortions Among Cosmetologists." *Epidemiology* 5 (1994): 147–55.

Johnson, M. L. "Skin Diseases." In *Cecil Textbook of Medicine*, vol. 2. Edited by J. B. Wyngaarden and J. B. Smith Jr. Philadelphia: W. B. Saunders, 1982.

Jones, J. "Labs Conjure Up Fragrances and Flavors to Add Allure." *New York Times*, New Jersey Section, New Jersey Weekly Desk, 26 December 1993, 1.

Kallmann, F. J. "Twin and Sibship Study of Overt Male Homosexuality." *American Journal of Human Genetics* 4 (1952): 136–46.

———. "Comparative Twin Study on the Genetic Aspects of Male Homosexuality." *Journal of Nervous Mental Diseases* 115 (1952): 283–98.

———. "Genetic Aspects of Sexual Determination and Sexual Maturation Potentials in Man." In *Determinants of Human Sexual Behavior*. Edited by G. Winokur. Springfield, Ill.: Charles G. Thomas, 1963.

Kano, T. and M. Mulavwa. "Feeding Ecology of the Pygmy Chimpanzees (*Pan paniscus*) of Wamba." In *The Pygmy Chimpanzee*. Edited by R. L. Susman. New York: Plenum Press, 1984.

Karlen, A. *Sexuality and Homosexuality: The Complete Account of Male and Female Sexual Behaviour and Deviation—With Case Histories*. London: MacDonald, 1971.

Karlson, P. and M. Luscher. "'Pheromones': A New Term for a Class of Biologically Active Substances." *Nature* 183 (1959): 55–6.

Keith, L., A. Dravicks, and B. Krotosyzinski. "Olfactory Study: Human Pheromones." *Archiv fur Gynakologie* 218 (1975): 203–4.

Keverne, E. B. "Chemical Communication in Primate Reproduction." In *Pheromones and Reproduction in Mammals*. Edited by J. G. Vandenbergh. New York: Academic Press, 1983.

——— and R. P. Michael. "Sex Attractant Properties of Ether Extracts of Vaginal Secretions from Rhesus Monkeys." *Journal of Endocrinology* 51(1971): 313–22.

Kimura, D. "Sex Differences in the Brain." *Scientific American* (September 1992): 119–25.

Kingston, B. H. "The Chemistry and Olfactory Properties of Musk, Civet and Castoreum." Proceedings of the 2d International Congress on Endocrinology, 1965. Int. Congr. Ser. No. 83 (1965): 209–214.

Klopfer, P. "Mother Love: What Turns It On? Studies of Maternal Arousal and Attachment in Ungulates May Have Implications for Man." *American Scientist* 59 (1971): 404–7.

Knobil, E. "Concluding Remarks." In *Control of the Onset of Puberty*. Edited by M. M. Grumback, P. C. Sizonenko, and M. L. Aubert. Baltimore: Williams and Wilkens, 1990.

———. "The GnRH Pulse Generator." *American Journal of Obstetrics and Gynecology* 163 (1990): 1721–26.

Koelega, H. S. and E. P. Koster. "Some Experiments on Sex Differences in Odor Perception." *Annals of New York Academy of Sciences* 237 (1974): 234–46.

Kohl, J. V. "Luteinizing Hormone: The Link Between Sex and the Sense of Smell." Paper Presented at the Annual Meeting of the Society for the Scientific Study of Sex, San Diego, California, 1992.

———. "Are Olfactory-Hormonal Relationships Primary Determinants of Human Sexual Behavior?" Poster Session at the Annual Meeting of the Society for the Scientific Study of Sex, Chicago, Illinois, 1993.

———. "Olfaction, the Endocrine System and Human Sexual Behavior?" Symposium Presentation at the Annual Meeting of the Society for the Scientific Study of Sex, Chicago, Illinois, 1993.

———. "Human Pheromones: The Link Between the Nature and the Nurture of Human Sexuality?" Presentation at the Annual Meeting of the Society for the Scientific Study of Sex, Miami, Florida, 1994.

Kohn, A. and F. Fish. "Wasted Resources/Missed Opportunities." *Journal of Irreproducible Results* 38, no. 1 (1993): 15.

Kolata, G. "From Fly to Man, Cells Obey Same Signal." *New York Times* 5 January 1993, C1, C10.

Kubie, J. L., A. Vagvolgyi, and M. Halpern. "The Roles of the Vomeronasal and Olfactory Systems in the Courtship Behavior of Male Garter Snakes." *Journal of Comparative and Physiological Psychology* 92 (1978): 627–41.

Kulin, H. and E. O. Reiter. "Gonadotropin and Testosterone Measurements After Estrogen Administration to Adult Men, Prepubertal and Pubertal Boys, and Men with Hypogonadism." *Pediatric Research* 10 (1976): 46–51.

Kuroda, S. "Interaction Over Food Among Pygmy Chimpanzees." In *The Pygmy Chimpanzee*. Edited by R. L. Susman. New York: Plenum Press, 1984.

Labows. J. N. and G. Preti. "Human Semiochemicals." In *Fragrance: The Psychology and Biology of Perfume*. Edited by S. Van Toller and G. H. Dodd. Amsterdam: Elsevier Applied Science, 1992.

Lacy, T. K. "Aromatheraphy." *Las Vegas Review-Journal* 13 June 1994, 1C, 3C.

Langley-Danysz, P. "La Truffe, un aphrodisiaque." *La Recherche* 136 (1982): 1059.

Larue, G. A. "Religious Traditions and Circumcision." *The Truth Seeker* 1 (1989): 4–8.

LeGuerer, A. *Scent: The Mysterious and Essential Powers of Smell*. New York: Turtle Bay Books, 1992.

LeVay, S. "A Difference in Hypothalamic Structure Between Heterosexual and Homosexual Men." *Science* 253 (1991): 1034–37.

———. *The Sexual Brain*. Cambridge, Mass.: MIT Press, 1993.

——— and D. H. Hamer. "Evidence for a Biological Influence in Male Homosexuality." *Scientific American* (May 1994): 44–9.

Licht, G. and M. Meredith. "Convergence of Main and Accessory Olfactory Pathways Onto Single Neurons in the Hamster Amygdala." *Experimental Brain Research* 69 (1987): 7–18.

Liebowitz, M. R. *The Chemistry of Love*. Boston: Little Brown, 1983.

Lincoln, D. W. "Translation of Hypothalamic Electrical Activity into Episodic Hormone Secretion." In *The Episodic Secretion of Hormones.* Edited by W. F. Crowley and J. G. Hofler. New York: John Wiley and Sons, 1987.

Lipsit, L. "Critical Conditions in Infancy: A Psychological Perspective." *American Psychologist* 34 (1979): 973–80.

Long, M. "Visions of a New Faith." *Science Digest* 89 (1981): 36–42.

MacFarlane, A. "Olfaction in the Development of Social Preferences in the Human Neonate." *Ciba Foundation Symposium* 33 (1975): 103–13.

MacLean, P. "The Brain's Generation Gap: Some Human Implications." *Zygon: Journal of Religion and Science* 8 (June 1973): 113–27.

———. "Brain Evolution: The Origins of Social and Cognitive Behaviors." In M. Frank, ed. 1984. *A Child's Brain: The Impact of Advanced Research on Cognitive and Social Behaviors.* New York: Haworth Press, 9–22. *Journal of Children in Contemporary Society* 16 (Fall/Winter 1983).

Mader, S. S. *Biology: Evolution, Diversity, and the Environment.* 2d ed. Dubuque, Iowa.: W. C. Brown, 1987.

Magrassi, L. and P. P. Graziadei. "Single Olfactory Organ Associated with Prosencephalic Malformation and Cyclopia in a *Xenopus laevis* Tadpole." *Brain Research* 412 (1987): 386–90.

Mallet, A. I., K. T. Holland, P. J. Rennie, W. J. Watkins, and D. B. Gower. "Applications of Gas Chromatography-Mass Spectrometry in the Study of Androgen and Odorous 16-androstene Metabolism by Human Axillary Bacteria." *Journal of Chromatography* 562 (1991): 647–58.

Malsbury, C. W. "Facilitation of Male Rat Copulatory Behavior by Electrical Stimulation of the Medial Preoptic Area." *Physiology and Behavior* 7 (1971): 797–805.

Marchetti, B., G. Pelletier, M. Cioni, M. Badr, G. Palumbo, and U. Scapagnini. "Age-Dependent Changes of LHRH Receptor Systems: Role of Central and Peripheral LHRH in the Decline of Reproductive Function." In *The Brain and Female Reproductive Function.* Edited by A. R. Genazzani, U. Montemagno, C. Nappi, and F. Petraglia. New Jersey: Parthenon, 1988.

Margolese, M. S. "Homosexuality: A New Endocrine Correlate." *Hormones and Behavior* 1 (1970): 151–55.

——— and O. Janiger. "Androsterone-Etiocholanolone Ratios in Male Homosexuals." *British Medical Journal* 207 (1973): 207–10.

Martin, E. "The Egg and Sperm: How Science has Constructed a Romance Based on Stereotypical Male-Female Roles." *Signs: Journal of Women in Culture and Society.* 13, no. 3 (Spring 1991).

Martin, L. "Finding Your Scents of Well-Being Through Aromatherapy." *Las Vegas Review-Journal/Sun,* 22 August 1993, 10J.

Mason, R. T., H. M. Fales, T. H. Jones, L., K. Pannell, J. W. Chinn, and D. Crews. "Sex Pheromones in Snakes." *Science* 245 (1989): 290–93.

McClintock, M. "Menstrual Synchrony and Suppression." *Nature* 229 (1979): 244–45.

McEwen, B. S. "Steroid Hormones and the Brain: Linking 'Nature and Nurture.'" *Neurochemical Research* 13(1988): 663–669.

McWhirter, K. "Ethnography of Specific Anosmia." *Canadian Journal of Genetics and Cytology* 11 (1969): 479.

Melrose, D. R., H. C. B. Reed, and R. L. S. Patterson. "Androgen Steroids Associated with Boar Odour as an Aid to the Detection of Oestrus in Pig Artificial Insemination." *British Veterinary Journal* 127 (1971): 497–502.

Mennella, J. A. and G. K. Beauchamp. "Olfactory Preferences in Children and Adults." In *The Human Sense of Smell.* Edited by D. G. Laing, R. L. Doty, and W. Breipohl. New York: Springer-Verlag, 1991.

Mennella, J. and A. H. Moltz. "Pheromonal Emission by Pregnant Rats Protects Against Infanticide by Nulliparous Conspecifics." *Physiology and Behavior* 46 (1989): 591–95.

Menter, M. "The Secret Messages of Scent." *Redbook* (January 1993): 30–2.

Meredith, M. "Patterned Response to Odor in Mammalian Olfactory Bulb: The Influence of Intensity." *Journal of Neurophysiology* 56 (1986): 572–97.

Meredith, M. "Sensory Processing in the Main and Accessory Olfactory Systems: Comparisons and Contrasts." *Journal of Steroid Biochemistry and Molecular Biology* 39 (1991): 601–14.

——— and G. Howard. "Intracerebroventricular LHRH Relieves Behavioral Deficits Due to Vomeronasal Organ Removal." *Brain Research Bulletin* 29 (1992): 75–9.

Meyer-Bahlburg, H.L. "Sex Hormones and Male Homosexuality in Comparative Perspective." *Archives of Sexual Behavior* 6 (1977): 297–325.

Michael, R. P. "Neuroendocrine Factors Regulating Primate Behaviour." In *Frontiers in Neuroendocrinology.* Edited by L. Martini and W. F. Ganong. New York: Oxford University Press, 1971.

——— and R. W. Bonsall. "Chemical Signals and Primate Behavior." In *Chemical Signals in Vertebrates.* Edited by D.Muller-Schwarze and M. M. Mozel. New York: Plenum Press, 1977.

——— and E. B. Keverne. "Primate Sex Pheromones of Vaginal Origin." *Nature* 225 (1975): 84–5.

———, R. W. Bonsall, and P. Warner. "Human Vaginal Secretions: Volatile Fatty Acid Content." *Science* 186 (1974): 1217–19.

Miller, S. M. "Saliva Testing—A Nontraditional Diagnostic Tool." *Clinical Laboratory Science* 7 (1994): 39–44.

Moncrieff, R. W. *Odour Preferences.* New York: John Wiley and Sons, 1966.

Money, J. *Love and Love Sickness: The Science of Sex, Gender Difference, and Pair-bonding.* Baltimore: Johns Hopkins, 1980.

———. *The Destroying Angel.* New York: Prometheus Books, 1985.

———. *Lovemaps.* New York: Irvington Publishers, 1986.

———. *Gay, Straight and In-Between.* New York: Oxford University Press, 1988.

Monmaney, T. "Are We Led by the Nose?" *Discover* 8 (September 1987): 48–55.

Montagna, W. "The Evolution of Human Skin." *Journal of Human Evolution* 14 (1985): 3–22.

Monti-Bloch, L. and B. I. Grosser. "Effect of Putative Pheromones on the Electrical Activity of the Human Vomeronasal Organ and Olfactory Epithelium." *Journal of Steroid Biochemistry and Molecular Biology* 39 (1991): 573–82.

Monti-Graziadei, A. G. and P. P. Graziadei. "Experimental Studies on the Olfactory Marker Protein. V. Olfactory Marker Protein in the Olfactory Neurons Transplanted With the Olfactory Bulb." *Brain Research* 484 (1989): 157–167.

————. "Sensory Reinnervation After Partial Removal of the Olfactory Bulb." *Journal of Comparative Neurology* 316 (1992): 32–44.

Moore, C. L. "Interaction of Species-Typical Environmental and Hormonal Factors in Sexual Differentiation of Behavior." *Annals of the New York Academy of Science* 474 (1986): 108–19.

Moore, K. L. and T. V. N. Persaud. *The Developing Human: Clinically Oriented Embryology.* 5th ed. Philadelphia: W. B. Saunders, 1993.

Moran, D. T., B. W. Jafek, and J. C. Rowley.) "The Ultrastructure of the Human Olfactory Mucosa." In *The Human Sense of Smell.* Edited by D. G. Laing, R. L. Doty, and W. Breipohl. New York: Springer-Verlag, 1991.

Morris, D. *The Naked Ape.* London: Jonathan Cape, 1967.

Muller-Schwarze, D. "Complex Mammalian Behavior and Pheromone Bioassay in the Field." In *Chemical Signals in Vertebrates.* Edited by D. Muller-Schwarze and M. M. Mozel. New York: Plenum Press, 1977.

Nelson, N. "Terribly Sensuous Woman." *Psychology Today* (July 1971): 68.

Neumann, F. and H. Steinbeck. "Influence of Sexual Hormones on the Differentiation of Neural Centers." *Archives of Sexual Behavior* 2 (1972): 147–62.

Ngai, J., M. M. Dowling, L. Buck, R. Axel, and A. Chess. "The Family of Genes Encoding Odorant Receptors in the Channel Catfish." *Cell* 72 (1993): 657–66.

Nicholson, B. "Does Kissing Aid Human Bonding by Semiochemical Addiction?" *British Journal of Dermatology* 111 (1984): 623–27.

Nicolaides, N. "Skin Lipids: Their Biochemical Uniqueness." *Science* 186 (1974): 19–26.

———— and J. M. B. Apron. "The Saturated Methyl Branched Fatty Acids of Adult Human Skin Surface Lipid." *Biomedicine and Mass Spectrometry* 4 (1977): 337–47.

Nilsson, L. *A Child is Born.* New York: Delacorte Press, 1990.

Nottelmann, E. D., G. Inoff-Germain, E. J. Susman, and G. P. Chrousos. "Hormones and Bhavior at Puberty." In *Adolescence and Puberty.* Edited by J. Bancroft and J. Machover-Reinisch. New York: Oxford University Press, 1990.

Numan, M. "Neuronal Basis of Maternal Behavior in the Rat." *Psychoneuroendocrinology* 13 (1988): 47–62.

Ogden, G. *Women Who Love Sex.* New York: Pocket Books, 1994.

Olds, J. and P. Milner. "Positive Reinforcement Produced by Electrical Stimulation of Septal Area and Other Regions of the Rat Brain." *Journal of Comparative and Physiological Psychology* 47 (1954): 419–27.

Olness, K. and R. Ader. "Conditioning As An Adjunct in the Pharmacotheraphy of Lupus Erythematosus." *Journal of Developmental and Behavioral Pediatrics* 13 (1992): 124–25.

Olsen, K. H., and N. R. Liley. "The Significance of Olfaction and Social Cues in Milt Availability, Sexual Hormone Status, and Spawning Behavior of Male Rainbow Trout (*Oncorhynchus mykiss*)." *General and Comparative Endocrinology* 89 (1993): 107–18.

Page, D. C., R. Mosher, E. M. Simpson, E. M. Fisher, G. Mardon, and J. Pollack. "The Sex-Determining Region of the Human Y Chromosome Encodes a Finger Protein." *Cell* 51 (1987): 1091–04.

Palmer, M. S., A. H. Sinclair, P. Berta, N. A. Ellis, P. N. Goodfellow, N. E. Abbas, and M. Fellous. "Genetic Evidence That ZFY is Not the Testis-Determining Factor." *Nature* 342, no. 6252 (1989): 937–39.

Parker, A. S. and H. M. Bruce. "Olfactory Stimuli in Mammalian Reproduction: Odor Excites Neurohormonal Responses Affecting Oestrus, Pseudopregnancy, and Pregnancy in the Mouse." *Science* 134 (1961): 1049–54.

Parrinder, G. *Sex in the World's Religions*. Ontario, Canada: Don Mills, 1980.

Perkins, A. "Hormones and the Behavioral Response of Male-Oriented Rams to Rams or Estrous Ewes." Symposium Presentation: Annual Meeting of the Society for the Scientific Study of Sex, Chicago, Illinois, 1993.

Perkins, A. and J. A. Fitzgerald. "Luteinizing Hormone, Testosterone, and Behavioral Response of Male-Oriented Rams to Estrous Ewes and Rams." *Journal of Animal Sciences* 70 (1992): 1787–94.

Perkins, A., J. A. Fitzgerald, and E. O. Price. "Luteinizing Hormone and Testosterone Response of Sexually Active and Inactive Rams." *Journal of Animal Sciences* 70 (1992): 2086–93.

Perper, T. *Sex Signals: The Biology of Love*. Philadelphia: iSi Press, 1985.

Persky, H. *Psychoendocrinology of Human Sexual Behavior*. New York: Praeger, 1987.

———, H. I. Lief, C. P. O'Brien, D. Straus, and W. Miller. "Reproductive Hormone Levels and Sexual Behavior of Young Couples During the Menstrual Cycle." In *Progress in Sexology: Selected Papers from the Proceedings of the 1976 International Congress of Sexology*. Edited by R. Genne and C. C. Wheeler. New York: Plenum Press, 1977.

Pfaff, D.W. and Y. Sakuma. "Deficit in the Lordosis Reflex of Female Rats Caused by Lesions in the Ventromedial Nucleus of the Hypothalamus." *Journal of Physiology* 288 (1979): 203–10.

Phillips, J. "Why Can't a Man Be More Like a Woman . . . and Vice Versa?" *Omni* 13 (October 1990): 42–68.

Pillard, R. C. and J. D. Weinrich. "Evidence of Familial Nature of Male Homosexuality." *Archives of General Psychiatry* 43 (1986): 808–12.

Pleim, E. T. and R. J. Barfield. "Progesterone Versus Estrogen Facilitation of Female Sexual Behavior by Intracranial Administration to Female Rats." *Hormones and Behavior* 22 (1988): 150-159.

Pool, R. E. *Eve's Rib: Searching for the Biological Roots of Sex Differences*. New York: Crown, 1994.

Porter, R. H., J. M. Cernoch, and R. D. Balogh. "Odor Signatures and Kin Recognition." *Physiology and Behavior* 34 (1985): 445–48.

Prescott. J. W. "Affectional Bonding for the Prevention of Violent Behaviors: Neurological, Psychological and Religious/Spiritual Determinants." In *Violent Behavior*. Vol. 1 of *Assessment and Intervention*. Edited by L. J. Hertzberg, G. F. Ostrum, and J. R. Field. New York: PMA Publishing, 1990.

Preti, G. and G. R. Huggins. "Cyclical Changes in Volatile Acidic Metabolites of Human Vaginal Secretions and Their Relation to Ovulation." *Journal of Chemical Ecology* 1 (1975): 316–26.

Preti, G., W. B. Cutler, C. R. Garcia, G. R. Huggins, and H. J. Lawley. "Human Axillary Secretions Influence Women's Menstrual Cycles: The Role of Donor Extract of Females." *Hormones and Behavior* 20 (1986): 474–82.

Quadagno, D. M., H. E. Shubeita, J. Deck, and D. Francoeur. "Influence of Male Social Contacts, Exercise and All-Female Living Conditions on the Menstrual Cycle." *Psychoneuroendocrinology* 6 (1981): 239–44.

Reamy, K. J. and S. E. White. "Sexuality in the Puerperium: A Review." *Archives of Sexual Behavior* 16 (1987): 165–86.

Redgrove, P. *The Black Goddess and the Sixth Sense*. London: Bloomsbury, 1987.

Reichlin, S. "Neuroendocrinology." In *Textbook of Endocrinology*. 8th ed. Edited by J. D. Wilson and D. W. Foster. Philadelphia: W.B. Saunders, 1992.

Ressler, K. J., S. L. Sullivan, and L. B. Buck. "A Zonal Organization of Odorant Receptor Gene Expression in the Olfactory Epithelium." *Cell* 73 (1993): 597–609.

Rist, D. Y. "Are Homosexuals Born That Way: Sex on the Brain." *The Nation* 255 (1992): 424–29.

Ross, R., L. Bernstein, H. Judd, R. Hanisch, M. Pike, and R. Henderson. "Serum Testosterone Levels in Healthy Young Black and White Men." *Journal of the National Cancer Institute* 76 (1986): 45–8.

Ross, R. K., L. Bernstein, R. A. Lobo, H. Shimizu, F. Z. Stanczyk, and M. C. Pike. "5-α-Reductase Activity and Risk of Prostate Cancer Among Japanese and U. S. Whie and Black Males." *Lancet* 339 (1992): 887–89.

Rossi, A. "Gender and Parenthood: American Sociological Association, 1983 Presidential Address." *American Sociological Review* 49 (1984): 1–19.

Rovesti, P. and E. Colombo. "Aromatherapy and Aerosols." *Soap, Perfumery and Cosmetics* 46 (1973): 475–78.

Rugarli, E. I. and A. B. Ballabio. "Kallmann Syndrome: from Genetics to Neurobiology." *Journal of the American Medical Association* 270 (1993): 2713–2716.

Russell, M. J. "Human Olfactory Communication." *Nature* 260 (1976): 520–22.

———, G. M. Switz, and K. Thompson. "Olfactory Influences on the Human Menstrual Cycle." *Pharmacology Biochemistry and Behavior* 13 (1980): 737–38.

Russell, R. J. H, P. A. Wells, and J. P. Rushton. "Evidence for Genetic Similarity Detection in Human Marriage." *Ethology and Sociobiology* 6 (1985): 183–87.

Rutter, M. *Maternal Deprivation Reassessed*. Middlesex, England: Penguin, 1972.

Sabelli, H. C. "Rapid Treatment of Depression with Selegiline-Phenylalanine Combination" (Letter to the editor). *Journal of Clinical Psychiatry* 52 (1991): 3.

Sabelli, H. C., A. Carlson-Sabelli, and J. I. Javaid. "The Thermodynamics of Bipolarity: A Bifurcation Model of Bipolar Illness and Bipolar Character and its Therapeutic Applications." *Psychiatry* 53 (1990): 346–68.

Sadler, T. W. *Langman's Medical Embryology*. 6th ed. Baltimore: Williams and Wilkins, 1990.

Sawahata, L. "The Sweet Smell of Success: Fragrance and Athletic Performance." *Self* (July 1994): 32.

Schiffman, S. S. "Taste and Smell in Disease." Second of Two Parts. *New England Journal of Medicine* 308 (1983): 1337–43.

———— and J. M. Siebert. "New Frontiers in Fragrance Use." *Cosmetics and Toiletries* 106 (June 1991): 39–45.

Schlegel, W. S. "Die Konstituitionbiologischen Grundlagen der Homosexualitat." Z. Mwnschl. Vererb. *Konstitutionshlehre* 36 (1993): 341–64.

Schleidt, M. "The Semiotic Relevance of Human Olfaction: A Biological Approach." In *Fragrance: The Psychology and Biology of Perfume*. Edited by S. Van Toller and G. H. Dodd. Amsterdam: Elsevier Applied Science, 1992.

Schleidt, M. and C. Genzel. "The Significance of Mother's Perfume for Infants in the First Weeks of Their Life." *Ethology and Sociobiology* 11 (1990): 145–54.

Schnarch, D. M. *Constructing the Sexual Crucible: An Integration of Sexual and Marital Therapy*. New York: W. W. Norton, 1991.

Schneider, R. A. "Anosmia: Verification and Etiologies." *Annals of Otology, Rhinology and Laryngology* 81(1972): 272–77.

————. "Newer Insights into the Role and Modifications of Olfaction in Man Through Clinical Studies." *Annals of the New York Academy of Sciences* 237 (1974): 217–23.

Schulz, S. and S. Toft. "Identification of a Sex Pheromone from a Spider." *Science* 260 (1993): 1635–37.

Schwenk, K. "Why Snakes have Forked Tongues." *Science* 263 (1994): 1573–77.

Shenker, A., L. Laue, S. Kosugi, J. J. Merendino Jr., T. Minegishi, and G. B. Cutler Jr. "A Constitutively Activating Mutation of the Luteinizing Hormone Receptor in Familial Male Precocious Puberty." *Nature* 365 (1993): 652–54.

Shipley, M. and P. Reyes. "Anatomy of the Human Olfactory Bulb and Central Olfactory Pathways." In *The Human Sense of Smell*. Edited by D. G. Laing, R. L. Doty, and W. Breipohl. New York: Springer-Verlag, 1991.

Shorey, H. H. *Animal Communication by Pheromones*. New York: Academic Press, 1976.

Shtarkshall, R. I. "Israel: Section of Kibbutz Movement." In *International Encyclopedia of Sexuality*. Edited by R. T. Francouer. New York: Continuum Press, in press.

Sinclair, A. H., P. Berta, M. S. Palmer, J. R. Hawkins, B. L. Griffiths, et al., "A Gene from the Human Sex-Determining Region Encodes a Protein with Homology to a Conserved DNA-Binding Motif." *Nature* 346 (1990): 240–44.

Small, M. F. "What's Love Got to do With it?" *Discover* 13 (June 1992): 46–51.

————. *Female Choices: Sexual Behavior of Female Primates*. Ithaca, N. Y.: Cornell University Press, 1993.

Smith, J. C. "Hedgehog, the Floor Plate, and the Zone of Polarizing Activity." *Cell* 76 (1994): 193–96.

Sokolov J. J., R. T. Harris, and M. R. Hecker. "Isolation of Substances from Human Vaginal Secretions Previously Shown to be Sex Attractant Pheromones in Higher Primates." *Archives of Sexual Behavior* 5 (1976): 269–74.

Soma, H., M. Takayama, T. Kiyokawa, T. Adaeda, and K. Tokoro. "Serum Gonadotropin Levels in Japanese Women." *Obstetrics and Gynecology* 46 (1975): 311.

Sorensen, P. W., T. J. Hara, N. E. Stacey, and F. W. Goetz. "F Prostaglandins Function as Potent Olfactory Stimulants that Comprise the Postovulatory Female Sex Pheromone in Goldfish." *Biology of Reproduction* 39 (1988): 1039–50.

Sparkes, R. S., R. W. Simpson, and C. A. Paulsen. "Familial Hypogonadotropic Hypogonadism with Anosmia." *Archives of Internal Medicine* 121 (1968): 534–38.

Sprague, G. F., L. C. Blair, and J. Thorner. "Cell Interactions and Regulation of Cell Type in the Yeast *Saccharomyces cerevisiae.*" *Annual Review of Microbiology* 37 (1983): 623–60.

Steel, D. *Heartbeat.* New York: Delacorte Press, 1991.

Steingarten, J. "The Sweet Smell of Sex?" *Vogue* (June 1993): 204–7.

Stensaas, L. J., R. M. Lavker, L. Monti-Bloch, B. I. Grosser, and D. L. Berliner. "Ultrastructure of the Human Vomeronasal Organ." *Journal of Steroid Biochemistry and Molecular Biology* 39 (1991): 553–60.

Stephens, K. "Pheromones Among the Procaryotes." *Critical Reviews of Microbiology* 13 (1986): 309–34.

Stephenson, F. "The Smell of Sex." Florida State University: *Research in Review* 9 (Fall/Winter 1991): 7.

Stoddart, D. M. *The Scented Ape: The Biology and Culture of Human Odour.* Cambridge: Cambridge University Press, 1990.

Takami, S., M. L. Getchell, Y. Chen, L. Monti-Bloch, D. L. Berliner, L. J. Stensaas, and T. V. Getchell. "Vomeronasal Epithelial Cells of the Adult Human Express Neuron-Specific Molecules." *Neuroreport* 4 (1993): 375–78.

Tavris, C. *The Mismeasure of Woman.* New York: Simon and Shuster, 1992.

Taylor, R. "Brave New Nose: Sniffing Out Human Sexual Chemistry." *Journal of NIH Research* 6 (1994): 47–51.

Thomas, L. "Notes of a Biology-Watcher. A Fear of Pheromones." *New England Journal of Medicine* 285 (1971): 392–93.

———. "Notes of a Biology-Watcher. On Smell." *New England Journal of Medicine* 302 (1980): 731–33.

Thompson-Handler, N., R. K. Malenky, and N. Badrian. "Sexual Behavior of Pan paniscus Under Natural Conditions in the Lomako Forest, Equateur, Zaire." In *The Pygmy Chimpanzee.* Edited by R. L. Susman. New York: Plenum Press, 1984.

Tiger, L. and R. Fox. *The Imperial Animal.* New York: Holt, Rinehart and Winston, 1971.

Van der Lee, S. and L. M. Boot. "Spontaneous Pseudopregnancy in Mice." *Acta Physiologica et Pharmacologica Neederlandica* 4 (1955): 442–44.

Van Toller, C., M. Kirk-Smith, N. Wood, J. Lombard, and G. H. Dodd. "Skin Conductance and Subjective Assessments Associated with the Odour of 5-a-androstan-3-one." *Biological Psychology* 16 (1983): 85–107.

Van Wimersma Greidanus, T. B. and D. DeWied. "Neuropeptides, Brain Function and Reproductive Behavior." In *The Brain and Female Reproductive Function*. Edited by A. R. Genazzani, U. Montemagno, C. Nappi, and F. Petraglia. Park Ridge, N. J.: Parthenon, 1987.

Veith, J. L., M. Buck, S. Getzlaf, P. Van Dalfsen, and S. Slade. "Exposure to Men Influences the Occurrence of Ovulation in Women." *Physiology and Behavior* 31 (1983): 313–15.

Vincent, J. D. *Biologie des Passions*. Paris: Odile Jacob, 1986.

Walker, A. and P Parmar. *Warrior Mark: Female Genital Mutilation and the Sexual Blinding of Women*. New York: Harcourt Brace Jovanovich, 1994.

Wallace, P. "Individual Discrimination of Humans by Odor." *Physiology and Behavior* 19 (1977): 577–79.

Walsh, A. *The Science of Love: Understanding Love and Its Effects on Mind and Body*. Buffalo, New York: Prometheus Books, 1991.

Watson, L. *Neophilia: The Tradition of the New*. London: Hodder and Soughton, 1989.

Weinrich, J. D. *Sexual Landscapes: Why We Are What We Are, Why We Love Whom We Love*. New York: Scribners, 1987.

Weitz, Ze'Ev W., A. J. Birnbaum, P. A. Sobotka, E. J. Zarling, and J. L. Skosey. "High Breath Pentane Concentrations During Acute Myocardial Infarction." *Lancet* 337 (1991): 933–35.

Wendt, H. *The Sex Life of the Animals*. New York: Simon and Shuster, 1965.

Whitam, F. L., M. Diamond, and J. Martin. "Homosexual Orientation in Twins: A Report on 61 Pairs and Three Triplet Sets." *Archives of Sexual Behavior* 22 (1993): 187–206.

Whitten, W. K. "Genetic Variation of Olfactory Function in Reproduction." *Journal Reproductive Fertility* 19 (1973): 405–10.

Wickler, W. *The Social Behavior of Animals and Men*. New York: Anchor/Doubleday, 1973.

Wilson, E. O. *Sociology: The New Synthesis*. Cambridge, Mass.: Harvard University Press, 1975.

Winter, R. *The Smell Book. Scent, Sex and Society*. New York: Lippincott 1976.

Wotman, S., I. D. Mandel, S. Khotim, R. H. Thompson, A. H. Kutsher, E. V. Zegarelli, and C. R. Denning. "Salt Thresholds and Cystic Fibrosis." *American Journal of Disease in Children*. 108 (1964): 372–74.

Wright, R. H. *The Sense of Smell*. Boca Raton, Flor.: C. R. C. Press, 1982,

Wright, K. "The Sniff of Legend. Human Pheromones: Chemical Sex Attractants? And a Sixth Sense Organ in the Nose? What Are We Animals?" *Discover* 15 (April 1994): 60–77.

Wysocki, C. J. and G. K. Beauchamp. "Ability to Smell Androstenone is Genetically Determined." *Proceedings of the National Academy of Science USA*. 81 (1984): 4899–902.

Wysocki, C. J.and A. N. Gilbert. "National Geographic Smell Survey: Effects of Age are Heterogenous." In *Nutrition and the Chemical Senses in Aging: Recent Advances and Current Research Needs.* Edited by C. Murphy, W. S. Cain, and D. M. Hegsted. New York: Academy of Sciences, 1989.

Wysocki, C. J., G. K. Beauchamp, H. L. Schmidt, and K. M. Dorries. "Changes in Olfactory Sensitivity to Androstenone with Age and Experience" (abstract). *Chemical Senses* 12 (1987): 710.

Wysocki, C. J., K. M. Dorries, and G. K. Beauchamp. "Ability to Perceive Androstenone Can be Acquired by Ostensibly Anosmic People." *Proceedings of the National Academy of Science USA* 86 (1989): 7976–78.

Yamazaki, K., M. Yamaguchi, L. Baranoski, J. Bard, E. A. Boyse, and L. Thomas. "Recognition Among Mice: Evidence from the Use of a Y-Maze Differentially Scented by Congenic Mice of Different Major Histocompatibility Types." *Journal of Experimental Medicine* 150 (1979): 755–60.

Yen, S. S. C. and A. Lein. "The Apparent Paradox of the Negative and Positive Feedback Control System on Gonadotropic Secretion." *American Journal of Obstetrics and Gynecology* 126 (1976): 942–54.

Yoshida, K., T. Hisatomi, and N. Yanagishima. "Sexual Behavior and its Pheromonal Regulation in Ascosporogenous Yeasts." *Journal of Basic Microbiology* 29 (1989): 99–128.

Young, M. "Attitudes and Behavior of College Students Relative to Oral-Genital Sexuality." *Archives of Sexual Behavior* 9 (1980): 61–7.

Zigova, T., P. P. Graziadei, and A. G. Monti-Graziadei. "Olfactory Bulb Transplantation into the Olfactory Bulb of Neonatal Rats." *Brain Research* 513 (1990): 315–19.

———. "Olfactory Bulb Transplanation Into the Olfactory Bulb of Neonatal Rats: An Autoradiographic Study." *Brain Research* 539 (1991): 51–8.

INDEX

EPILOGUE

HUMAN PHEROMONES IN THE NEW MILLENIUM

"...a new scientific truth does not triumph by convincing its opponents and making them see the light, but rather because its opponents eventually die, and a new generation grows up that is familiar with it." – Max Planck[1]

More than a century ago, in 1900, Max Planck, one of the greatest physicists of all time, announced his revolutionary new scientific theory of an energy constant in quantum mechanics. Eighteen years later he was awarded a Nobel Prize.[2] Evidently, 18 years was sufficient time for opponents of Planck's theory to die, and for a new generation (also enlightened by Albert Einstein and Sigmund Freud) to become familiar with quantum theory. Planck's "constant" became an established new scientific truth.

A decade ago, anatomists and embryologists were convinced that pheromones could not possibly affect human sexual behavior for two reasons. Embryology texts clearly stated that, while the vomeronasal organ (VNO) could be found in human embryos, this pheromone-sensing organ degenerated and disappeared before birth. Since humans lacked the VNO, they could not detect pheromones. More crucial, researchers argued, human sexual behavior was too sophisticated to be influenced by anything as primitive or animalistic as pheromones.

Now you know the real story. In 1995, we wrote *The Scent of Eros,* to propose and defend a new scientific theory: We were convinced that pheromones are more important to human sexuality that any other form of sensory input. We were convinced that this theory would soon be documented, and then accepted as a new scientific truth! Since no one can accurately predict how long it will take to establish a new scientific truth, let us step back in time to our first presentation of this new theory at a scientific meeting. That happened at the 1992 annual meeting of the Society for the Scientific Study of Sexuality in San Diego, when Kohl presented and defended the logic of his hypothesis about "Luteinizing Hormone (LH): The Link Between Sex and the Sense of Smell?"[3] Just before Kohl's 1992 presentation, researchers reported that, indeed, humans do have a well developed VNO (see pages 63-66). Today, within the ten years after Kohl's first presentation, many researchers recognize convincing evidence that human pheromones do in fact alter levels of LH in other humans. [4][5][6][7]

This hormone: LH, affects many aspects of human sexuality, including ovulation and sperm production. The link between LH and the human sense of smell is no longer speculative; it is a scientific truth. LH *is* the link between sex and the human sense of smell.

Evidence that pheromones can and do alter LH production helps us understand how sensory input from our social environment, our "nurture" interacts with our genetic "nature" to affect human behavior.[8] This evidence also confirms that animal models connecting pheromones and behavior also apply to people, and that animal models of behavioral development can be extended to a developmental model for human physical attraction, and for sexual behavior.

Before the connection between human pheromones and LH was established, any attempt to explain how pheromones influence the development of human sexuality suffered from a fatal flaw: namely, that results from research on other animals do not always apply well to human behavior. Since we now know that pheromones influence human hormone levels, the fatal flaw no longer exists. We can now move from human pheromones to LH and other hormones, and from the effect human pheromones have on these hormones to the effect these hormones have on our behavior. Today we can trace the path we have so clearly documented in animals and use that path to explain behavioral development in humans.[9]

LH: LINKING SEX AND THE SENSE OF SMELL

Since few readers will be interested in the intricacies of how hormones like LH affect human behavior, we will give only a brief summary here. As we saw in Chapter 7, GnRH is produced in the hypothalamus and then directs mechanisms in the pituitary that control the levels of LH and of follicle stimulating hormone (FSH). The ratio of LH to FSH determines and alters levels of our sex hormones like estrogen and testosterone. The effect of GnRH on LH/FSH ratios and on levels of sex hormones begins long before we are born, and causes sex differences in the sense of smell.

The sexual differentiation that results in sex differences in the sense of smell also results in physical differences in males and females. Scientists describe these differences as sexually dimorphic. The human olfactory system is sexually dimorphic from early in pregnancy (see pages 93-94). At birth, a sexually dimorphic sense of smell enables males and females to respond differently to pheromones. This means that from birth on, and throughout life, the effect of male and female pheromones on GnRH production is different in males and females.

Although we cannot directly measure GnRH in humans, we can be sure that human pheromones influence it. There is no doubt that changes in GnRH production cause changes in the production of LH, FSH, estrogen, and testosterone in other animals. Research on the behavior of other mammals shows that pheromones affect these hormones, and that these hormones alter sexual behavior. The link from pheromones to GnRH, to LH, FSH, to estrogen and testosterone, and to our sexual behavior is now both clear and obvious in animals, including humans.

Nevertheless, some of our readers, even our scientific colleagues, may wonder how pheromones can possibly be involved in human sexual attraction, especially when we find ourselves attracted to someone from across a crowded room. Few people fully realize that pheromones influence our experiences during development, and long before we reach sexual maturity. Equally significant is the fact that human pheromones operate below the level of our conscious world. Small wonder that some people discount the effects of pheromones on our hormones and on our behavior. We hope the evidence we presented in 1995, when we wrote The Scent of Eros, and the more recent research findings we add in this Epilogue will convince you of the link between sex and the sense of smell.

ODORS AND PERSONAL PREFERENCES

Our choices of food and a mate are two behaviors essential for the survival of a species. This similarity and connection makes for an interesting illustration: While we commonly think that food and mate choice are based on attractive visual appeal, it is well known that food preferences are based more on appealing odor than on visual appeal. Our taste buds are limited to sweet, sour, bitter and salty. The rest of taste is odor. We quickly turn down food that looks great, if it smells wrong. Understanding the importance of odors in our choice of food makes it easier to understand the major importance of odors in mate selection, even when these odors are pheromones that operate below the level of consciousness. Whether or not we are aware of pheromones they affect mate choice just as much, or more, than food odors affect what we eat.

THE HUMAN ANIMAL

Species survival depends primarily on the majority of individuals within the species choosing a fertile mate. Wrong or poor choices in this area will endanger a species' ability to survive. As noted earlier, the sense of smell started as an elementary but incredibly sensitive and effective means of chemical communication at a distance. Chemical communication at a distance is as essential for survival of the first and most ancient forms of life, as it is to humans.

Why then, are people so quick to think that the sexual attraction we humans experience is primarily based on visual appeal, when the eye is a much more recent development in the evolutionary process? The simple answer is that survival mechanisms like pheromonal communication, which evolved in the most primitive forms of life, operate below the conscious level. The circuits of our conscious brain are easily swept away by a colorful and powerful vision, whether that vision is of a well-endowed voluptuous female, or a tawny muscular male. Visual input feeds into the optic lobes of our conscious brain where lusty fantasies take over. Distracted by this seemingly irresistible conscious seduction, we are oblivious to the fact that the pheromones from that male or female body have triggered production of GnRH in the hard-wired (unconscious) survival circuits of our brain. We are equally oblivious of the hard-wired second phase, in which GnRH regulates the production of LH, FSH, estrogen, and testosterone. These hormones circulate throughout the body and brain, firing up our sexual appetite and arousal mechanisms in the conscious brain. Whether we know it, and whether we like it or not, pheromones are a more powerful influence on our behavior than any other type of sensory input. Pheromones affect the hormones that direct our behavior.

Earlier, we explained how odor cues vary with hair color, and with healthy physical features. If we reject the role of pheromonal messengers, there is no comprehensive explanation for the development of personal preferences based on hair color or physical "body" type. Whether you prefer a blond to a brunette, dark skin to light skin, men to women; all these preferences develop as our behavior responds to hormones, while it is also responding to pheromones. In addition, there is no mammalian model that even hints at why we would base any type of sexual behavior on visual input. Sexual behavior is dependent on pheromones in other mammals. Pheromones attract or repel to ensure successful mating. Why would this not be true in humans? [10]

SEX DIFFERENCES

Just as our early experiences with food chemistry can alter our food choice later in life, our initial experience with the chemistry of other people—their pheromones, can alter our mate choice later in life. Current research, for example, tells us, with relative certainty, that a mother's pheromones alter LH and testosterone levels in infant sons, but not in her infant daughters. The olfactory system of a son reacts to his mother's pheromones because they come from the "opposite" sex. When the mother's pheromones induce a change in the infant male's level of testosterone, and when this change is associated with a pleasurable sensation—a reward, the son's emotional brain will readily associate that pleasurable sensation with the pheromones. Again, this association is made automatically, without rising to the level of consciousness. A good example is an experiment involving adding lemon scent to a mother rat's nipples and vagina. When they grow up, her male offspring will prefer to mate with lemon-scented females.[11]

Since, the mother's breast is the source of pheromones and food, an infant son's visual response to the breast is readily linked to the effect of her pheromones on his hormones. Psychologists call this a conditioned response. It occurs when one form of sensory input, our sense of smell for instance, affects a response associated with another form of sensory input, in this case, vision. Odor-driven changes in a male infant's hormone levels condition him to respond with pleasure to the sight of his mother's breast. What causes this connection? The obvious answer is the effect of the mother's pheromones on her son's hormones.[12]

Since we know that human pheromones influence levels of hormones in other humans, we can now ask how a son's response to pheromones from his mother's lactating breast might influence his adult fixation with women's breasts. After all, a mother's lactating breast appears relatively large. This visual stimulus, coupled with the pheromones from the breast, early in life—will be repeatedly associated with the very pleasurable experiences of food, touch, and warmth. That's why nearly every mother's son will, as he matures, begin to find large-breasted women more attractive than women with smaller breasts.

In Chapter 6, we suggested an explanation for the development of pendulous breasts in women, which was also based on what we know about pheromones. The pendulous breasts of women are modified scent-producing glands. Larger breasts contain more scent glands to secrete more pheromones. Increased pheromone production means more potent effects on male hormones, like testosterone. Might this scent-testosterone connection also cause males to prefer large-breasted women. Although this multi-tiered explanation is somewhat complicated, biological realities tell us that any visually-based explanation both for breast development, and for attraction to larger breasts, is not as convincing as our olfactory-based explanation.[13]

The association between large breasts and sexuality is very basic. One might even describe it as instinctive. It remains in the subconscious mind, only to be demonstrated when the hormones of puberty begin to kick in.[14] Long before the hormones of puberty trigger profound differences in the behavior of adolescent males and females, pheromones are triggering hormonal changes in the infant. Good and bad associations, including visual associations, conditioned by pheromones, are being made from birth—even though they do not show up until the onset of puberty

HUMAN PHEROMONES AND PUBERTY

We also now have evidence that pheromones alter the timing of the onset of puberty in human females. Apparently, the presence or absence of a biological father's pheromones makes a difference. When the father is present, his daughter does not advance into puberty as quickly as she does when he is not present. [15] If a stepfather or mother's boyfriend is present, young women advance into puberty faster.[16] Other factors like nutrition also influence the onset of puberty. However, evidence that exposure to the pheromones of biologically related or unrelated males affects the onset of puberty has been documented in the females of many different species.

For humans, an earlier onset of puberty, coupled with still developing emotional controls, can increase the risk of psychologically premature sexual experiences, unwanted pregnancies, and exposure to sexually transmitted diseases. In other animals, early pregnancy and offspring are linked to survival of the species. To date, we know of no research that explores the impact of human pheromones on earlier puberty and its consequences of earlier sexual intercourse, unwanted pregnancy, abortion, and sexually transmitted diseases.

This absence of research and the likelihood that no researcher will be willing to enter such a sensitive area suggests some speculation and some questions that might be worth mentioning here. For instance, what results might we expect if mothers collected pheromones from their daughter's biological father, and used them to delay puberty, in the event that the biological father leaves home prematurely? We might also ask whether it might be wise to begin sex education earlier in families where the father is absent, and especially if a stepfather or mother's boyfriend is present. Provocative questions like these are very unlikely to be pursued in any clinical test.

Meanwhile, many mothers have reported that maintaining a "bank" of their own pheromones can be helpful with cantankerous infants and young children. Most mothers are aware that placing a article of clothing they have worn in the crib with an infant will help sooth the infant when they are absent. Maternal clothing, or the nesting material of other animals, contains the mother's natural scent; her pheromones, which play a major role in mother-infant bond. This connection to the scent of one's mother is crucial for bonding in all mammals.[17]

Some observers of human culture have suggested that we humans try to distance our own sexuality from that of animals so that we can continue to delude ourselves that we are somehow different, and therefore superior. We don't deny that humans are different, and that, typically, we are able to make superior choices. Still, we fail to understand why there is such resistance to recognizing our animalistic heritage, and particularly to recognizing the role that pheromones and hormones play in our behavior.[18] Regardless of this resistance, pheromones leave their hormonally driven mark on every human born with a sense of smell.

I CAN'T SMELL ANYTHING

What about people who are born with no sense of smell? If pheromones are so important to our sexual lives, we should expect to see some delay in puberty for in those who are not affected by pheromones. Earlier, on page 59 and page 167, we mentioned Kallmann's syndrome, where a gene affects the development of our reproductive system, our levels of hormones, and our ability to smell. People with Kallmann's syndrome are born with no sense of smell, and experience delayed puberty. Affected males reportedly lack interest in the opposite sex; and sexual firsts—if any—occur many years later than in people whose sense of smell is functional. Can you imagine how your life might be changed by an inability to smell?

Our sense of smell plays a primary role in our ability to bond with others, because pheromones alter levels of hormones, like oxytocin, that are linked to these bonds. People with Kallmann's syndrome have repeatedly reported a failure to bond, and with surprising specifics. For example, several have reported their concern that they did not cry at their mother's funeral. "What's wrong with me?" is a common question. We believe that the lack of the sense of smell and subsequent lack of the bonding between mother and child best explains this commonly reported problem. Unfortunately, we cannot cite any scientific study that proves this, since this information comes from internet postings and discussions on a listserver for people interested in Kallmann's syndrome. Nonetheless, we know that the sense of smell is the link that establishes the mother-infant bond in other animals, and that this bond is very important.[19]

PHEROMONES AND DESIRE

We also know that people who lose their sense of smell later in life, due to head injury or viral infection, are affected by the loss. Food odors no longer activate the hypothalamus. People who lose their sense of smell tend to gain weight, because no chemical signal gets through to the hypothalamus to tell their brain they have had enough to eat. More important, sexual desire declines with the loss of the sense of smell in humans, just as it does in other animals. Other animals can be manipulated in experiments to show how much difference their response to pheromones makes in their sexual interest and behavior.[20] When people lose their sense of smell, the effect mimics the results of animal experiments. With no sense of smell, there are no longer any pheromonal associations on which to base sexual behavior and mate choice; sexual desire declines. Even gradual loss of the sense of smell creates problems. With age, our ability to detect odors declines and so does sexual desire. Smoking cigarettes also reduces our ability to detect odors,[21] and has been linked to increased rates of impotence in men.[22]

PHEROMONES AND TALL MEN

Surges in testosterone levels during puberty accelerate bone growth and increased density of bones. This is reflected in sex differences in height and in bone density (e.g., taller men with the stronger male jaw). Increased testosterone levels also increase male pheromone production. So, simply put, taller men with strong jaws produce more masculine pheromones.[23] When women select a tall man, their selection is readily linked to an increase in male pheromone production.

PHEROMONES AND "DARK" MEN

Women in the ovulatory phase of their menstrual cycle are in the most fertile phase. The fairer skinned of the "fairer sex" have lighter complexions as a result of reduced melanin and hemoglobin levels in the skin's outer layers. The difference between the male's darker and the female's lighter complexion arises at puberty, since sex hormones influence melanin production, hemoglobin levels, and thus, skin color. The production of these sex hormones is also responsible for sex differences in pheromone production. So, keep in mind, ovulatory women prefer the scent of men with darker complexions.[24]

It makes good pheromonal sense that women who are at the most fertile phase of their menstrual cycle would prefer what is visually perceived to be a darker complexion in males, since darker skin is linked to increased production both of testosterone and of male pheromones. Accordingly, the preference for darker skin is not a visual preference. Rather, it is a subconscious olfactory preference that we attribute to a visual preference. Similarly, the effect tanned skin may have on visual aspects of physical attraction can be linked with the testosterone-influenced pheromone production in men.

Vitamin D, a steroid hormone activated by light, has been used to correct deficiencies in testosterone in vitamin D-deficient male rats.[25] A "good" tan may provide a visual signal of higher testosterone levels. At the same time, this visual signal is accompanied by a chemical signal that is linked to higher testosterone levels and increased masculine pheromone output. This may be why natural sun tanning and tanning parlors remain popular, regardless of the associated risk between tanning and skin cancer. Others might argue that tanned skin continues to be viewed as a sign of health and a leisurely lifestyle. So, perhaps it is not merely a pheromone connection that makes darker skin more attractive to women.

PHEROMONES AND HANDSOME MEN

Bilateral symmetry can be described as the equal balance of two halves.[26] A line drawn from the middle of your forehead to the middle of your chin, would help to establish the degree to which your face is bilaterally symmetrical. If both sides of the line can be precisely matched, you are perfectly symmetrical, and for whatever reason, symmetry is widely considered attractive. Less of a match, asymmetry, is less attractive. Symmetry is believed to be a visual sign of hormonally determined reproductive fitness, which is basically the testosterone-linked ability to impregnate a woman, or the estrogen-linked ability of a woman to become pregnant.[27]

Ovulatory women find the scent of symmetrical men most attractive.[28] A woman's ability to detect musky male pheromones also peaks at this stage of her cycle, when she is most fertile. Thus, she is most sensitive to, and responds best to male pheromones that are genetically linked to the development of symmetrical features and male reproductive fitness. There is even one report that women have more orgasms when they select men with symmetrical features.[29] Orgasm has a powerful conditioning effect on future behavior; it will be sought after because of the pleasure associated with the endorphins produced during orgasm. The combination of scent, symmetry, and orgasm helps to reinforce an ovulating woman's sexual behavior and help her to unconsciously select for the "handsome" pheromones of reproductive fitness when she is most likely to get pregnant.

PHEROMONES AND GENETIC DIVERSITY

Ovulatory women also find the scent of men more attractive when they are most genetically unrelated.[30] It is important that all animals select mates who are not closely related. Failure to do so results in inbreeding, which brings increased genetic defects and susceptibility to infections that accumulate and affect the species ability to survive. Species survival depends on the ability of animals to use their sense of smell to detect extremely subtle differences in the genetically determined odor of a potential mate. Both men and women can detect these differences, and use this ability to select genetically diverse mates.[31] We hinted at this when we reported that children raised in an Israeli kibbutz invariably married outside their group, and that the Hutterite women selected men who were the most genetically diverse from those who were available to them for marriage (see pages 137-138). There is now stronger evidence for this claim. Whether this evidence proves beyond any shadow of a doubt that women use their sense of smell to chose genetically diverse mates is a matter of opinion. However, the evidence shows that women maintain the ability found in other mammals to select for chemical cues of genetic diversity.[32]

PHEROMONES AND FEMALE FERTILITY

Men find the scent of women who are near the most fertile stage of the menstrual cycle to be most attractive.[33] When a woman is most fertile (e.g., when she is in the ovulatory phase of her menstrual cycle), her estrogen level reaches its peak. There is evidence that strongly suggests estrogen levels affect the active pheromones she secretes, and that these pheromones also have a profound effect on levels of testosterone in men. For example, testosterone levels peak 15 minutes after exposure to a chemical mixture, which mimics the natural vaginal odor that is present when a woman is most fertile.[34] The result of this testosterone peak is expected to be an increased desire to become sexually active with the fertile female, who is most likely to become pregnant as a result.

In other mammalian females, chemical signals alert the male to her readiness for mating and her ovulation. The "bitch in heat" for example sends her chemical signals to male dogs that can pick up her scent from a long distance away and respond with mating overtures. Like other mammalian males, men seem to prefer the scent of a woman who is most fertile.

PHEROMONES AND THE WAIST-TO-HIP RATIO

Men generally prefer women whose body type, specifically, their waist to hip ratio, is linked to fertility. Dividing your hip measurement by your waist measurement provides a waist-to-hip ratio (WHR) that is characteristic of sex differences in post-pubertal males and females. An attractive male WHR is 1.0, which when compared to the most attractive female WHR: 0.7, simply reflects that women have a thinner waist and wider hips than men. This sex difference is primarily the result of sex hormones, and the way that these hormones affect fat distribution. Women tend to distribute fat on their hips; men tend to distribute fat on their mid-section.

Why would a study show that 0.7 is consistently preferred as the most visually attractive WHR of women,[35] while 1.0 is preferred in men? There is no biological basis for the development of this visual preference—unless it is a conditioned response to pheromones. We can fully expect that women with the most desirable WHR also emit pheromones linked to the hormones that correlate well with their fat distribution and with their WHR. These pheromones are the most likely reason women with a 0.7 WHR are more visually appealing to men, and men with a 1.0 WHR are most appealing to women.

PHEROMONES AND SEXUAL ORIENTATION

Currently, sexual orientation cannot be explained using the hypothesis that physical attraction is primarily visual. Any explanation of human sexual behavior must account for variations in behavior, like bisexuality and homosexuality. It is not enough, for example, to say that we develop visual preferences that drive our sexual behavior, without explaining how men become visually attracted to men, and how women become visually attracted to women. Since homosexual attraction is common among many mammals, and pheromones drive the sexual behavior of other mammals, it seems more likely that pheromones can better explain homosexuality than any other approach involving visual stimuli.

If the development of a male rat's sense of smell is altered by a drug that limits sexual differentiation of his olfactory system, as an adult, the male will exhibit bi-sexual behavior.[36] The male rat will respond to the odors of a female by mounting her, but he will also respond to the odors of a male by exhibiting a posture that allows him to be mounted.

Homosexual rams respond with increased testosterone to the odors of other males.[37] The homosexual rams also have differences in an olfactory processing center in the brain: the amygdala. Male rats that exhibit the posture that allows other males to mount them have similar differences in their hypothalamus.[38] So do homosexual human males.[39, 40] The hypothalamus and the amygdala are integral parts of the limbic system, the "emotional center" of the human brain. Accordingly, pheromones also may be involved in variations of sexual behavior.

PHEROMONES AND OTHER ATTRACTIVE FEATURES

A colleague who has studied facial beauty was having trouble with the concept of human pheromones and how they are involved with determining what men perceive to be attractive. "I like all women," he said. First question: "Do you like fat women, or thin women?" His answer indicated a preference for the estrogen component that determines body fat distribution. Estrogen is closely associated with the pheromones that women produce. Second question: "Do you prefer blondes, brunettes, or redheads?" Natural hair color is also linked with both the genetic components of pheromone production and with pheromone distribution. Brunettes, for example, trap more pheromones in their hair, because their hair is typically thicker than blond hair. The genes that determine hair (and eye) color are also linked to pheromone production (see pages 159-160).

Our colleague preferred red hair and green eyes. In fact, his first "true love," and his last three lovers were red-heads, and one even had green eyes.

"What about symmetrical features; the balance that most people find attractive?" Symmetry also is determined in part by hormones linked to pheromone production. No answer from the colleague.

"Do you prefer a woman with broad shoulders, or narrow shoulders; a strong jaw, or more feminine features like high cheekbones and a small jaw?" It didn't take long for our colleague to discover that all the features for which he stated a visual preference had connections to women's differences in genes, hormones, and pheromones. During the course of a weekend conference, he was relatively convinced that he had developed preferences for different characteristics of women based on pheromones. Of course, it helped to convince him that his preferences for women were based on pheromones when women's preferences were explained. Simply put, women prefer tall, dark, and handsome men because these traits are visual signals of fertile masculinity. As we indicated earlier, tall, dark, and handsome is a visual description of a masculine pheromone signature.

A few years later, both Kohl and this colleague were filmed for separate segments of a television special on "Survival of the Prettiest." Finally, it seemed that Kohl had an opportunity to tell a large television audience about the role pheromones play in sexual attraction, while also comparing the role of visual input. We waited for the broadcast in anxious anticipation. Francoeur, on the East Coast, was one of the first to learn that Kohl's interview, filmed in the laboratory, had been left on the cutting room floor. What happened?

The producers substituted a segment on cosmetic surgery, which they felt was more appropriate given the title of the show. Everything else in the show was related to visual aspects of physical attraction, with no room for our olfactory approach. This is somewhat typical of the mass media approach to human sexuality. The olfactory connection is difficult to present on television, which of course is designed for visual stimulation. Besides, some people think the real mysteries of odor in human sexuality are best left unexplained.

Soon after the 1995 release of "The Scent of Eros," Kohl was interviewed for an article for *Newsweek*. Also interviewed were Devendra Singh (of WHR fame) and Randy Thornhill, (of facial symmetry fame). The article was to be entitled "The Biology of Love." Nothing from the interview with Kohl was included. When asked why, the journalist said his editor realized that the article was so focussed on visual appeal, that anything about olfactory appeal contradicted *Newsweek*'s approach to the biology of love. We were disappointed, because when it comes to biology, there is no non-olfactory basis for visually perceived physical attraction. That's why pheromones are more important than what we see, biologically speaking.

PHEROMONES, NATURAL AND SYNTHETIC

We are frequently asked about what pheromone-containing product works best to attract the opposite sex. However, evidence of a human pheromone-hormone connection does not support the marketing claims for the plethora of products that supposedly contain human pheromones guaranteed to attract the other sex. Despite marketing claims that human pheromones will trigger sexual attraction and desire in another person, we are not like other animals. Unlike most animals, most people typically think before they act on some hormonally driven sexual impulse.

At the same time, no one can predict what physical characteristics will be most important to sexual attraction in any other person. Nor can anyone predict what pheromones will be most important to sexual attraction in another person. These preferences develop over a lifetime of unpredictable life experiences.

Wearing a pheromone-containing fragrance is not likely to "drive women wild" or to make every man "want" you, unless that person has had an sexually-rewarding experience or relationship with a particular pheromone or fragrance. The other person's reaction and our own are just as likely to be associated negatively as positively, based upon life's experience. A woman who has been raped, for example, might even find that the natural male scent of a loving spouse triggers her memory of the rape, and repulses her.

Women who learn to love the increased male odor associated with testosterone-charged men in outlaw motorcycle clubs, are less likely to enjoy a more docile and less odorous man.

DHEA

When human pheromones are discussed at scientific conferences, or just among friends, the most obvious and frequently asked question is whether we have discovered a human pheromone. Kohl believes he has. While others have experimented with putative human pheromones like androstenone and androstenol, or synthesized chemicals that appear to have genuine effects on others: the "vomeropherins" and the "copulins," Kohl has focussed on a different approach.

Any human male pheromone is likely to have a variety of functions. Those that are linked closely to testosterone levels would also be linked to signals of dominance, of attractive physical features, and might possibly be used in establishing territory—if only the amount of personal space preferred. Increased production of a male pheromone is also likely to be linked to a rapid response so that when a signal of dominance is required to attract a female, the signal will be manifest quickly, before she walks away. Pheromones linked to testosterone production in the male pig, androstenone and androstenol, are primarily linked to a response cycle that, in men, takes 15 minutes to achieve. To us, 15 minutes means an opportunity lost.

A much quicker response mechanism is required, something akin to the fight or flight response, which is also related to testosterone levels. This kind of near immediate response one finds in the adrenal glands, which we know contribute to pheromone production in mice.[41]

The primary adrenal hormone linked to testosterone production is dehydroepiandrosterone (DHEA). This hormone has been marketed as a human pheromone for use as an additive in a product marketed by the Athena Institute, as we mentioned in Chapter 14. A form of DHEA, its sulfate: DHEA-S, ranks second only to cholesterol as the most abundantly produced steroid hormone in men and women.[42]

Is DHEA, or DHEA-S a human pheromone? For a variety of reasons, this is unlikely. To start with, the levels of DHEA vary little between men and women. If DHEA were a human pheromone, it would be hard to imagine how it could effectively signal any particular distinguishing quality of a male, or of a female. Certainly, DHEA would not act as a signal of male hormone levels or of female hormone levels. Hormone-related signals should clearly distinguish a male from a female, and clearly distinguish the menstrual cycle phase of a female. DHEA lacks this sexually dimorphic quality.

When attempting to find a true human pheromone, it is best to take into account the differences between men and women; and, in this case between boys and girls. Pheromone production in boys and girls begins with maturation of the adrenal glands, slightly before the onset of puberty. Adrenal gland maturation also is linked to the early stages of visible axillary and pubic hair, which help to distribute pheromones. Once the adrenal glands are mature, there also is a sex difference in the productions of the two primary metabolites of DHEA: androsterone (A) and etiocholanolone (E).

Without burdening the reader with the technical details of steroid hormone biochemistry, we need to note that A/E ratios are different in men and women. For this reason A may signal masculinity, and either lesser concentrations of A, or greater concentrations of E, may signal femininity.

Accordingly, the A/E ratio may reflect the degree of masculinity or femininity. More A probably means a higher A/E ratio and more masculine pheromone production. Less A probably means more feminine pheromone production. The A/E ratio also changes in response to fight or flight situations, because the stress hormone: cortisol, suppresses DHEA production. Stressful situations could lead to a more feminine A/E ratio in men due to DHEA suppression. Dominant males who control their environment are less likely to experience stress than subordinate males who may even be stressed by the presence of other males. Dominant males are also more likely to have higher A/E ratios that could pheromonally signal their dominance.

Homosexual males are reported to have A/E ratios characteristic of females. In one experiment, a scientist who measured A/E ratios in urine samples was able to predict with 100 percent accuracy whether or not the man who submitted the specimen was homosexual.[43] This research is particularly interesting because in 1992, just prior to Kohl's first scientific presentation on this topic, Dr. William G. Turner, an octogenarian psychiatrist, turned geneticist, contacted Kohl. Turner wrote that during the 1950's, several aging, gay, male patients responded to his request for information on how they found other gay males. He repeatedly was told: "we smell each other." During the 1950's a man who made a mistake about another man's sexual orientation would probably have been lucky if he escaped with a beating. Perhaps the atypical A/E ratio, manifest in chemical cues, helped avoid such problems.

Is something like this happening in homosexual rams? Back in 1992, before Kohl's first presentation to the Society for the Scientific Study of Sexuality, Dr. Anne Perkins was listening to Kohl explain his model to Dr. F. Robert Brush. However, she didn't listen for very long. She interrupted and said, quite simply: "That's exactly what's happening in my sheep." Her homosexual rams would approach and sniff the genitals of other males, and exhibit a hormone response characteristic of other rams when they sniffed the genitals of an estrus ewe.

Schizophrenics have unusual DHEA levels when compared to non-schizophrenics. They also produce an odor that has been said to be characteristic of schizophrenia. This odor could be related to their level of DHEA and subsequently their A/E ratio. DHEA levels also are linked to age-related sexual problems.[44] Do the metabolites of DHEA become pheromonal signals? If so, it may take a few more years of research to prove. It will also take a few more years of research to prove that human pheromones are the primary driving force behind all of human sexual behavior. Meanwhile, Kohl has begun marketing of a product containing androsterone that seems to enhance masculine appeal.

WHY HASN'T ANYONE ELSE TOLD YOU ABOUT THIS?

Researchers have many reasons to avoid discussing topics they consider insignificant, improbable, not worth their time, or simply something they cannot integrate into their overall scientific picture. When it comes to human behavior, especially sexual behavior, a hypothesis that makes sense can also make for controversy in institutions that require political correctness for funding or other support. It is sometimes as dangerous today, as it was in the days of Charles Darwin, to propose strong links between animals and humans—especially when it comes to sexual behavior. Professors seeking tenure may be passed over for promotion, lose tenure-track positions, or be "black-balled" for making claims that are considered too controversial. Right or wrong makes less difference in a politically correct world filled with litigious pitfalls.

Research on the menstrual cycle of women or simply the claim that male pheromones can alter the menstrual cycle and the sexual behavior of women can be twisted into a charge of sexual harassment when it is linked with sexual differences.

Perhaps it is for the best that human sexuality research only be discussed in scientific forums, or in scientific journal articles. Journalists can then interpret this information and reduce its technical content down to something more people can better understand and talk about. We have seen this happen with the arrival of nearly every new report that mentions human pheromones. And yet, the journalists aren't telling the whole story, and many people don't understand.

This does not surprise us, and will not surprise you given a recent report of sex differences in the response to the estrogenic (i.e., female) compound oestra-1,3,5(10),16-tetraen-3-ol (EST) and the androgenic (i.e., male) compound 4,16-androstadien-3-one (AND). Hypothalamic activation with AND was significantly greater in women, while hypothalamic activation by EST was greater in men. EST induced activity in the olfactory regions of women, while AND induced activity in the olfactory regions of men.[45] What, you and the mass media journalists, may ask, does this mean? It means that there is no longer any question about whether human pheromones exist, and that it is time to fully examine the effects of human pheromones on our behavior.

Kohl was recently enlisted by colleagues from Vienna, to detail the link between pheromones and hormones for publication in a scientific journal. "Human Pheromones: Linking Neuroendocrinology and Ethology," will help other scientists to better understand the link between pheromones and behavior.[46] Another recent article links pheromones and male sexual orientation.[47] But, as Max Planck indicated in the quote we used to begin this epilogue, it is not necessarily scientists who will help the majority of people understand the importance of human pheromones. Instead, it is likely that people like you, who have read this book, will help a new generation become familiar with the scientific truth about human pheromones.

The authors of this volume hope that you now have a better understanding of human pheromones and how they influence your life. The picture we have tried to present is like a two-sided coin. One side is the pheromones of others that affect your life. The other side is the effect your pheromones have on the lives of others.

Since we started this epilogue with a quote, it seems fitting to end this update on pheromone research, and its relevance to what we perceive to be visual attraction, to end with another quote borrowed from our first chapter on The Mystery of Odor.

"I should think that we might fairly gauge the future of biological science, centuries ahead, by estimating the time it will take to reach a complete comprehensive understanding of odor. It may not seem a profound enough problem to dominate all the life sciences, but it contains, piece by piece, all the mysteries." Lewis Thomas [48]

1 In: "The Structure of Scientific Revolutions" Third edition, Thomas S. Kuhn, p. 151, paperback. From Max Planck, "Scientific Autobiography and other Papers", trans. F. Gaynor (New York, 1949), pp. 33-34.

2 Planck was the first prominent physicist to support Albert Einstein's theory of special relativity.

3 Kohl was persuaded by a reviewer to include the question mark at the end of his presentation title, due to the theoretical nature of his presentation.

4 Stern K, McClintock MK (1998). Regulation of ovulation by human pheromones. Nature 392: 177-179.

5 Shinohara K, Morofushi M, Funabashi T, Mitsushima D, Kimura F. (2000). Effects of 5alpha-androst-16-en-3alpha-ol on the pulsatile secretion of luteinizing hormone in human females. Chemical Senses 25: 465-467.

6 Preti G, Wysocki CJ, Barnhart K, Sonheimer SJ, Leyden JJ, (2001) Male axillary extracts effect lutenizing hormone (LH) pulsing in female recipients. Poster presentation at the 23rd Association for Chemoreception Sciences Annual Meeting, Sarasota, Florida.

7 Shinohara K, Morofushi M, Funabashi T, Kimura, F. (2000) Axillary pheromones modulate pulsatile LH secretion in humans. Neuroreport 12: 893-895.

8 Diamond M, Binstock T, Kohl JV. (1996) From fertilization to adult sexual behavior. Hormones and Behavior 30:333-53.

9 Nevertheless, we don't expect to receive a Nobel Prize. Actually, anyone who became overly familiar with the relationship between pheromones and hormones in other mammals could also have predicted that human pheromones would be the primary sensory influence on human behavior.

10 It is necessary here to move from an animal model to a more specific mammalian model. Otherwise, someone will invariably focus their attention on avian, i.e., bird models of sexual attraction. This leads to a discussion about the male peacock's tail being visually attractive to the female—and a number of other examples of how birds use visual characteristics in mate choice. So, in moving from animal models to mammalian models, we can also simply

say that humans are mammals, we are not birds—and birds are not good models for the behavior of mammals.

11 Fillion TJ, Blass EM (1986). Infantile experience with suckling odors determines adult sexual behavior in male rats. Science 231: 729-31.

12 We know that women react to the pheromones of other women, as is the case with menstrual synchrony, but so far there is no evidence that infant daughters react to the pheromones of their mother. Typically, it is the effect of pheromones from the other sex that increase LH and levels of testosterone in males.

13 There is a popular theory of why the pendulous breasts of women are unique among female mammals. Desmond Morris suggests that pendulous breasts developed to mimic the fleshy buttocks of women, and provide a visual cue of sexual maturation and fertility, as we developed our frontal approach to sexual inter-course. Again, we see how the focus changes from the effect of pheromones on hormones and behavior, to the effect of visual input, without mention of how visual input affects hormones.

14 So as not to discourage breast feeding by mothers who are appalled that they may be providing sexual stimulation to their infant sons, we note that their infant sons, like infant male rats, have no concept of sexual stimulation. Though most mothers know that infant males exhibit erections that are hormonally driven by increased testosterone (a typical male response to pheromones from the opposite sex), there is no reason to believe that an infant son has sexual thoughts about his mother.

15 Ellis BJ, McFadyen-Ketchum S, Dodge KA, Pettit GS, Bates JE. (1999). Quality of early family relationships and individual differences in the timing of pubertal maturation in girls: a longitudinal

test of an evolutionary model. Journal of Perssonal and Social Psychology 77: 387-401.

16 Ellis BJ, Garber J. (2000). Psychosocial antecedents of variation in girls' pubertal timing: maternal depression, stepfather presence, and marital and family stress. Child Development 71: 485-501

17 In 1997, after a conference presentation, Kohl met with Mindy Rothstein, who had conceptualized a "Bonding Blanket" based upon what she had learned about human pheromones from reading *The Scent of Eros*. Though it has taken several years for her to bring her new product to market, we can be relatively sure of its success.

18 Weiderman M. Personal correspondence, Kohl: July 2001.

19 Winberg J, Porter RH (1998). Olfaction and human neonatal behaviour: clinical implications. Acta Paediatrics 87: 6-10.

20 One recent study showed that anosmic ferrets could not recognize the difference between males and females. Kelliher KR, Baum MJ (2001). Nares occlusion eliminates heterosexual partner selection without disrupting coitus in ferrets of both sexes. Journal of Neuroscience 1;21:5832-40.

21 Frye RE, Schwartz BS, Doty RL (1990) Dose-related effects of cigarette smoking on olfactory function. JAMA 263: 1233-6.

22 Mannino DM., Klevens RM, Flanders D (1994). Cigarette smoking: An independent risk factor for impotence. American Journal of Epidemiology 140: 1003-1008.

23 When levels of testosterone are too high, however, maximum height may not be achieved.

24 Frost P. (1994) Preference for darker faces in photographs at different phases of the menstrual cycle: preliminary assessment of

evidence for a hormonal relationship. Perceptual and Motor Skills 79: 507-514.

25 Sonnenberg J, Luine VN, Krey LC, Christakos S (1986) 1,25-dihydroxyvitamin D3 treatment results in increased cholinacetyltransferase activity in specific brain nuclei. Endocrinology 118: 1433-1439.

26 Rikowski A., Grammer K. (1999) Human body odour, symmetry and attractiveness. Proceedings of the Royal Society of London 266: 869-874.

27 Tom Cruise has nearly perfect symmetry in facial features; Lyle Lovett has very assymetrical facial features.

28 Rikowski A, Grammer K. (1999) Human body odour, symmetry and attractiveness. Proc R Soc Lond B Biol Sci. 266: 869-74.

29 Thornhill R, Gangestad SW, Comer R. (1995) Human female orgasm and male fluctuating asymmetry. Animal Behavior 50: 1601-1615.

30 Wedekind C, Seebeck T, Bettens F, Paepke AJ. (1995) MHC-dependent mate preferences in humans. Proc R Soc Lond B. 260: 245-9.

31 Ober C, Weitkamp LR, Cox N, Dytch H, Kostyu DD, Elias S (1997) HLA and mate choice in humans. American Journal of Human Genetics 61: 6-14.

32 Wedekind C, Seebeck T, Bettens F, Paepke AJ (1995) MHC-dependent mate preferences in humans. Pro Roy Soc Lond, 260, 1359 (Jun 22), 245-249.

33 Singh D, Bronstad PM. (2001) Female body odour is a potential cue to ovulation. Proc R Soc Lond B Biol Sci 268: 797-801.

34 Juette A (1995) Weibliche Pheromone - Wirkung und Rolle von synthetischen "Kopulinen" bei der versteckten Ovulation des Menschen. Diplomarbeit an der Universität Wien.

35 Singh D. (1993) Adaptive significance of female physical attractiveness: role of waist-to-hip ratio. Journal of Personality and Social Psychology 65: 293-307.

36 Bakker J, Baum MJ, & Slob AK (1996) Neonatal inhibition of brain estrogen synthesis alters adult neural Fos responses to mating and pheromonal stimulation in the male rat. Neuroscience 74: 251-260. Neonatal treatment with 1,4,5-androstatriene-3,17-dione (ATD), which blocks the aromatization of T to E, affects sexual differentiation of olfactory pathways and causes male rats to respond with bi-sexual behavior in the presence of chemosensory stimuli either from females or from other males.

37 Perkins A, Fitzgerald JA, Moss GE (1995) A comparison of LH secretion and brain estradiol receptors in heterosexual and homosexual rams and female sheep. Hormones and Behavior 29: 31-41.

38 Samama B, Aron C (1989) Changes in estrogen receptors in the mediobasal hypothalamus mediate the facilitory effects exerted by the male's olfactory cues and progesterone on feminine behavior in the male rat. Journal of Steroid Biochemistry 32: 525-529.

39 LeVay S. (1991)A difference in hypothalamic structure between heterosexual and homosexual men. Science 253: 1034-37.

40 Byne W, Lasco MS, Kemether E, Shinwari A, Edgar MA, Morgello S, Jones LB, Tobet S. (2000). The interstitial nuclei of the human anterior hypothalamus: an investigation of sexual variation in volume and cell size, number and density. Brain Research 856: 254-8.

41 Ma W, Miao Z, Novotny MV (1998) Role of the adrenal gland and adrenal-mediated chemosignals in suppression of estrus in the house mouse: the lee-boot effect revisited. Biology of Reproduction 59:1317-1320.

42 Davis SR and Burger HG (1996) Androgens and the post-menopausal woman. J clinical Endocrinol Metab 81:2759-2764

43 Margolese MS, Janiger O. (1973) Androsterone-etio-cholanolone ratios in male homosexuals. British Medical Journal 207: 207-210.

44 Reiter WJ, Pycha A, Schatzl G, Klingler HC, Mark I, Auterith A, Marberger M. (2000) Serum dehydroepiandrosterone sulfate concentrations in men with erectile dysfunction. Urology 55:755-8.

45 Savic I, Berglund H, Gulyas B, Roland P. (2001) Smelling of odorous sex hormone-like compounds causes sex-differentiated hypothalamic activations in humans. Neuron. 31:661-8.

46 Kohl JV, Atzmueller M, Fink B, Grammer K. (2001). Human Pheromones: Integrating Neuroendocrinology and Ethology. Neuroendocrinology Letters 22: 309-321.

47 Kohl, JV (2002) Homosexual Orientation in Males: Human Pheromones and Neuroscience. The ASCAP Bulletin 3 (2), 19-24.

48 Thomas, L. (1980) Notes of a biology-watcher: On Smell. New England Journal of Medicine 302,13:732.